Welcome

Foreword

To date, the five volumes of the *Modelling British Railways* series have all looked at various types of rolling stock, be it wagons, parcels vehicles or departmental stock. This sixth entry takes a different approach by moving to the front of the trains to examine the locomotives used to haul such vehicles. Although motive power is the most popular aspect of model railways, there is still plenty of scope to take the subject further, such as showcasing how to make the most of ready-to-run models or detailing appropriate coaches and freight stock to run behind the locos.

As with pretty much any other aspect of the railways, the subject of locomotives is a vast one that could fill numerous publications so the focus here is on the diesel and electric classes that were operating in the final decade of the 20th century. The 1990s saw the greatest change to the UK's railway system since the end of steam with British Rail broken up and privatised by the government. While this is not the place to discuss the merits of the policy, the effect on the locomotive fleet was profound with an explosion of new operators, all keen to put their stamp on this brave new railway system.

By the end of the decade, the railway looked very different to how it had been ten years earlier with a number of popular BR loco types either completely gone or reduced to a mere handful of examples while the General Motors invasion had begun in earnest with regular shipments of Class 66s across the Atlantic, not to mention Class 67s arriving from Spain. However, the focus here is on the loco types that existed under the auspices of British Rail in its final years and their subsequent development.

To detail the history of every loco type during this ten-year period would be impossible in the space available though, let alone to model them all, so instead a snapshot approach has been taken whereby key class and livery combinations from throughout the 1990s are considered and modelled. The detailing and weathering techniques discussed can then be transferred across to other locos in the same colours for example.

The chosen projects are drawn from four groups, including older BR liveries that could still be found early in the decade along with the new schemes that were introduced by the national operator in its last years. The shadow privatisation period is then considered, which is when the re-structured freight companies came to the fore, before examining the new looks of the fully privatised train operators.

Thanks are due to the modellers whose work is featured here, particularly James Makin but also Gareth Bayer, Alex Carpenter, Timara Easter, Mark Lambert, and Paul Wade. As ever, the support of the many photographers credited throughout these pages is much appreciated along with that of selected manufacturers and retailers. Particular thanks are due to Accurascale for early access to a Class 92 and to Hornby for providing a Class 91 upon release.

Simon Bendall
Editor

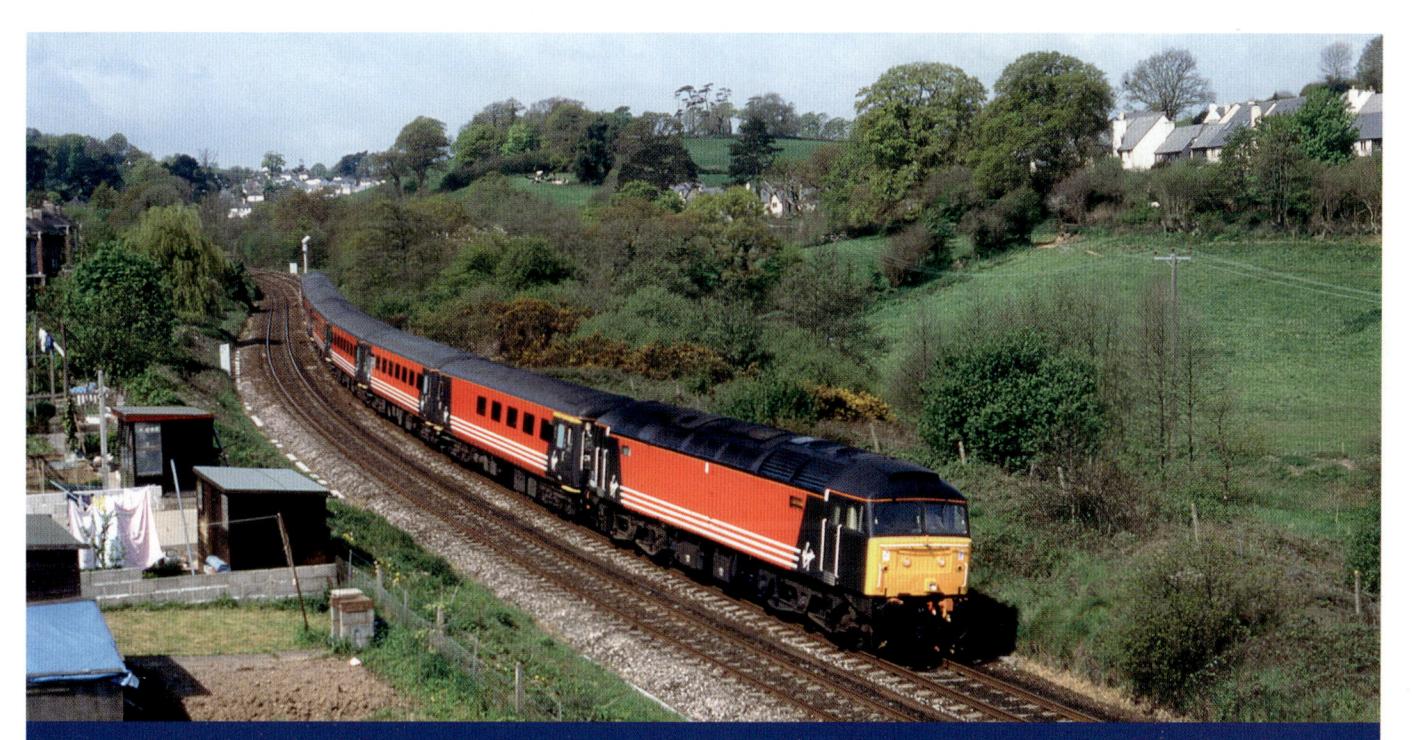

ABOVE: Privatisation was a boon for paint and vinyl suppliers to the rail industry as the raft of new companies all introduced bold new looks to the various passenger and freight operations. While opinion was split on some schemes, Virgin Trains was widely commended for the red and dark grey livery utilised on its West Coast and CrossCountry franchises. Representing the latter, a sparkling 47806 passes through Totnes on May 5, 1998, with a Plymouth to Manchester Piccadilly working, which is formed of a seven-coach set of air-conditioned Mk.2e/f coaches. In recent years, Hornby has released the Mk.2e in Virgin colours in OO gauge with Bachmann providing the Mk.2f in the same livery. However, the Mk.2f Restaurant First Buffet (RFB) leading the formation and required for all CrossCountry formations of this period is only available from Bachmann. Simon Bendall Collection

◀ COVER: During the early 1990s, the Class 91s were the flagships of British Rail and its InterCity services. On May 2, 1992, 91029 *Queen Elizabeth II* powers away from Newark Northgate under a threatening sky with the 13.10 King's Cross to Leeds. Paul Robertson

Go to www.keymodelworld.com for the best model railway news, features, and reviews.

Modelling BR Locomotives of the 1990s 3

MAGAZINE SPECIALS

ESSENTIAL READING FROM KEY PUBLISHING

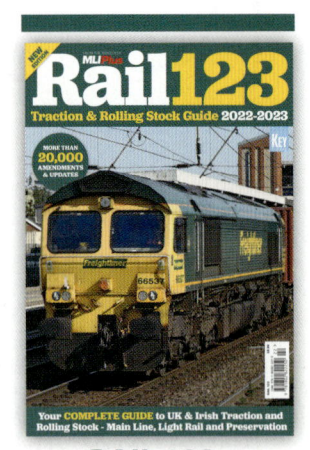

RAIL 123
Traction & Rolling Stock Guide 2022 - 2023

£9.99 inc FREE P&P*

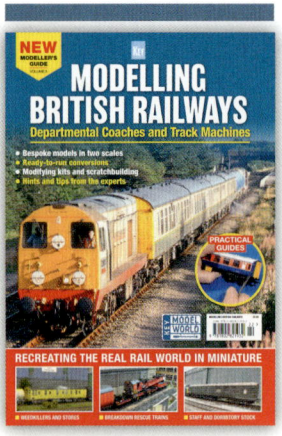

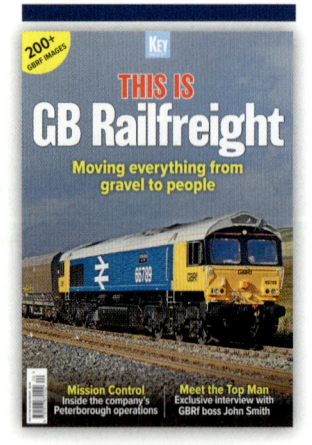

MODELLING BRITISH RAILWAYS
Departmental Coaches & Track Machines

£8.99 inc FREE P&P*

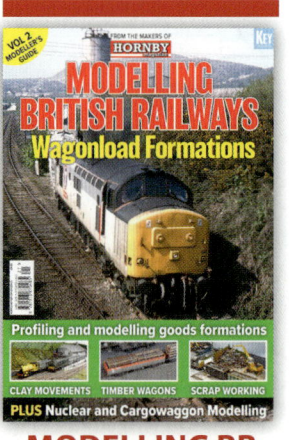

MODELLING BR WAGONLOAD FORMATIONS
The new modeller's guide.

£8.99 inc FREE P&P*

BRITISH RAILWAYS THE PRIVATISATION YEARS

£8.99 inc FREE P&P*

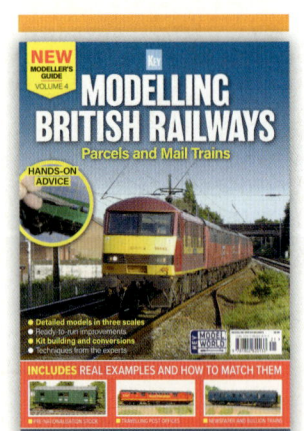

MODELLING BRITISH RAILWAYS 4 - PARCELS AND MAIL TRAINS

£8.99 inc FREE P&P*

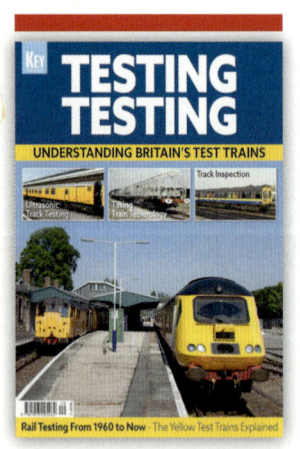

TESTING, TESTING
Understanding Britain's Test Trains.

£8.99 inc FREE P&P*

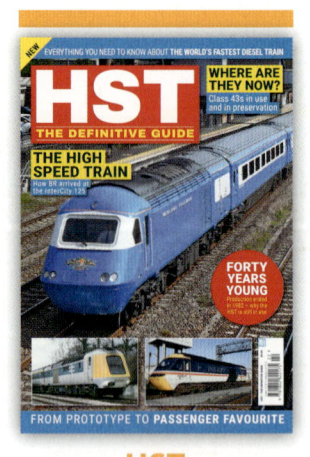

HST - THE DEFINITIVE GUIDE
A must for all rail enthusiasts

£9.99 inc FREE P&P*

THIS IS GB RAILFREIGHT
Moving everything from gravel to people

£8.99 inc FREE P&P*

MAGAZINE SPECIALS

ESSENTIAL reading from the teams behind your FAVOURITE magazines

HOW TO ORDER

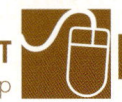

VISIT
www.keypublishing.com/shop

PHONE
UK: 01780 480404
ROW: (+44)1780 480404

*Prices correct at time of going to press. Free 2nd class P&P on all UK & BFPO orders. Overseas charges apply. Postage charges vary depending on total order value.

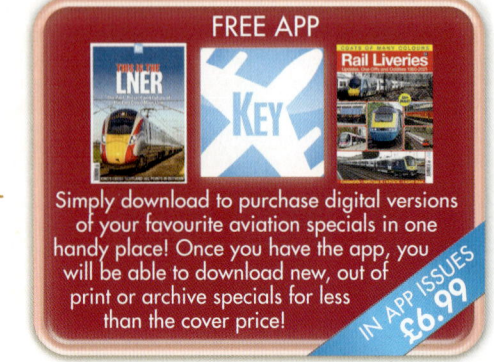

FREE APP

Simply download to purchase digital versions of your favourite aviation specials in one handy place! Once you have the app, you will be able to download new, out of print or archive specials for less than the cover price!

IN APP ISSUES £6.99

205/22

Contents

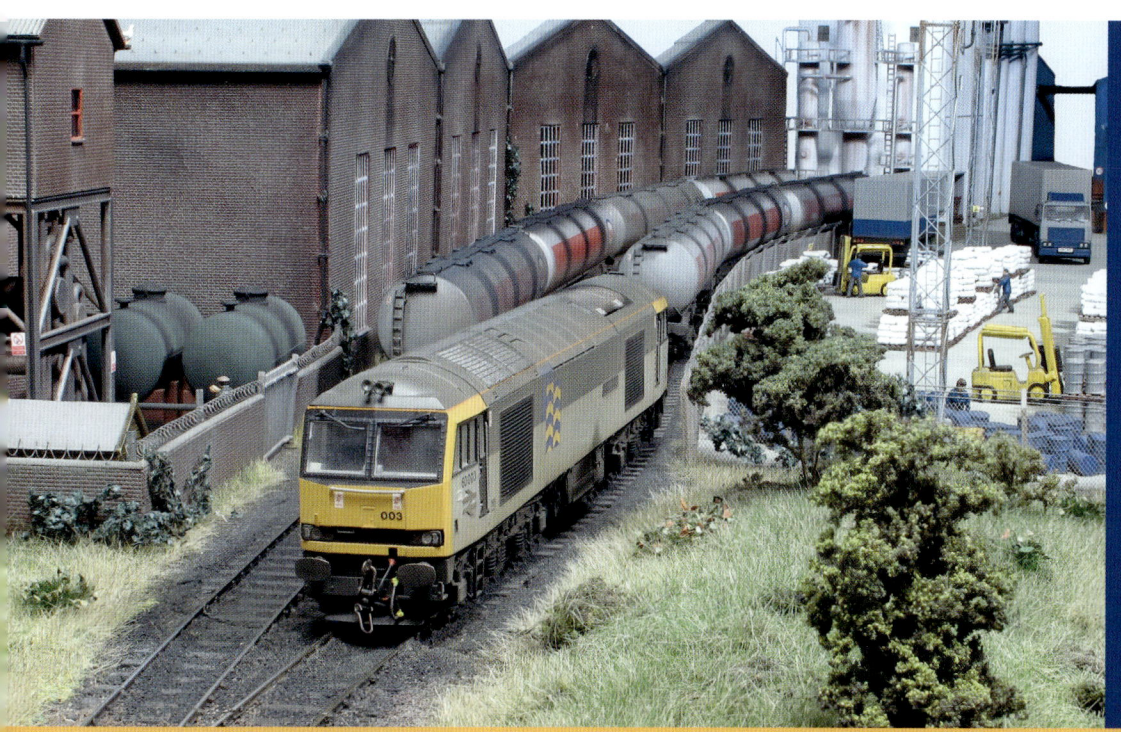

LEFT: Although 60001 was unveiled in June 1989, such was the delay in getting the Class 60s into traffic with their numerous teething troubles that they were very much locomotives of the 1990s. The Brush-built machines would come to dominate heavy freight workings throughout the decade, first with Railfreight and then the three shadow freight companies before being reunited under the control of EWS. For over 15 years, Hornby has been the go to option for a model in OO gauge and some time spent on weathering and livery enhancements will result in scenes such as this as 60003 *Christopher Wren* shunts the oil terminal on Farkham, then owned by the Mickleover Model Railway Group but since sold into private ownership.
Ian Manderson

6 A legacy continued
As the 1990s began, there was still corporate BR blue in evidence along with other obsolete liveries such as the early Railfreight grey schemes. Other late 1980s designs were purposefully continued, such as the Railfreight sub-sectors.

34 New looks for the decade
The early 1990s saw several of the sectors update their image, none more so than Parcels which morphed into Rail Express Systems while Provincial became Regional Railways. Both adapted their looks while the Civil Engineers went 'Dutch'.

58 Out of the shadows
With BR broken up into saleable business units, the shadow privatisation period of the mid-1990s was one of great upheaval. This was particularly true in the freight sector where the regional operators adopted bold but ultimately short-lived new looks.

90 The railway reborn
The decade ended with freight and passenger companies under private ownership and new identities being unveiled as consolidation and takeovers took place. While the network was undoubtedly more colourful, the variety of loco types was in decline.

ISBN: 978 1 80282 227 4

Editor: Simon Bendall

Senior editor, specials: Roger Mortimer

Email: roger.mortimer@keypublishing.com
Design: SJmagic DESIGN SERVICES, India
Cover: Dan Hilliard
Advertising Sales Manager: Brodie Baxter
Email: brodie.baxter@keypublishing.com
Tel: 01780 755131
Advertising Production: Debi McGowan
Email: debi.mcgowan@keypublishing.com

Subscription/Mail Order
Key Publishing Ltd, PO Box 300, Stamford, Lincs, PE9 1NA

Tel: 01780 480404 **Fax:** 01780 757812
Subscriptions email: subs@keypublishing.com
Mail Order email: orders@keypublishing.com
Website: www.keypublishing.com/shop

Publishing
Group CEO: Adrian Cox
Publisher: Jonathan Jackson
Head of Publishing: Finbarr O'Reilly
Head of Marketing: Shaun Binnington
Key Publishing Ltd, PO Box 100, Stamford, Lincs, PE9 1XP
Tel: 01780 755131
Website: www.keypublishing.com

Printing
Precision Colour Printing Ltd, Haldane, Halesfield 1, Telford, Shropshire. TF7 4QQ

Distribution
Seymour Distribution Ltd, 2 Poultry Avenue, London, EC1A 9PU
Enquiries Line: 02074 294000.

We are unable to guarantee the bonafides of any of our advertisers. Readers are strongly recommended to take their own precautions before parting with any information or item of value, including, but not limited to money, manuscripts, photographs, or personal information in response to any advertisements within this publication.

© Key Publishing Ltd 2022
All rights reserved. No part of this magazine may be reproduced or transmitted in any form by any means, electronic or mechanical, including photocopying, recording or by any information storage and retrieval system, without prior permission in writing from the copyright owner. Multiple copying of the contents of the magazine without prior written approval is not permitted.

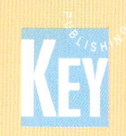

Modelling BR Locomotives of the 1990s **5**

A legacy continued

A legacy continued

The 1990s began with British Rail still in the throes of modernisation, both in terms of infrastructure and rolling stock. The effect of this investment would have a significant impact on the size and composition of the locomotive fleet as would less welcome outside influences, as Simon Bendall details.

ABOVE: **With less than two months to go until withdrawal, a shabby 50003 *Temeraire* powers away from Yeovil Junction with the 10.20 Exeter St Davids to Waterloo on May 25, 1991. Indeed, it would soon be all change for Network SouthEast's West of England services with the Class 47/7s arriving to largely replace the 'Hoovers'. The formation is entirely typical of the route with the nine coaches consisting of three Mk.2a/b/c Tourist Standard Opens (TSO) at each end, these sandwiching a Mk.2c micro-buffet (TSOT) and two Mk.2a/c Brake First Corridors (BFK). The Mk.2a coaches are available in both 2mm and 4mm scale from Bachmann, the former under its Graham Farish brand, while Accurascale is in the process of developing a range of Mk.2b/c in OO gauge. As for the Class 50, Hornby produces a OO model with the best N gauge rendering coming from Dapol and a 7mm offering from Heljan.** Simon Bendall Collection

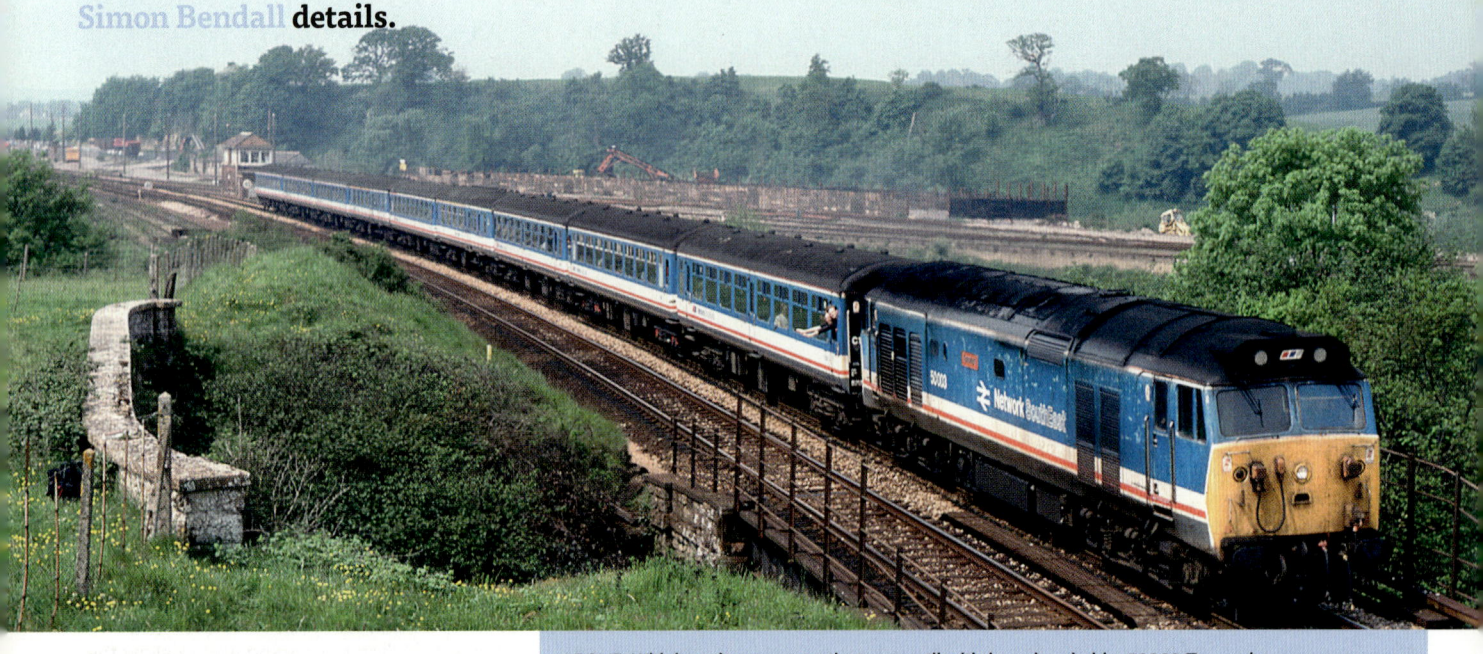

British Rail commenced the 1990s with its structure of business units, known as sectors, still in place, these consisting of the InterCity, Network SouthEast, and Provincial passenger operations along with Railfreight and Parcels. This arrangement had served BR relatively well for much of the preceding decade and would remain in place until the break-up of the company commenced in 1994.

Operating conditions were far from favourable though as a recession was in effect, leading to an already indifferent government cutting investment in the network, forcing above-inflation fare rises to be introduced. At this point, InterCity and Railfreight were the only sectors returning a profit, the other three all operating at an overall loss, especially Provincial where the costs and revenue support needed to keep rural services going were resulting in a deficit of well over £400m per year.

For InterCity, the most notable event of the start of the decade was the completion of the electrification of the East Coast Main Line with full electric services to Leeds commencing in the spring of 1990 while the revamped Edinburgh timetable was inaugurated in July 1991. This gave the sector and BR a new flagship route to market with services operated by the new Class 91 and Mk.4 formations, collectively known as InterCity 225s.

On the West Coast Main Line along with the Great Eastern route between London and Norwich, similar operating efficiencies were achieved by expanding fixed-formation

RIGHT: **One of the most significant changes for InterCity services at the beginning of the 1990s was the introduction of push-pull operation on the West Coast Main Line. Achieved using the Time Division Multiplex (TDM) control system, it brought a standardisation of coaching stock formations to the route and more efficient operation by removing the need for loco changes at terminus stations. By 1992 the changeover was largely complete as an un-manned 90002 propels a Mk.3 set through Motherwell on June 26 under the control of the Mk.3b DVT at the other end of the train. The Class 90s were originally delivered with their TDM cables stowed in the recess below the air horn grille, but this left them vulnerable to damage by bird strikes and other objects, the loco showing the revised storage location on the sides of the bufferbeam.** Simon Bendall Collection

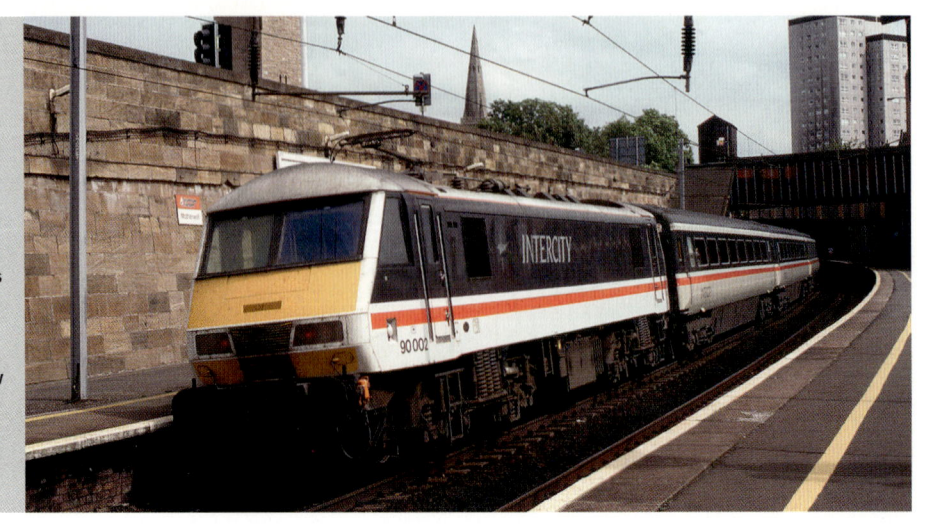

A legacy continued

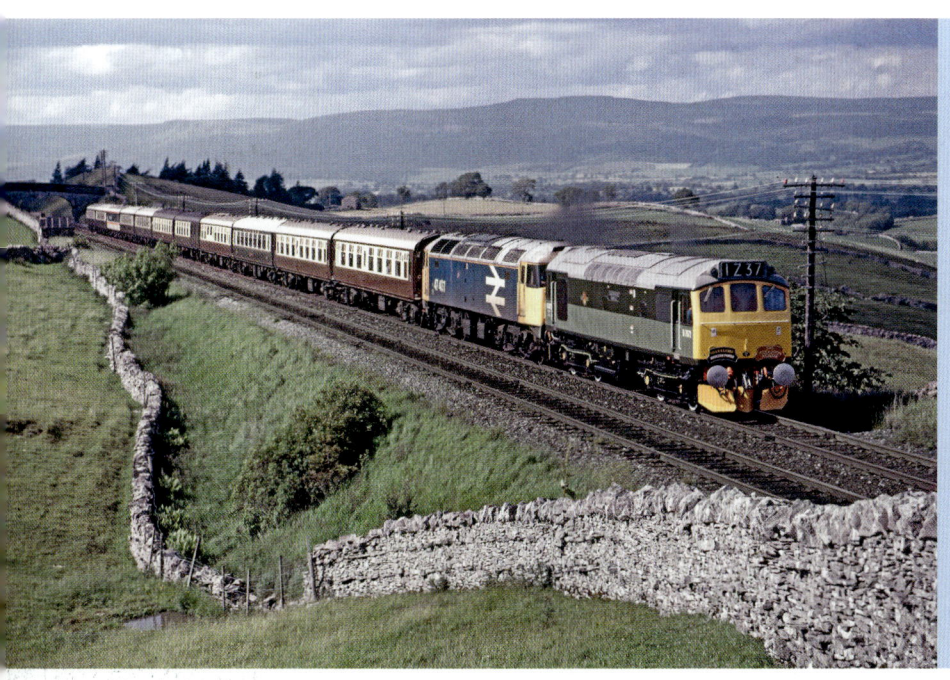

LEFT: The 1980s and early 1990s saw a number of locos returned to interpretations of their original green liveries for a variety of reasons, many becoming firm favourites for use on railtours and charter trains. Having been retained as a training loco at Leeds Holbeck depot, 25912 *Tamworth Castle* was later returned to main line use for special duties, gaining a coat of two-tone green in March 1989. In this form, it gave the Class 25s a last hurrah on the network before being withdrawn again in September 1991 and passing into preservation. On June 23, 1990, the Type 2 tops 47407 at Greengate with the 1Z37 16.38 Carlisle to King's Cross 'The Middleton Pioneer', which was originally due to have been steam-hauled. The stock is a mix of privately-owned standard and Pullman Mk.1 coaches operating at this point under the Pullman Rail banner with only a Mk.1 Restaurant Buffet (RBR) from the InterCity Charter Unit disrupting the umber and cream set. In OO gauge, the Class 25s have become fertile ground in recent years with Heljan releasing a new model in 2021 and both Bachmann and Rail Exclusive having versions under development. The Farish range is again the source in 2mm with Heljan producing O gauge incarnations.
Bob Lumley

push-pull operation. This saw coaching stock sets become much more standardised in their make-up with an AC electric loco provided at one end and an unpowered driving vehicle at the other. This not only reduced dwell times at terminus stations by allowing faster turn-round times, but also enabled the number of locos required to be reduced. On the West Coast, new build Mk.3b Driving Van Trailers (DVTs) provided the requisite remote driving facilities partnered with the still new Class 90s along with progressively modified Class 86s and Class 87s while services out of Liverpool Street had to make do with refurbished and modified Mk.2f Driving Brake Standard Opens (DBSOs) working with Class 86s.

Across the other InterCity routes of the Great Western, Midland Main Line and Cross-Country, High Speed Trains (HSTs), or InterCity 125s if you prefer, continued to reign supreme supported by loco-hauled sets that were invariably Class 47-powered. While the introduction of the InterCity 225s allowed some displacement of HSTs from the ECML, a reduced fleet had to be retained to cover services to Inverness, Aberdeen and the east coast destinations that had been omitted from electrification.

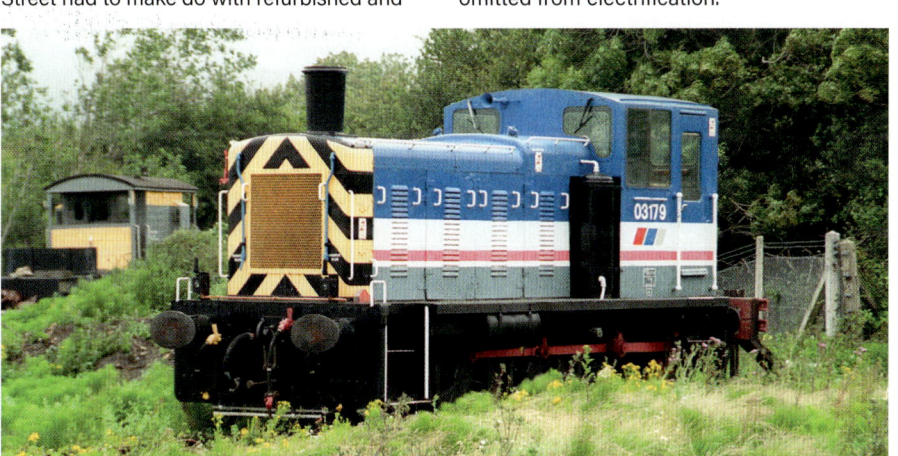

Down south

For Network SouthEast (NSE), the 1990s began with continued investment in new multiple units and, in some cases, the infrastructure required to operate them. This included electrification to King's Lynn, the completion of Thameslink through Central London and the extension of the third rail system to infill various gaps, such as the Solent Link around Southampton and Portsmouth.

A key goal of this spending was to allow the sector to completely eliminate the operation of loco-hauled trains, which were both costly and prone to unreliability, in favour of an efficient unit-based railway. The first route to lose such trains was Liverpool Street to Cambridge, where Class 86s sourced from InterCity had reigned since completion of electrification to the university city in 1987 with a small fleet of NSE Class 47s retained for through workings to King's Lynn. Newly-built Class 321s had ousted the Class 86s from May 1989 and the Class 47s went the same way 12 months later, initially in favour of a DMU shuttle service to the Norfolk coast until the wires were completed.

May 1990 also saw the AC electric-hauled and largely peak-hour 'Cobbler' services withdrawn between Euston and Northampton as further Class 321s entered traffic. This allowed the hire of Class 85s and Class 86s from InterCity to again cease.

ABOVE AND RIGHT: The variety of shunter types that once existed in the BR fleet was long gone by the start of the 1990s with just Class 08s and Class 09s remaining for virtually all work, and even the former were in decline. One exception was on the Isle of Wight where two Class 03s were specially retained, the type having otherwise disappeared from service in 1989. One of the pair, 03179 is seen at Sandown in April 1990, having received NSE colours five months earlier. The current RTR offerings in N and OO are again from Bachmann with this particular colourful example having previously been produced for the company's collectors' club in 4mm while a limited edition 2mm version was released by Kernow Model Rail Centre in March 2022 and is illustrated here.
Simon Bendall Collection

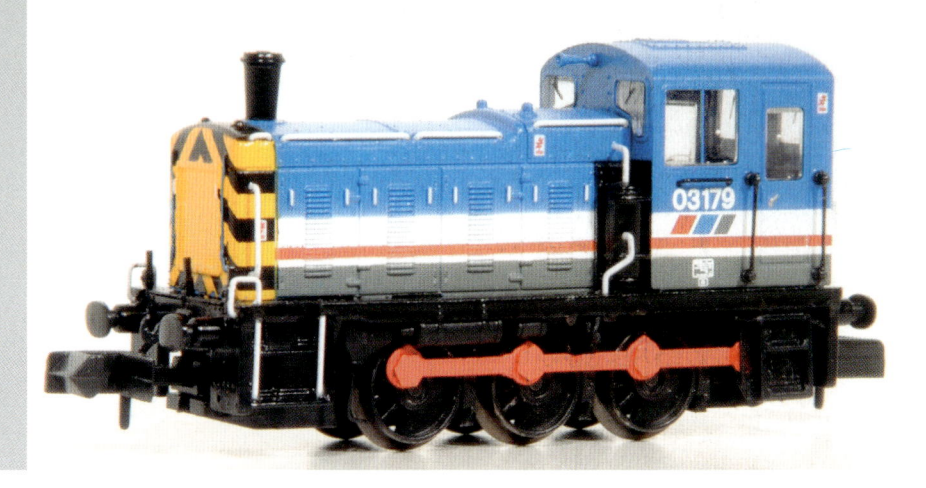

A legacy continued

Change also came to the Thames route that extended from Paddington to principally Oxford and Newbury along with the limited number of loco-hauled trains along the Chiltern line to High Wycombe and Banbury. Class 47s had already begun to replace Class 50s on the services in the late 1980s and this process was completed by the summer of 1990 as reliability of the latter began to become particularly troublesome. The replacements initially featured Class 47/4s displaced from the King's Lynn workings and Class 47/7s transferred south from Scotland following the belated introduction of the Class 158 DMUs.

By the end of 1990, NSE's share of the former push-pull Class 47/7 fleet had all arrived, several being rushed into service still carrying ScotRail colours. However, the sub-class' time on the Thames route was short-lived as during the summer of 1991, they were transferred en masse to the West of England line. This left NSE with a significant issue as with the Class 50s gone and many of the ex-King's Lynn Class 47/4s having been released to the Parcels sector, there was a loco shortfall for Thames services.

The solution was to acquire a motley collection of long-in-the-tooth Class 47/4s, most coming from Railfreight Distribution having been declared surplus following the termination of the Speedlink network. This rag-tag fleet of mainly plain blue and large logo machines was just about sufficient to tide services over until July 1992, by when enough new Class 165 'Turbos' had been delivered to allow the elimination of loco-hauled services on the Thames route, the last Chiltern line train having already run in January the same year.

The longest-lived of the NSE loco-hauled services were those on the West of England line from Waterloo to Exeter via Salisbury and Yeovil Junction, these having been powered by Class 50s since 1980 and backed up by Class 33s as required. The 'Hoovers' dominance remained largely unchallenged until a combination of factors caused a drop in reliability as the 1990s dawned. From the summer of 1990, the ailing Laira-based examples were bolstered by classmates displaced from the Thames route, but it was not enough, the following summer seeing the mass arrival of the Class 47/7s as replacements. This included not only the NSE machines but the balance of the sub-class that had initially gone to Parcels on leaving Scotland, including the infamously tatty ScotRail-liveried 47706.

Five Class 50s made it into 1992 although 50029 and 50030 dropped by the wayside soon afterwards, leaving 50007/33/50 to soldier on until the end of regular Class 50 operations that May with ultimate withdrawal coming in March 1994. This left the Class 47/7s to carry the burden of Waterloo-Exeter services and in the event, they fared little better, leading to regular Class 33 substitutions once again. Relief finally came in 1993 with the arrival of the Class 159 DMUs, the final loco-hauled services running that July.

Provincial woes

The decade started badly for Provincial with construction of its new BREL Class 158 fleet mired in production delays caused by faults and poor build quality. This in turn delayed a cascade of stock, such as Class 156s, to other routes and forced the sector to keep ageing first generation DMUs in traffic while others had to be withdrawn as they were overdue for overhaul, this bringing loco-hauled substitutes on some lines, particularly in the northwest. When the Class 158s did eventually enter squadron service in 1991/92, it was at the expense of the remaining loco-hauled trains in many areas, particularly Scotland, the northeast, central England, and East Anglia.

The Parcels sector continued to slowly bleed traffic in the same period, 1990 seeing the total loss of weekend Royal Mail trains while unremunerative cross-country and secondary routes were progressively cut. Traffic out of London termini was not immune either as all services from London Bridge and Waterloo were withdrawn in May 1990.

While Railfreight was overall profitable as the decade began, the Speedlink wagonload network was not, and it was decreed that this would be withdrawn from June 1991. Its demise had a significant impact on the loco fleet with Railfreight Distribution ending its use of Class 85s on the West Coast and Class 20s in Scotland for example while other types were pruned, most notably Class 47s. Already targeted for reduction, the Class 08 shunters suffered further casualties, particularly among older examples and those that were still vacuum-braked only.

Outside factors also played a significant role in the fortunes of the freight sector, such as the closure of Ravenscraig steelworks in 1991 and then the decimation of the UK coal industry over the following two years. The latter plus the introduction of the Class 60s meant that Class 20s ceased to be used on power station coal workings during 1993 while Class 56s were also impacted for the first time with a number of the unfavoured Romanian-built examples stood down for good. The traffic losses also meant Class 37s were now available in significant numbers for use by the Civil Engineers, with Class 26s, 31s and 33s all suffering casualties as a result. These would prove terminal in the case of the Scottish Type 2s with the last survivors withdrawn en masse in October 1993.

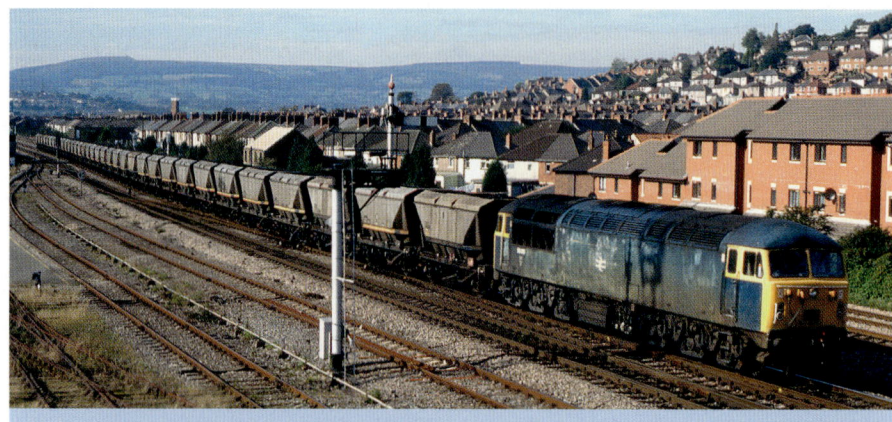

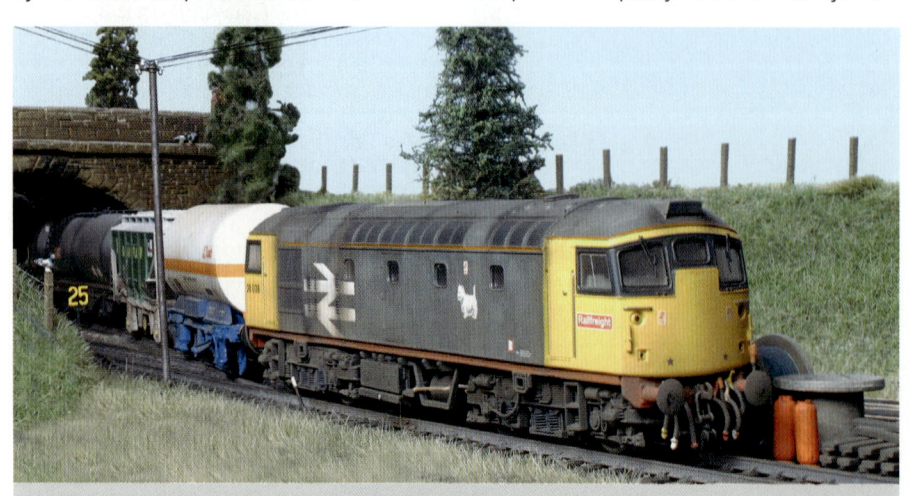

ABOVE: By 1994, main line locos retaining BR blue were increasingly uncommon as withdrawals of older types and overhauls progressively thinned the ranks. Having escaped a call to works for some years, a shabby 56010 rumbles past East Usk Yard on October 7 as it nears Llanwern steelworks with one of the daily coal trans from Port Talbot. By this date, it was owned by Transrail and would go on to receive the company's triple grey colours the following year. The entire rake of merry-go-round coal hoppers have received aerodynamic canopies, making them HFA, with most having yellow-painted cradles and Railfreight Coal logos. In 4mm scale, both Accurascale and Cavalex have newly released highly-detailed models of the iconic wagons, joining the older Hornby version, while both Farish and Peco offer N gauge recreations and Dapol a 7mm version. Simon Bendall Collection

ABOVE: Although very much a 1980s livery, Railfreight Red Stripe could still be seen into the following decade. The scheme particularly suited the Class 26s as shown by 26038 on the 4mm scale layout Ringburn Yard, then owned by Alex Hall but now sold on. This is the rather nice Heljan model, the manufacturer also producing a 7mm version with Dapol covering the N gauge market. This loco would be withdrawn in October 1992 by when it was carrying Civil Engineers grey/yellow but several of its classmates would go their graves in this livery. Ian Manderson

A legacy continued

Choppers cut down

The early 1990s were not kind to the remaining English Electric Type 1s as the Class 60s arrived to take over merry-go-round coal trains while the closure of Speedlink and collieries along with other traffic losses also made significant inroads into the fleet. Simon Bendall **recounts the final years while** Alex Carpenter **creates a couple of former Thornaby machines.**

At the beginning of 1990, there were 133 Class 20s in active service, these being spread across four Railfreight sub-sectors with a lesser number allocated to departmental use. Unsurprisingly, the largest allocation was to Railfreight Coal where the class was still frontline traction for power station merry-go-round (MGR) workings in the traditional pairs. Based entirely at Toton depot, the 76 Type 1s were almost equally split between two pools, one covering the Nottinghamshire area while the other was for traffic in the northwest of England.

Taking the local Nottinghamshire pool first, this featured disc headcode examples 20004/07/26/40/47/52/53/59/73/75/78 /81/ 84/85/88/94 and 20103/04/05/08 along with headcode box equipped 20129/ 36/42/43/51/57/63/66/70/77/86/87/90 / 96 and 20210/14/15. Livery highlights included Railfreight Red Stripe 20059, 20104/08/63/70 and 20215 along with the sole member of the class to receive Railfreight triple grey 20088.

The northwest allocation at the same point featured 20006/10/13/16/19-21/23/28/45/55/ 57/71/80/82/90 and 20106/13/17/20/21/28 with disc headcodes while 20130-33/35/40/41/ 54/59/68/69/72/75/82/94/95/97 were from those built with headcode boxes. In amongst the plain blue examples were ex Thornaby duo 20028 and 20172 with red stripe additions while 20010/23/90 and 20132/41/75 were in Railfreight Red Stripe.

Elsewhere, Immingham was host to 20046/61/93/98 and 20107/12 for steel traffic while Thornaby had 20118/19/22/24/37/38/44/56/65 for similar purposes, although these could feature on other commodities as well. Of the latter, only 20119/24/44 retained BR blue, the others all being in Railfreight Red Stripe. In Scotland, 20066, 20148 and 20185 were assigned to Eastfield for petroleum traffic and 20198, 20211 and 20212 for Railfreight Distribution duties.

Completing matters were those in use with the Civil Engineers department, Immingham being home to 20025/30/64/96, the middle pair being the former Tinsley celebrities that were clinging to their now filthy BR green livery. Toton was home to a sizeable fleet which was assigned to work across a wide area stretching from Birmingham to Crewe, Manchester and Liverpool and reaching across to Nottingham and the Midland Main Line, the locos being 20029/31/32/34/35/4 2/43/48/56/63/69/70/72/92/95, 20102/10/1 4/27/39/45/60/76/88/89/99 and 20227/28. Liveries of note here were 20070 in blue with red solebars and Railfreight Red Stripe 202227. Completing matters were 20206 and 20213 assigned to Eastfield for the Mechanical and Electrical Engineers and 20058 and 20087 to the BR Research department, although the latter pair spent much of their time working passenger trains for Provincial.

Downsizing

Within a year, 31 locos had been withdrawn with Immingham losing all of its Class 20s, be they revenue or departmental examples. Toton was also stripped of its Civil Engineers allocation, some transferring to the more logical depot of Bescot in Birmingham while others re-joined Railfreight, and the rest were condemned. Changes in the Eastfield Distribution fleet also saw all of 20118/19/22/24/37/38/56/65 arrive from Thornaby.

This was just the tip of the decimation that followed though, 1992 beginning with just 52 Class 20s remaining as the arrival of the Class 60s was felt. The axing of Speedlink in June 1991 had seen the Eastfield allocation abolished and the locos returned south, although not all to Thornaby, while all of the class in engineers use except the Research examples (now comprising 20058/66/87 and 20119/38) were withdrawn. This left 20007/32/55/57/71/72/75/78/82/96, 20104/06/17/21/28/35/42/43/63/68/69/85-87/90 and 20210/14/15 on Nottinghamshire area MGRs with 20016/59/73/81/90/94 and 20131/32/40/51/54/77/95/96 likewise engaged in the northwest. The Railfreight Metals fleet was down to just 20046/92 and 20118/37/65, all based at Thornaby.

The destruction of the British coal industry during 1992 delivered the final blow to Class 20s in use with any Railfreight sub-sector, the Nottinghamshire MGR pool being abolished as was the Teesside steel allocation. Only 20016/57/59/81 and 20154/68 were retained into the spring of 1993 to cover the northwest workings, after which the future of those Class 20s that remained lay with newly created engineering divisions and ultimately, Direct Rail Services.

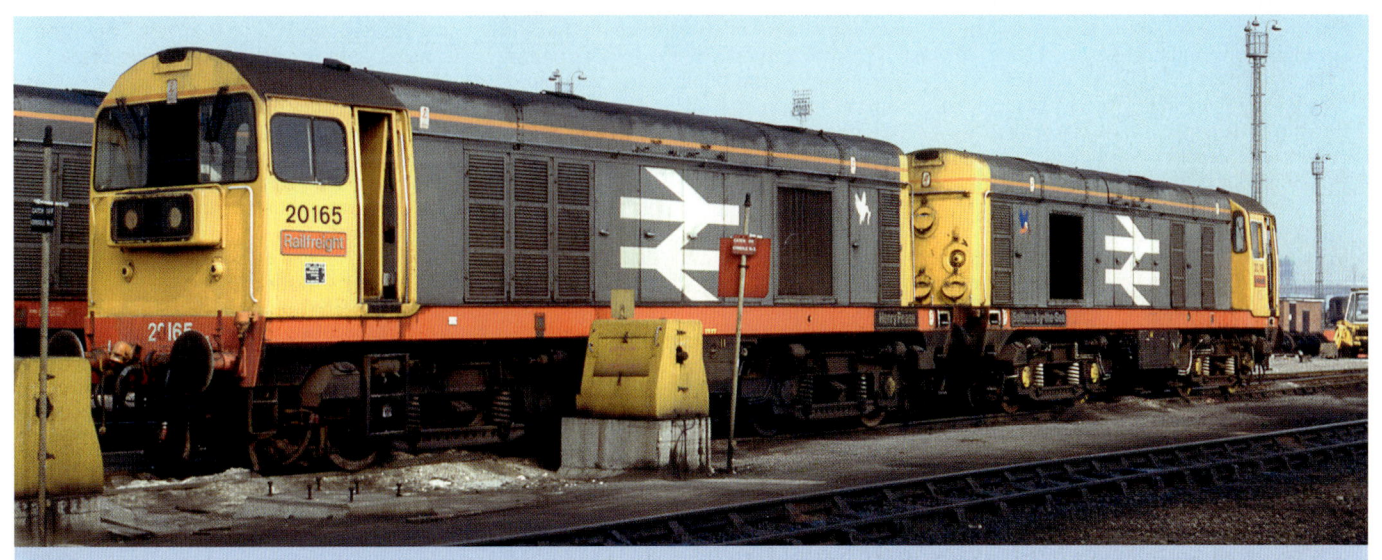

ABOVE: While Class 20s are best associated with coal traffic, Railfreight Metals also retained a much smaller fleet into the early 1990s. On March 31, 1990, Thornaby favourites 20165 *Henry Pease* and 20118 *Saltburn-by-the-Sea* are seen at their much-missed home depot. Two months later, they would join an exodus to Eastfield to work for Railfreight Distribution in Scotland, but they were returned south following the closure of Speedlink, initially to Toton in July 1991 but they were back on Teesside three months later. Simon Bendall Collection

Modelling BR Locomotives of the 1990s **9**

A legacy continued

A red stripe duo

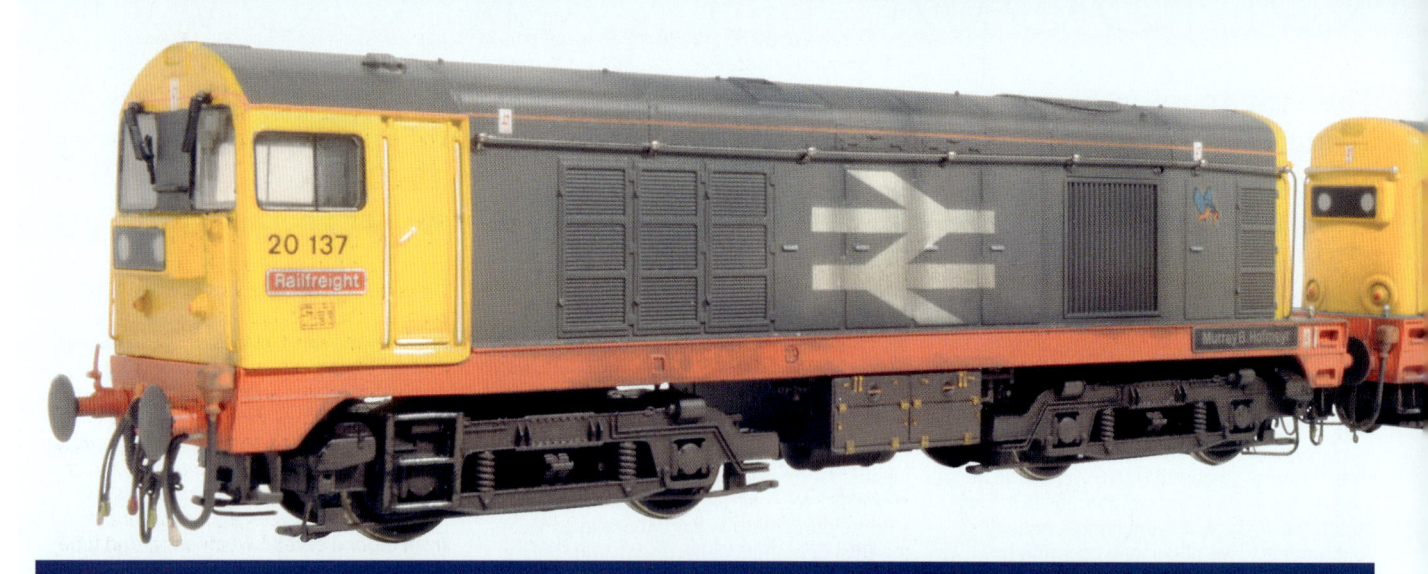

ABOVE: The former Thornaby stablemates pose together still sporting their depot customisation. Although now superseded, the older Bachmann tooling still has merit especially if you are not concerned about working lights.

This project used the older version of Bachmann's OO gauge Class 20 as it was completed prior to the release of the current all-new model in 2021. This now somewhat obsolete but still useful model underwent a couple of upgrades during its lifetime, these improving both the roof fan grille and the exhaust ports externally.

For those owing the older tooling, such as the Railfreight Red Stripe-liveried duo of 20023 and 20132, the most significant upgrade than can be made is the replacement of the roof fan grille with the etch from Shawplan's Extreme Etchings range. For this, it is best to fit the lower spacer rings first and do any filling to ensure a good fit but leave adding the fragile mesh and upper cross-frame until just before painting to avoid damaging them during handling of the bodyshell. Sticking with the roof for a moment, the prominent mould lines on the cab roof ventilators can also be pared away.

Many of the other upgrades undertaken here concern the ends. Chief amongst them was the replacement of the plastic sprung buffers with the black-finished turned brass Oleo buffers produced by Markits. Not only do these offer a visual improvement, but they also overcome the curious decision to fit buffers with different shank types to the disc headcode and centre box models. Once these were in place, lamp brackets fabricated from brass strip were added on top of the shanks, although not all of the Type 1s carried a full set of four by this period. The inverted 'L' shaped handrails on the cab front were also replaced by brass wire to give a finer appearance while Bachmann's meagre selection of bufferbeam pipework was supplemented by Hornby spares intended for the Class 50.

Bogie modifications

The real 20172 was notable for carrying a mixed set of bogie equalising beams, it

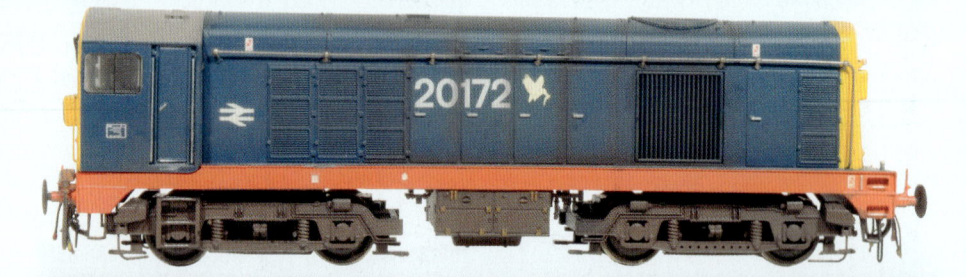

ABOVE: The former *Redmire* shows off its mismatched bogie sideframes, the equalising beam under the bonnet having the weight relieving holes while that under the cab lacks this feature. This is the sort of customisation that can help a model stand out and rewards the careful study of photos during research.

having three with the weight relieving holes but the fourth was of the solid fluted type. Plasticard rod was used to fill the holes in the relevant sideframe moulding before applying filler to ensure a smooth finish. In 20137's case, the donor model was already riding on the right bogie type so required no work in this area. While further Extreme Etchings parts could have been added,

such as the replacement bonnet doors, the need for the locos to survive the rigours of exhibition use meant that a certain robustness was required, rather than full showcase standard.

As for 20172's livery, it was one of five Thornaby-allocated Class 20s to be customised with red solebars, white or light grey cab roofs, unofficial names, and the

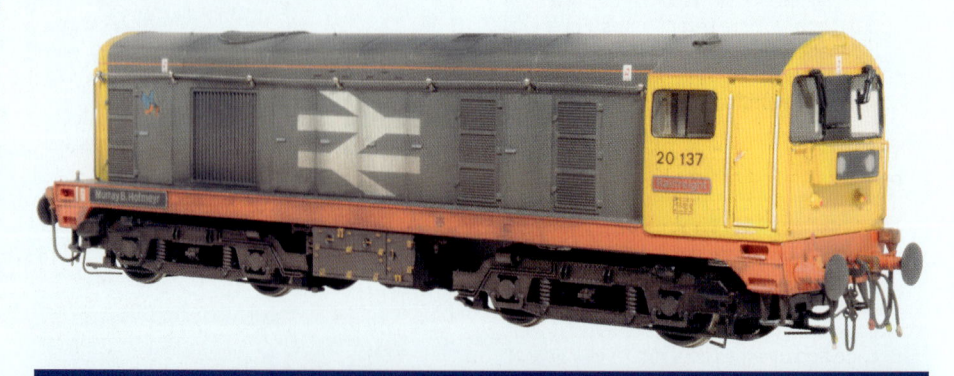

ABOVE: Thornaby had a quartet of Railfreight Red Stripe Class 20s that were given official cast nameplates and Railfreight plaques along with depot logos. This helped them stand out from their classmates and no layout set around Teesside in the late 1980s or early 1990s should be without at least one of them, in this case 20137 *Murray B. Hofmeyr*.

A legacy continued

In the case of 20172, its *Redmire* name would be removed by late 1988 ahead of transfer to Toton at the beginning of the following year while its depot logos would also be painted over a few months later. However, the large numbers and paintwork enhancements remained in place to withdrawal in November 1990.

Finished in Railfreight Red Stripe, 20137 also carried Thornaby kingfisher embellishments alongside its *Murray B. Hofmeyr* nameplates but these were initially all left alone when the loco transferred to Eastfield depot in May 1990 so are in place here.

Painting for two

In terms of painting, Halfords grey primer was used as a base, followed by a coat of Railmatch Rail blue or Railfreight grey as appropriate to the loco. The solebars and bufferbeams were masked off and sprayed white, this giving the Rail red topcoat a light base so as to avoid multiple coats. This technique was also used for the yellow ends with the black window surround on 20137 then masked and painted. The solebar tops were touched in with blue or grey afterwards as it was impossible to mask off the yellow at the bonnet end in one piece without some over-spray. Finally, the cab roof of 20172 was painted with Railmatch diesel roof grey.

For the blue example, custom transfers were provided by Precision Decals, these being supplied as a complete pack for the loco, including data panels, ready-made numbersets, kingfishers and depot stickers, while 20137 utilised Replica numbers and Fox BR arrows and kingfishers with etched nameplates and Railfreight plaques coming from Shawplan. The transfers were applied and sealed in with the usual layers of gloss and satin varnish. A Class 20 will always benefit from a good careful weathering and time spent here really pays off. Little touches like picking out the horn grilles in black and adding the grime build up and fading on the bodyside doors really brings the locos to life.

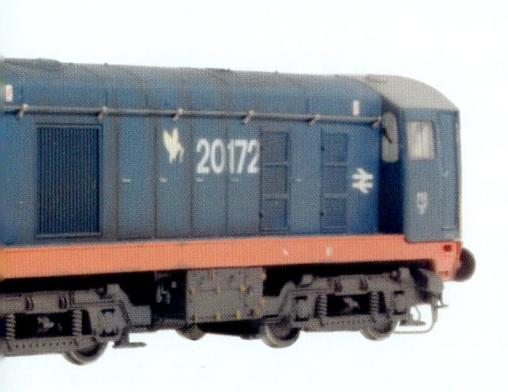

trademark kingfisher emblems from 1987. Joining it were 20028 *Bedale*, 20070 *Leyburn*, 20173 *Wensleydale* and, the odd one out in name terms, 20174 *Captain James Cook RN*.

Model availability

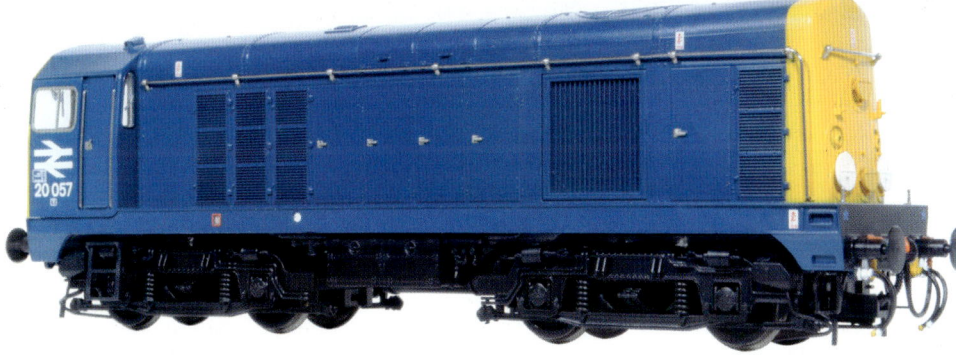

Ready-to-run models of the Class 20s have been plentiful over the years, if not always accurate when going back to Hornby Dublo and Wrenn days. For OO gauge, Lima was the go to model during the 1980s and 1990s and this tooling now resides with Hornby, where it has made the occasional appearance in more recent times. For the last two decades though, Bachmann has had the class sewn up, the first iteration serving the company well until the surprise appearance of the completely retooled model in 2021. This not only allowed a full lighting suite to be provided for the first time but also delivered a bodyshell with an improved shape and enhanced tooling options to cater for a wider range of detail variations.

It is a similar story in N gauge where the Poole-era Graham Farish Class 20 served the market for many years until it was replaced a decade ago by an all new model developed by Bachmann under the same brand name. In 7mm, it is Heljan that dominates the market with its popular rendering which, like in the other scales, caters for both disc and headcode box variants.

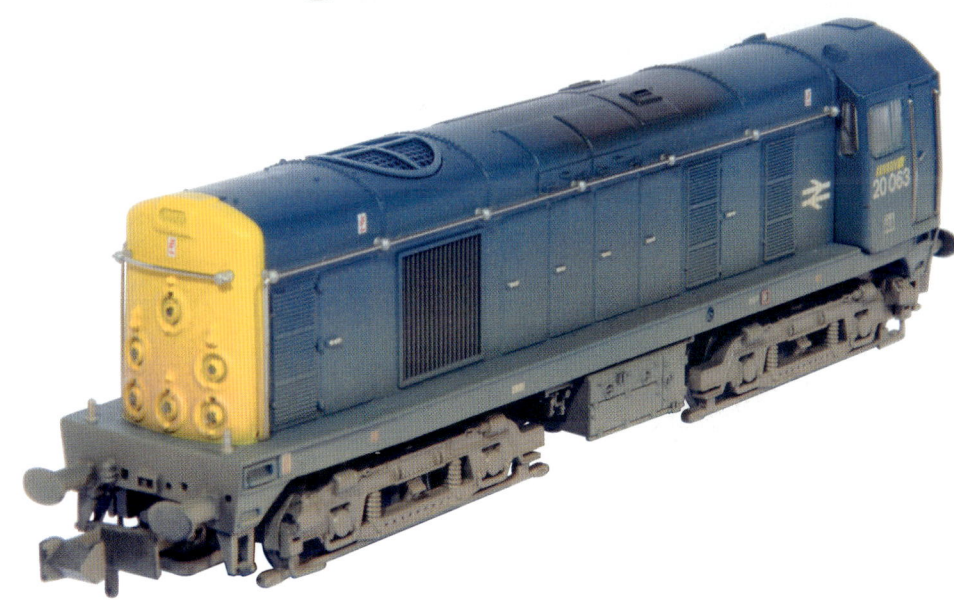

LEFT: **Bachmann's current generation Class 20 was released last year and delivered a model in line with today's expected standards in 4mm scale.**

ABOVE: **The retooled Farish Class 20 was a step change in quality when released ten years ago, it makes the original N gauge tooling redundant.**

Modelling BR Locomotives of the 1990s

A legacy continued

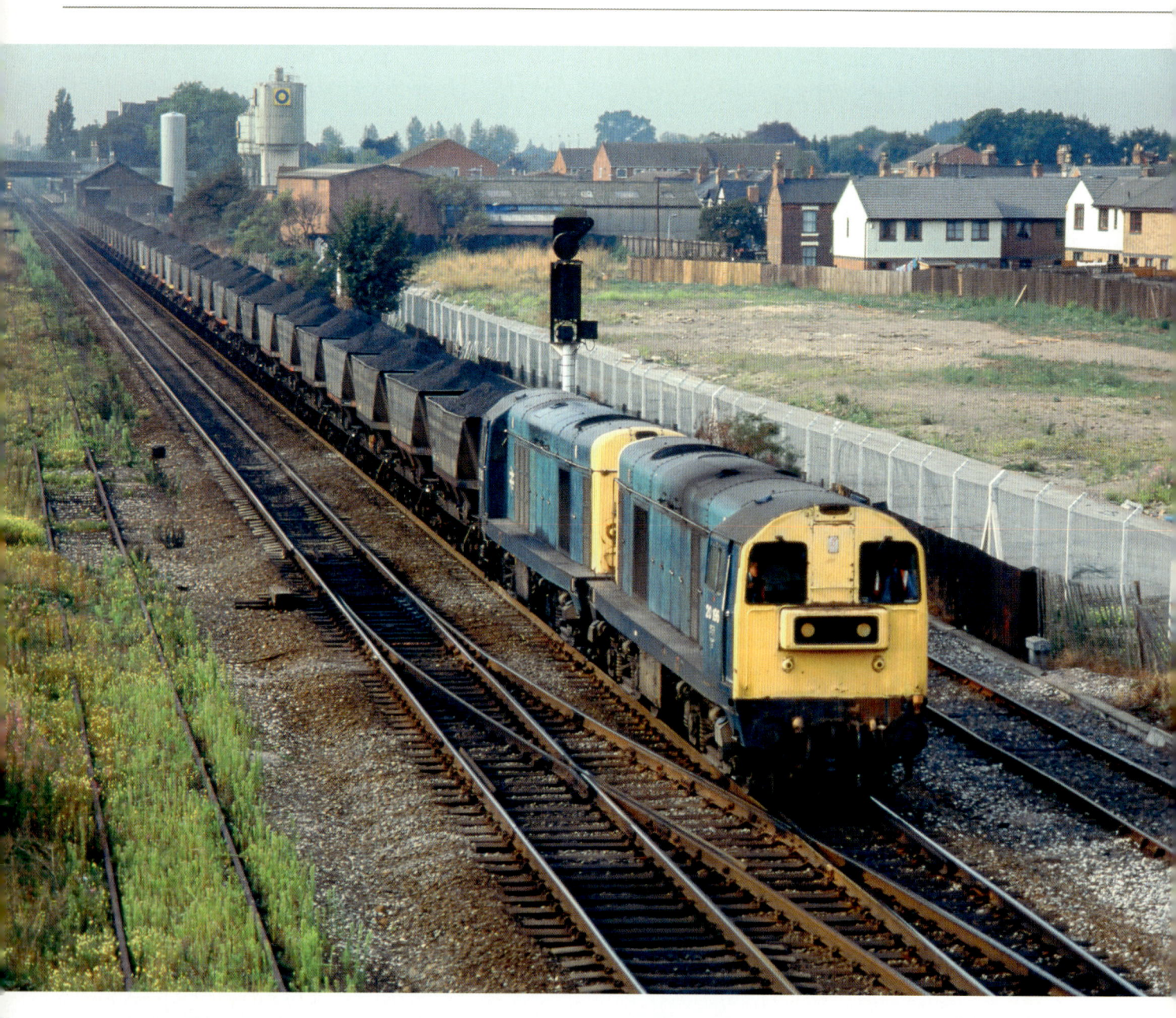

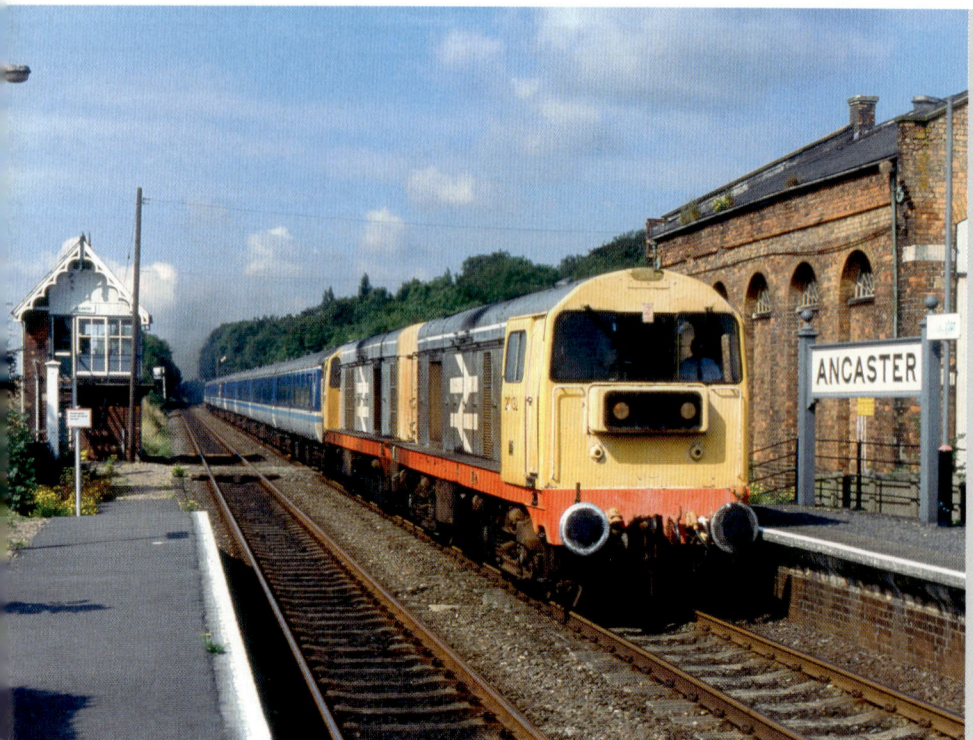

ABOVE: The traditional employment of pairs of Class 20s was still prominent in the early 1990s, finally ending in the spring of 1993. On September 11, 1990, the blue duo of 20196 and 20105, both from Toton's Nottinghamshire area allocation, are appropriately local as they pass Beeston with a well-loaded northbound MGR working. Modellers in OO gauge now have considerable choice for models of the HAA hoppers and derivatives following the release of new highly-detailed offerings from both Accurascale and Cavalex Models, these joining the well-established Hornby version. There is a choice of suppliers in N gauge too courtesy of Graham Farish and Peco while 7mm is covered by Dapol. Martin Loader

LEFT: Despite having no booked passenger work, Class 20s were common enough on such work in the Midlands during warmer months, especially at weekends. This included the famed workings to Skegness which on October 21, 1992, saw the Railfreight-liveried duo of 20132 and 20090 passing through Ancaster with the 1E86 09.25 from Derby to the east coast resort. In tow is a set of recently-painted Regional Railways coaches, which would be predominately Etches Park-based Mk.2a but with a small number of Mk.1 and Mk.2c also in the fleet. The Bachmann and Graham Farish ranges have featured suitable stock in the respective scales over the years.
Martin Loader

A legacy continued

RIGHT: From Immingham's soon to be abolished Railfreight Metals allocation, 20112 and 20098 whistle along near Melton Ross on July 12, 1990, with a Scunthorpe to Immingham trip working of steel slab. The mix of flats is led by four BMA, as converted from BDA bogie bolsters and BPA Boplates. Next comes a BDA with its distinctive low red sides and, after another BMA, are three BBA, these being examples equipped with both coil cradles and stanchions. Another BMA and more BDAs round out the visible portion. In 4mm scale, Bachmann produces the BDA, Cavalex does the BBA and Cambrian a kit for the BMA along with the BBA and BDA in the same form. In N gauge, Farish offers the BDA while Chivers Finelines does a kit for the BBA. *John Chalcraft/Rail Photoprints*

BELOW: A key duty of the Class 20s based at Eastfield for Railfreight Distribution was to work trip freights to the Fife area from Mossend as part of Speedlink. On May 30, 1990, Thornaby exile 20137 *Murray B. Hofmeyr* was newly arrived north of the border as it partners 20198 at Lochgelly on a working from the Glasgow yard to Thornton. The consist includes Grainflow Polybulks and carbon dioxide tanks for the distillery at Cameron Bridge along with VEA vans and a Warwell for the military dockyard at Rosyth. In 4mm, the available models are limited to the Bachmann VEA and Hattons or Oxford Rail Warwell while in N gauge, the VEA has been produced by Sonic Models in conjunction with Revolution Trains. The N Gauge Society also offers kits for the Polybulks and Warwells. *John Chalcraft/Rail Photoprints*

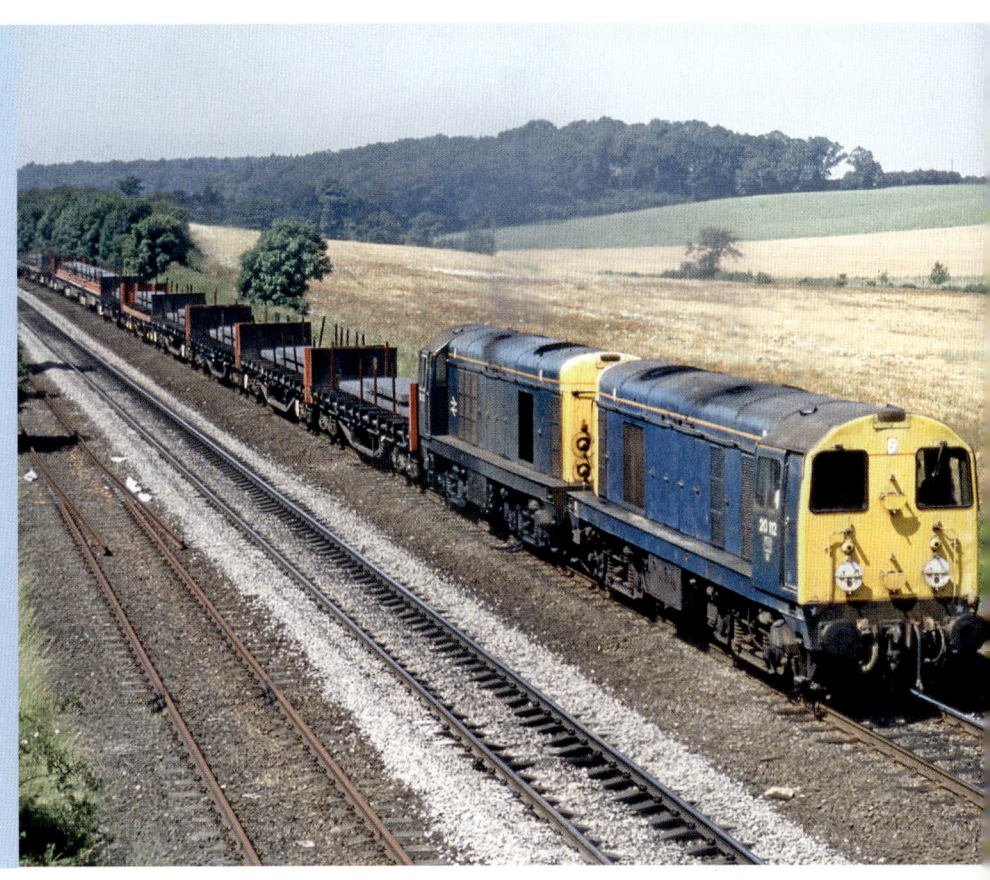

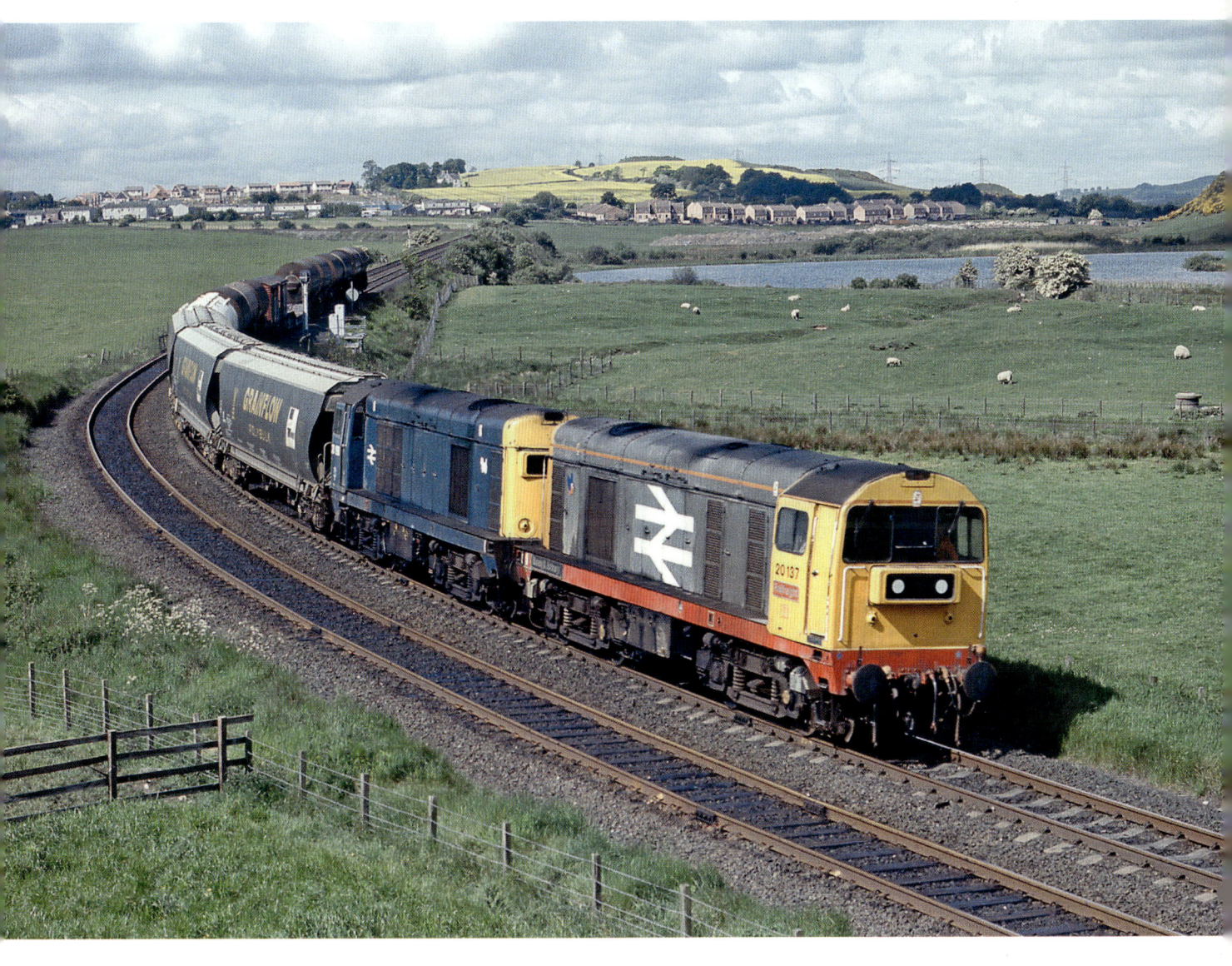

A legacy continued

Electrics fade away

The last of the first generation AC electrics to be withdrawn were the Class 85s, particularly those that spent their final few years dedicated to freight work with Railfreight Distribution. Simon Bendall recounts the history of the sub-class while Alex Carpenter tweaks the OO gauge Bachmann model.

The story of the Class 85/1s began in the spring of 1989 when ten members of the class, 85006/09/10/12/16/21/24/32/35/36, were identified as 'long-life' locomotives for use solely on freight duties. Given a 75mph speed restriction, the electric train supply (ETS) jumper cables were also removed, leaving the bufferbeam fittings behind. This modification was partly carried out to reduce maintenance costs, but it also meant that the locos were less likely to be purloined at short notice for InterCity passenger duties, although it was by no means an unknown occurrence! To reflect the alterations, the ten machines were renumbered in order as 85101-10 during June and July 1989 and found use on all manner of freight traffic along the West Coast Main Line.

Despite the 'long-life' designation, there was a limit on the amount of money that would be expended on the sub-class so when 85107 combusted near Penrith on September 2, 1989, it was immediately stored. Having worked for less than three months with its new identity, it would eventually be condemned the following spring. Meanwhile, October 19 found 85101 arriving at Ripple Lane with a car train from Garston, this being the first visit of a Class 85/1 to the area.

Extra conversions

Early November saw 85004 become 85111 to take the place of the doomed 85107 but it fared just as badly, succumbing to transformer damage in February 1990 and almost immediate condemnation. Again, a replacement was quickly provided with 85112 being renumbered from 85007. For much of the rest of the year, the sub-class continued with its regular diet of freight work with the odd passenger and parcels turn thrown in for variety. October saw two further Class 85s renumbered, 85003 and 85011 becoming 85113/14 respectively, just days before 85106 went up in flames at Soho followed by the inevitable withdrawal. 1990 ended with 85112 and 85113 both in store at Crewe, the former never working again.

January 1991 brought another first for 85101 when the sub-class pioneer was deployed on Project Mercury engineers' duties in Belsize Tunnel, this being located on the Midland Main Line near Kentish Town. The loco would later stable at St Pancras, becoming only the second AC electric and first Class 85 to visit the famous London terminus. However, the sub-class was facing extinction by the middle of the year as the Speedlink wagonload network was abandoned from July 8, making the Class 85/1s surplus to requirements. Condemned prior to this date, in May, were 85102 and 85103, the latter having suffered collision damage, whilst 85104/05/08/09/12-14 were all withdrawn within the first eight days of July.

InterCity comeback

However, this was not quite the end for the Class 85/1s as 85101 and 85110 were claimed by InterCity during July for 40mph local empty stock movements, the former being re-allocated to Willesden and the latter to Longsight, although it actually worked off Liverpool Edge Hill. Prior to taking up their new duties, both machines had their ETS cables reinstated at Crewe Electric. Along with 85105, 85101 had taken part in the 'Roarer Requiem' railtour on June 30, this heading to the unlikely locations of Shoeburyness, Liverpool Street, Colchester St. Botolph's and Walton-on-the-Naze from Manchester Piccadilly. For this duty, 85101 had received a makeover, this including red bufferbeams and the application of original E3061 numbers on the secondman's cabsides.

Despite having spent the first half of 1991 in store, the withdrawal of 85113 was reversed, it too joining the InterCity fleet at Willesden for Euston stock movements with its ETS capability suitably reinstated. Its arrival also saw off the last remaining pair of Class 81s, 81012 and 81017 being condemned in late July. However, the reprieve for this trio of Class 85/1s was only ever a short-term duty as, with Class 86s becoming available from the autumn as push-pull working took fuller effect, 85110 was condemned in October with 85101 and 85113 joining it the following month.

That should have been it for the Class 85/1s under British Rail but, curiously, 85101 was reinstated to the Railfreight Distribution stored fleet in May 1992 pending possible conversion to a mobile load bank for testing the new Class 92s. In the event, no work took place, and it was withdrawn again six months later, becoming the sole example of the class to be preserved.

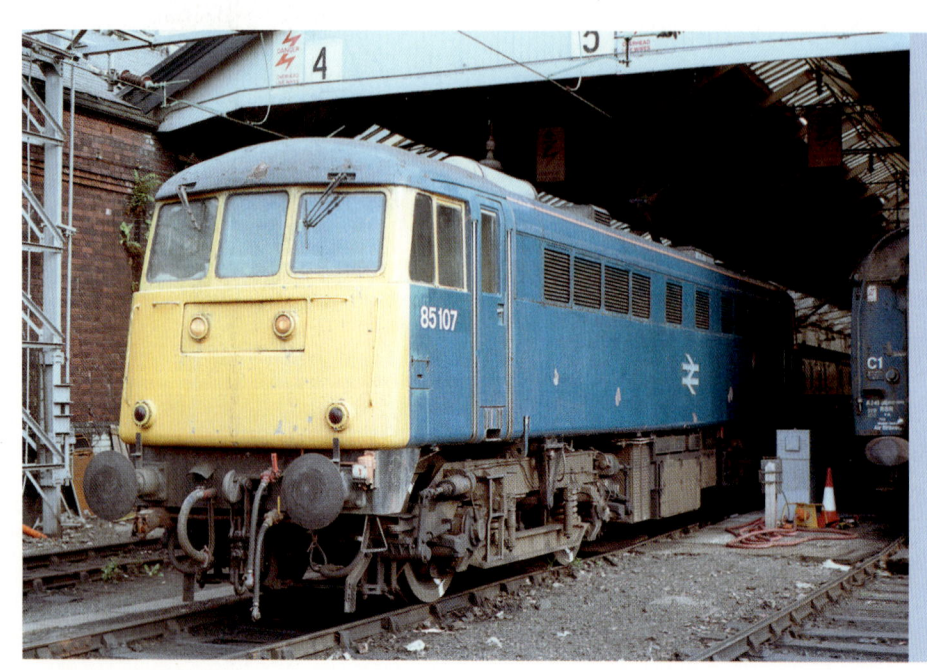

LEFT: Renumbered in June 1989, 85107 was the shortest-lived of the Class 85/1 sub-class, suffering terminal fire damage three months later although official withdrawal did not come until May 1990. The ill-fated machine is seen at Longsight that summer showing the simple 'modification' that created the freight-only machines with the ETS cable removed from the bufferbeam but with the jumper boxes left in place. Simon Bendall Collection

A legacy continued

A freight-only electric

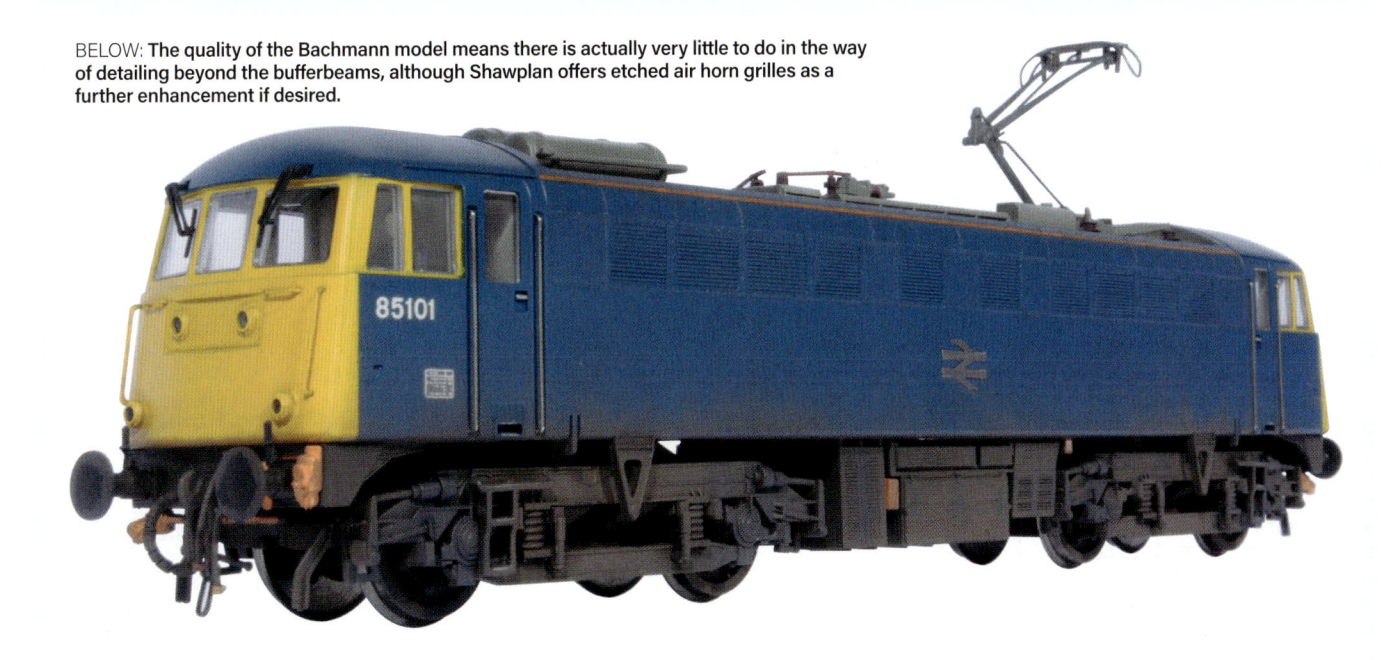

BELOW: The quality of the Bachmann model means there is actually very little to do in the way of detailing beyond the bufferbeams, although Shawplan offers etched air horn grilles as a further enhancement if desired.

The Class 85 was Bachmann's first venture into the world of AC electric locos in OO gauge and helped pave the way for the other models that have since followed. The manufacturer did an excellent job of capturing the look of these locos, which makes subsequent customisation much easier as there are no major faults to correct, and the work can be concentrated on detailing and weathering.

Firstly, I had to choose a loco. I wanted to represent a Class 85 at the end of its career as the main period I model is the very early 1990s, so I opted for one of the freight-dedicated '85/1' sub-class. This in turn led me to 85101 (ex 85006), which I decided to model before it gained the garish red bufferbeams and pre-TOPS numbers for its final months in traffic.

Detail wise, the Class 85/1s were outwardly identical to the standard class members except for the removal of the ETS cable in the vast majority of cases, the corresponding sockets being left in place. As no major work was required, I decided to keep the original paint as the colours were pretty much spot on, just giving it an all over coat of satin varnish to tone it down a bit and remove the shine. White TOPS numbers came from Fox Transfers and Replica Railways supplied the data panels, while the BR cast arrows that came with the model were also fitted with sparing amounts of superglue. This was all sealed in with another coat of satin varnish.

The Class 85 bufferbeam equipment is straightforward with cast air and vacuum pipes coming from Shawplan and the ETS receptacles from Heljan Class 47 spares. The screw couplings along with the ETS pipework and jumpers are Bachmann as supplied as they look the part after a lick of paint.

Attention was next turned to the weathering, which really does bring the Class 85 to life and highlight all the little details. Railmatch acrylic 'sleeper grime' was applied liberally to the underframe and bodysides, then mostly washed off with a cotton bud soaked in acrylic thinners, giving the streaking effect. Once the loco was suitably 'cleaned', a light coat of 'fresh' dirt was applied.

The roof was weathered with 'roof dirt' using the same technique and was made significantly grubbier, including the light brown staining from the pantograph and overhead wires. The underframe and bogies were picked out in various shades to represent the oily patches typical of the class. Lastly, the wheels were weathered separately to highlight the detail of the final drive linkage on the wheel face, this being a neatly modelled touch.

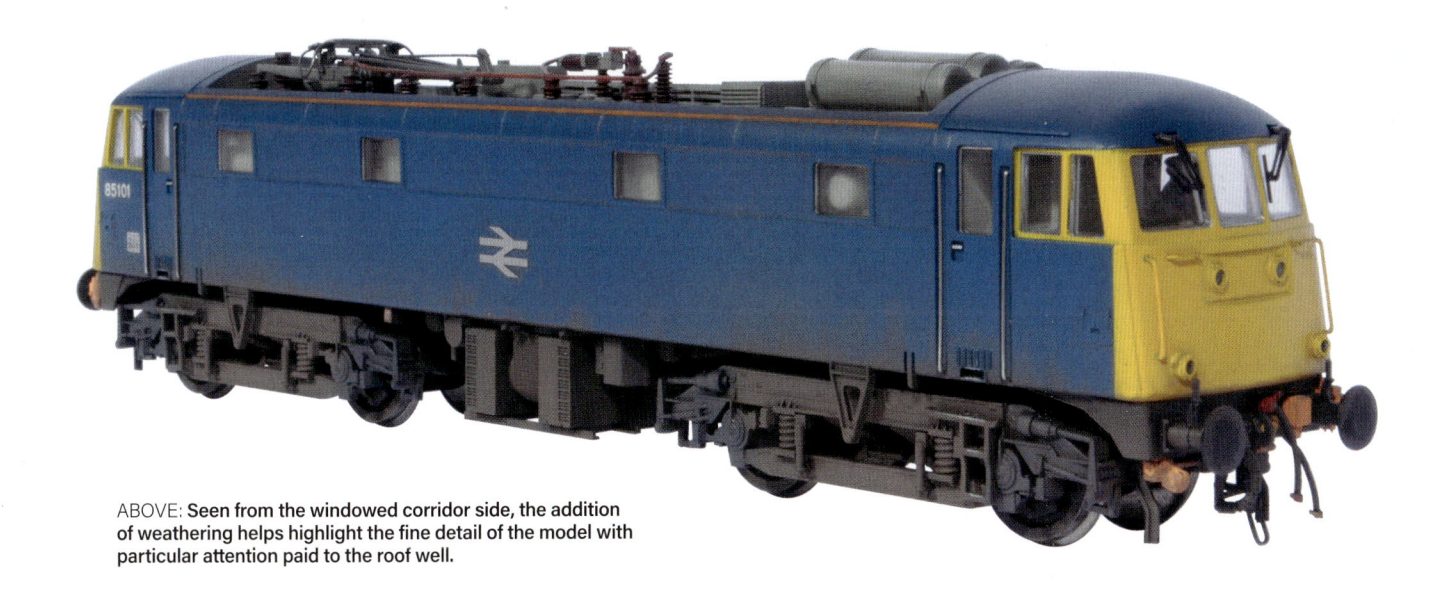

ABOVE: Seen from the windowed corridor side, the addition of weathering helps highlight the fine detail of the model with particular attention paid to the roof well.

Modelling BR Locomotives of the 1990s

A legacy continued

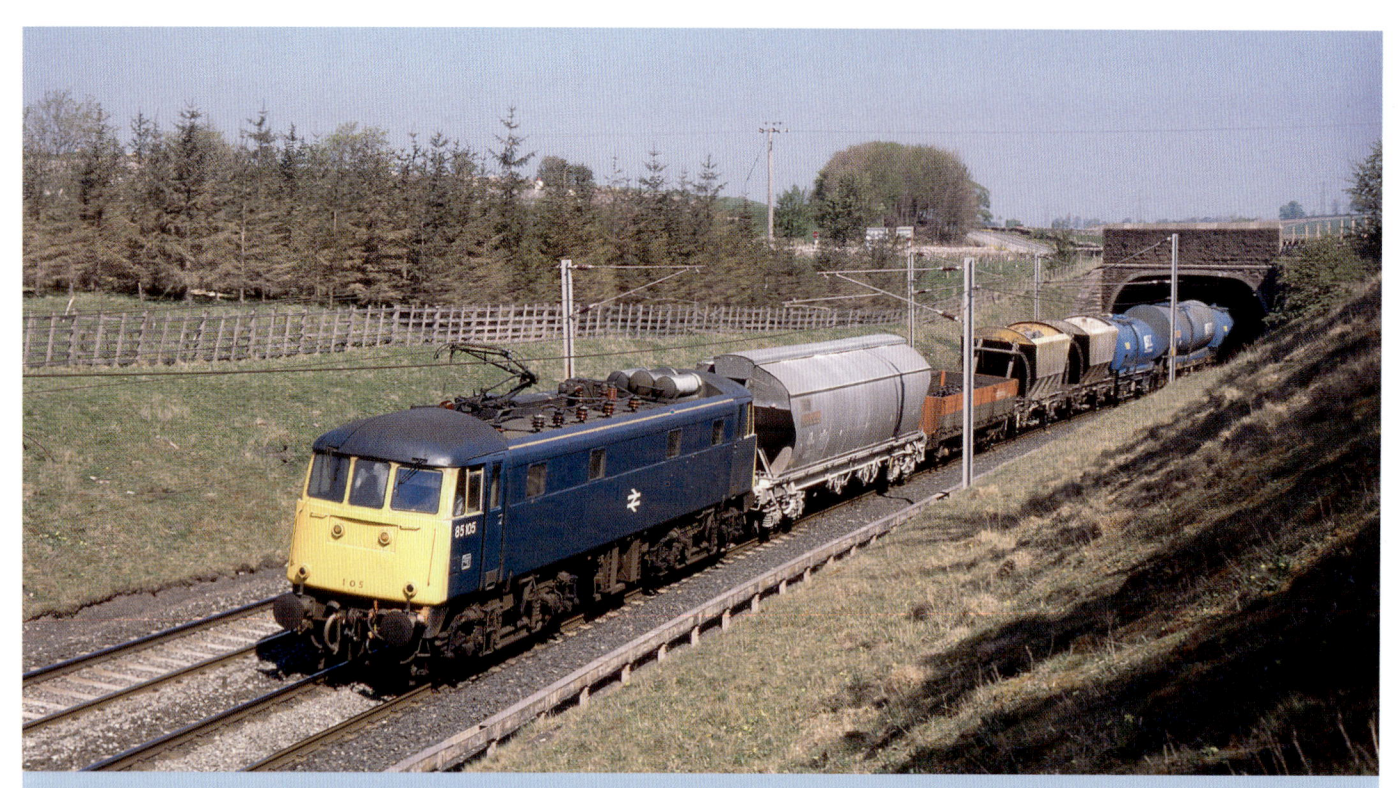

ABOVE: The Class 85/1s could be found atop a variety of freight services on the West Coast Main Line, including Speedlink wagonload services. On May 1, 1990, 85105 has just passed beneath the A6 at Shap Beck as it hums south with the 08.20 Mossend-Stoke Gifford. Leading the formation is a Polybulk covered hopper, as produced in both 2mm and 4mm by Bachmann, followed by an OAA open, which is available in N gauge from the same source and with a modern OO gauge model due from Rapido later in 2022. The rest of the visible consist is all for china clay traffic with the two ex-salt PGA hoppers being unavailable in any scale as is the bogie TIA slurry tank. However, the smaller TUAs will be a welcome release in OO gauge later this year from Rainbow Railways and Revolution Trains. Dave McAlone

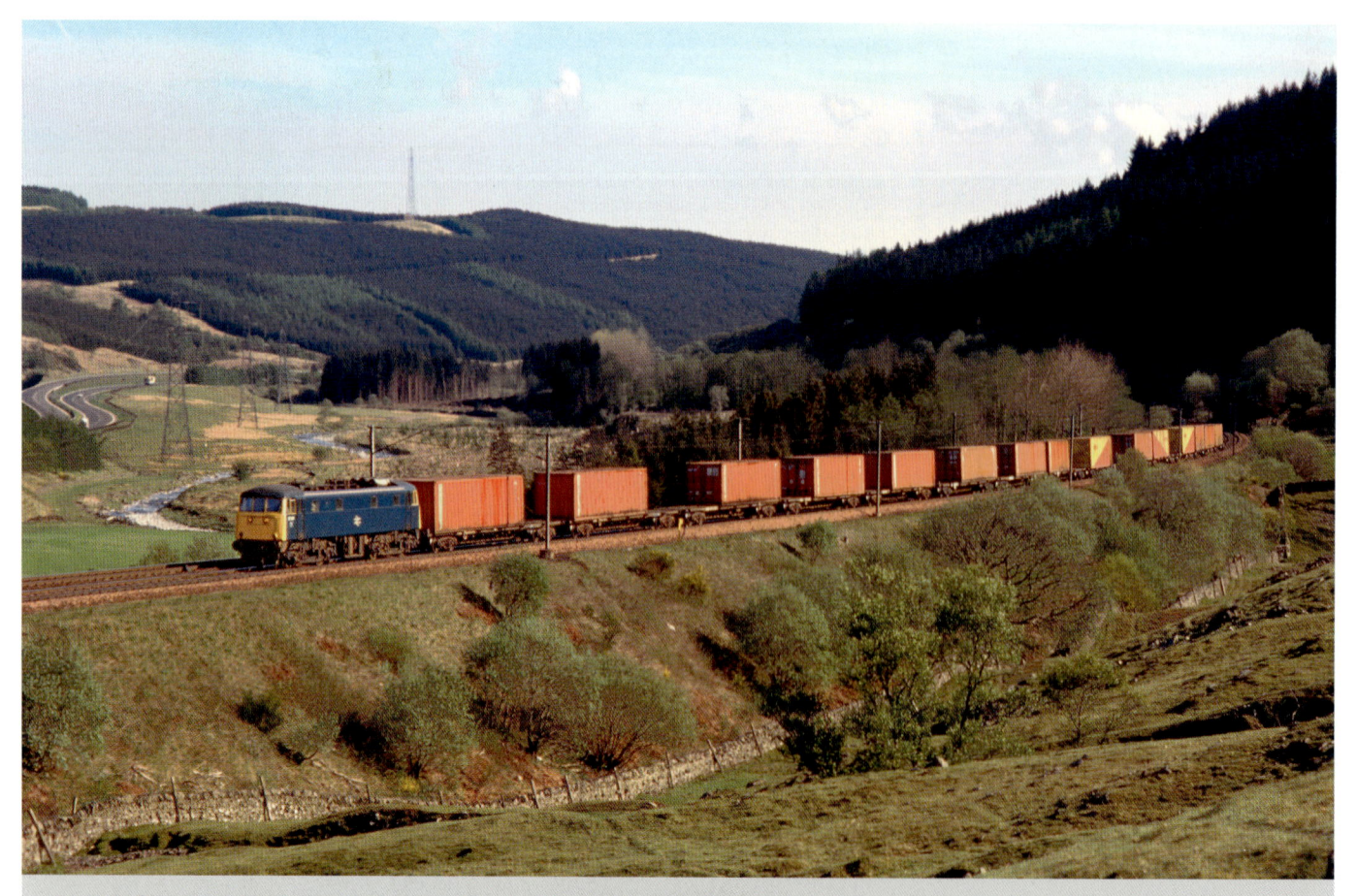

ABOVE: At this point, Freightliner services were under the remit of Railfreight Distribution as 85106 climbs Beattock at Harthope Bank with a Glasgow-bound service on May 5, 1990. With a predominance of 40ft-long boxes, the 15-wagon train is formed entirely of FFA inner, and FGA outer Freightliner flats as produced in 4mm scale to current standards by Bachmann, while a somewhat older model resides in the company's Farish range. C-Rail Intermodal is a good source of the necessary containers in both scales. Dave McAlone

A legacy continued

Channel Tunnel 'Cromptons'

The late 1980s saw a pool of Class 33s allocated to the Construction sub-sector, these being largely dedicated to transporting materials for the building of the Channel Tunnel. Simon Bendall recounts the history of the pool while Paul Wade describes how to upgrade the 'Slim Jim' variant of the OO gauge Heljan model.

The construction of the Channel Tunnel during the late 1980s and early 1990s created a need for a fleet of locos to deliver the multitude of building materials to the construction sites, most notably tunnel lining segments from the Isle of Grain to Shakespeare Cliff. Much of this traffic was contained within Kent making Class 33s, either singly or in pairs, the natural choice for the work.

By the beginning of 1990, no less than 25 of the 32 remaining Class 33/0s were allocated to Railfreight Construction, encompassing 33 004/09/12/19/20/21/23/27/29/33/40/42/46-48/50-53/56-58/60/63/64 along with 33202, 33204 and 33207 from the narrow-bodied Class 33/2s. Of these, 33050 and 33051 had been repainted in Railfreight triple grey with Construction logos in May 1988 to mark the start of the contract with Trans-Manche Link.

A further ten 'Cromptons' would be similarly repainted between October 1988 and August 1989 as they passed through Eastleigh Works for overhaul, these being 33021/33/42/53/56/63/64 and the trio of Class 33/2s. The rest of the pool remained in BR blue though.

Other related workings for the locos included hauling Yeoman PGA hoppers containing stone from Grain to Sevington, further tunnel segments to Ashford Kimberley Sidings, minestone from Snowdown Colliery, spoil from Shakespeare Cliff to Sevington, and some trains of steel items. The Construction-allocated Class 33s could also be found working more widely across the southeast on other aggregates duties and could be borrowed for weekend engineering work as well.

Rapid rundown

As construction of the Channel Tunnel progressed and the need for building materials and spoil removal wound down, the number of 'Cromptons' assigned to Railfreight Construction decreased drastically. By the start of 1992, just seven locos, 33021/42/50/53/63/64 and 33207, remained, with the rest either transferred to the Civil Engineers or withdrawn.

During the course of 1992, these seven remaining locos were also relinquished by Railfreight Construction, most transferring to what was now the Network SouthEast-managed infrastructure fleet but with 33207 going to Railfreight Distribution for use shunting the Dover train ferry. Of the dozen that received the sub-sector's colours, 33033/42/50/53/56/64 would all be withdrawn without another change of livery while 33204 was rebadged to Distribution and 33021, 33063 and 33207 altered to the coloured version of the Mainline Freight logo as they remained in triple grey. Only 33051 and 33202 were repainted again, both into Civil Engineers 'Dutch'.

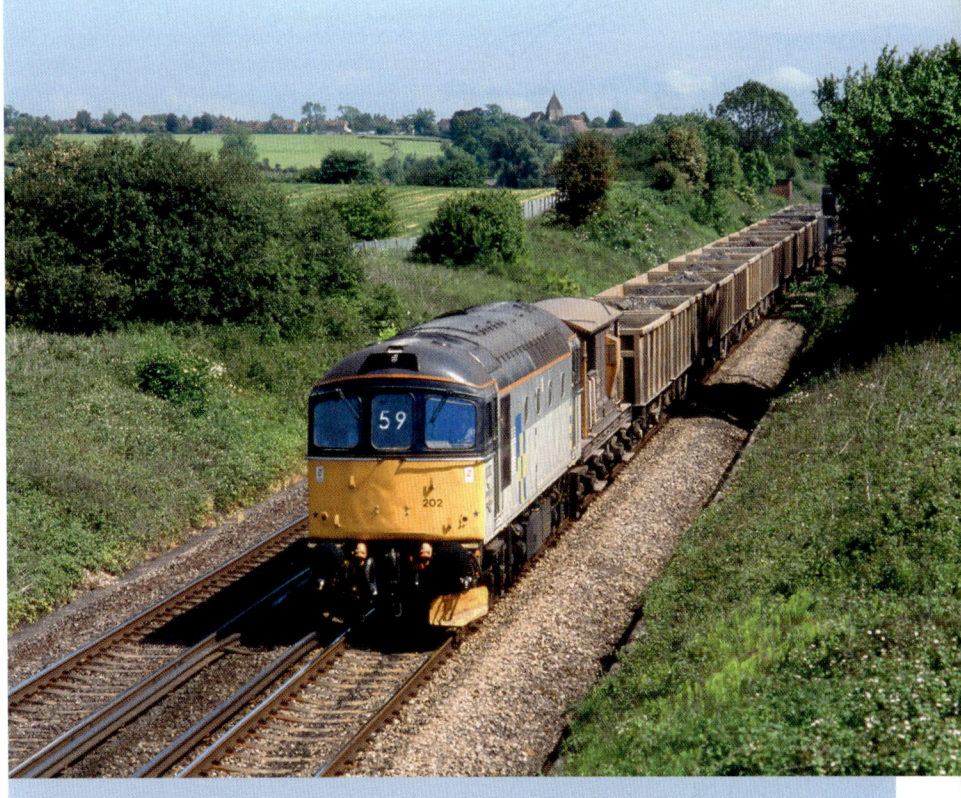

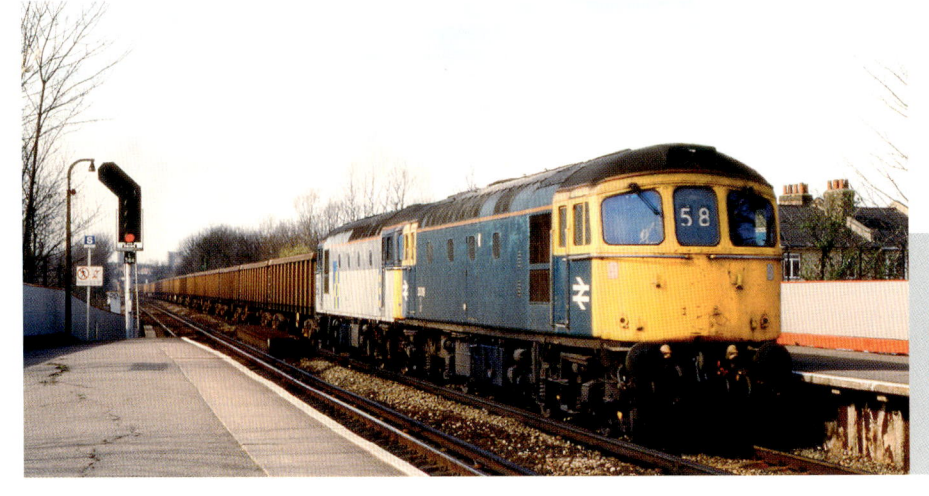

ABOVE: Narrow-bodied 33202 nears the end of its short journey on June 2, 1989, as it passes Sevington with a spoil train from Shakespeare Cliff. This was destined for the sidings of the same name on the outskirts of Ashford and was conveying waste from the excavation of the Channel Tunnel. The wagons are two-axle POA/PNA aggregate boxes as produced by Bachmann in both 2mm and 4mm while the Queen Mary bogie brake van was required as trains propelled out of the sidings onto the main line. *Martin Loader*

LEFT: The mixed livery and sub-class pairing of 33019 and 33204 power through southeast London at Lee on March 9, 1990, with the 10.17 from Shakespeare Cliff to Grain. The lengthy rake of bogie box wagons, then coded PXA, were returning empty for another load of tunnel lining segments. These had only been built in 1987/88 and utilised bogies recovered from scrapped tank wagons. *Simon Bendall Collection*

A legacy continued

Fine-tuning for Heljan's 'Slim Jims'

Current day models for the 'Cromptons' include the Dapol offering in N gauge along with Heljan's 7mm rendering. The Danish manufacturer is also the source of all three sub-classes in OO gauge, it having had two stabs at producing the most common Class 33/0 variant, although both suffer from errors around the cabs or roof that are difficult to correct.

Therefore, the easiest route to modelling some Construction Class 33s for use on my layout Tonbridge West Yard was to alter the then new Railfreight Distribution-liveried 'Slim Jims'. This version was chosen as it required the least changes, but the model still contained an error in the placement of the Distribution repeater logo on one side, it being positioned by the left hand cab door instead of the right hand one. As the logos needed to be removed anyway, this was not a significant issue. A more recent Distribution release features cab front headlights if your chosen example requires them but it still has the same repeater stripe error.

I began by removing all the Railfreight logos, numbers, BR double arrows and cab front blue star multiple working symbols by using a curved knife blade to scratch off the printing. This was done very carefully to minimise the damage to the base colours.

Other methods of removal could be used if preferred but I have had success with using a blade.

Using photographs, I then carved the distinctive cab front dents that are typically found above the coupling hooks, these being caused by the screw coupling striking the bodywork when lifted on or off. These dents varied in shape and size while they were occasionally repaired during works visits; the chosen pair of 33204 and 33207 having no discernible damage on the No.1 (radiator fan) end for example. At the same time, the redundant tail lights were carved off and filled on the same cab of 33207, these often being removed as a result of bodywork repairs.

Cosmetic mods

The next job was to touch up the Rail grey on the lower bodysides where it had been nicked while removing the logos and other printing. The engine roof hatch section was then painted with Executive dark grey as the glass fibre panel weathered with time, while the underframe, bogies and bufferbeams were painted with track colour brown.

Other detail painting included adding silver to the buffer shanks, orange on the bufferbeam fittings where needed, and black for the jumper cables and buffer heads. The cab front lamp irons and newly added dents were painted yellow as were the catches on the battery boxes. The air tanks tucked in above the fuel tank were picked out in white as were the fuel tank gauges. Once the latter were dry, the capacity needles were drawn on with a black 0.1mm edding pen.

Fox transfers were employed for the Construction logos and door repeaters along with the blue star symbols and black data panels, while the Replica range provided the black rub-on loco numbers. Photos should be checked for the correct locations of the smaller items as there were many variations between the various locos. Finally, matt varnish was applied to protect the transfers.

The two locos were lightly weathered with water colours while the area around the exhaust port on each loco was covered in black. Etched double arrows were fitted on the driver's cabsides while Hither Green depot plaques were added to the secondman's cabsides on 33207 only. Both locos also gained etched shedplates (73A) centrally on the cab fronts, the background colour first being changed from black to red. Finally, the etched nameplates and crests on 33207 were fixed in place with Deluxe Materials 'Glue 'n' Glaze'. This is white when applied but dries clear and any excess can then be pulled off with tweezers.

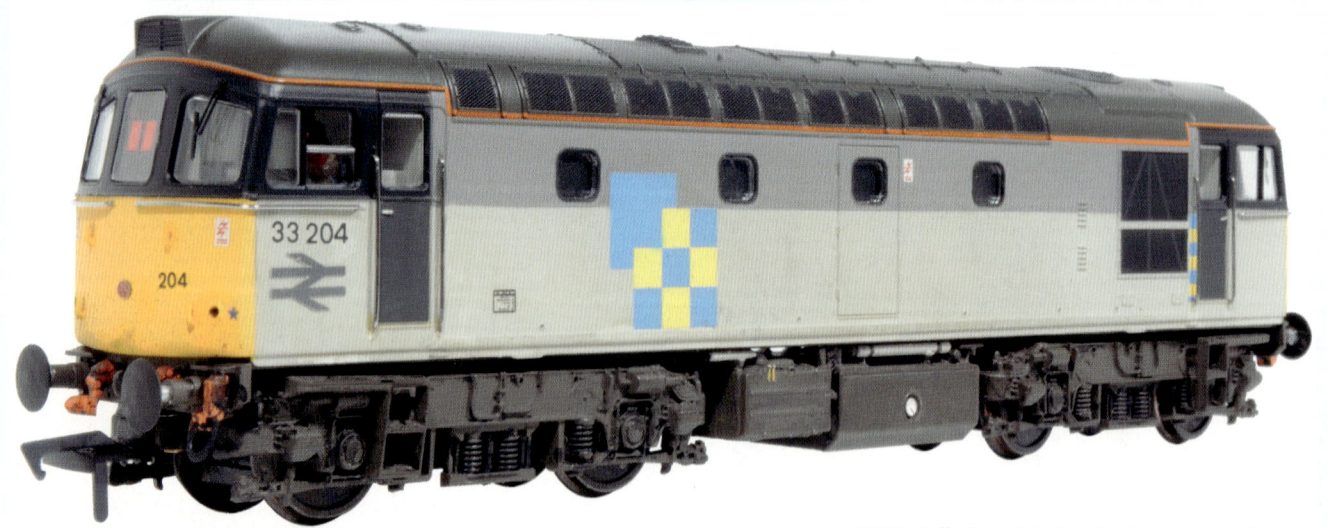

ABOVE: Heljan's model of the Hastings-gauge Class 33/2s is the best of its OO gauge 'Cromptons' and rewards some additional detailing. This example, 33204, was painted at Eastleigh Works during overhaul in February 1989 and would spend just over two more years with the sub-sector before switching to train ferry duties.

LEFT: 33207 *Earl Mountbatten of Burma* was something of a photographer's favourite on the Channel Tunnel workings thanks to its colourful nameplates and full set of cast arrows and depot plaques. It looks just as good in model form and would serve with Railfreight Construction until May 1992.

A legacy continued

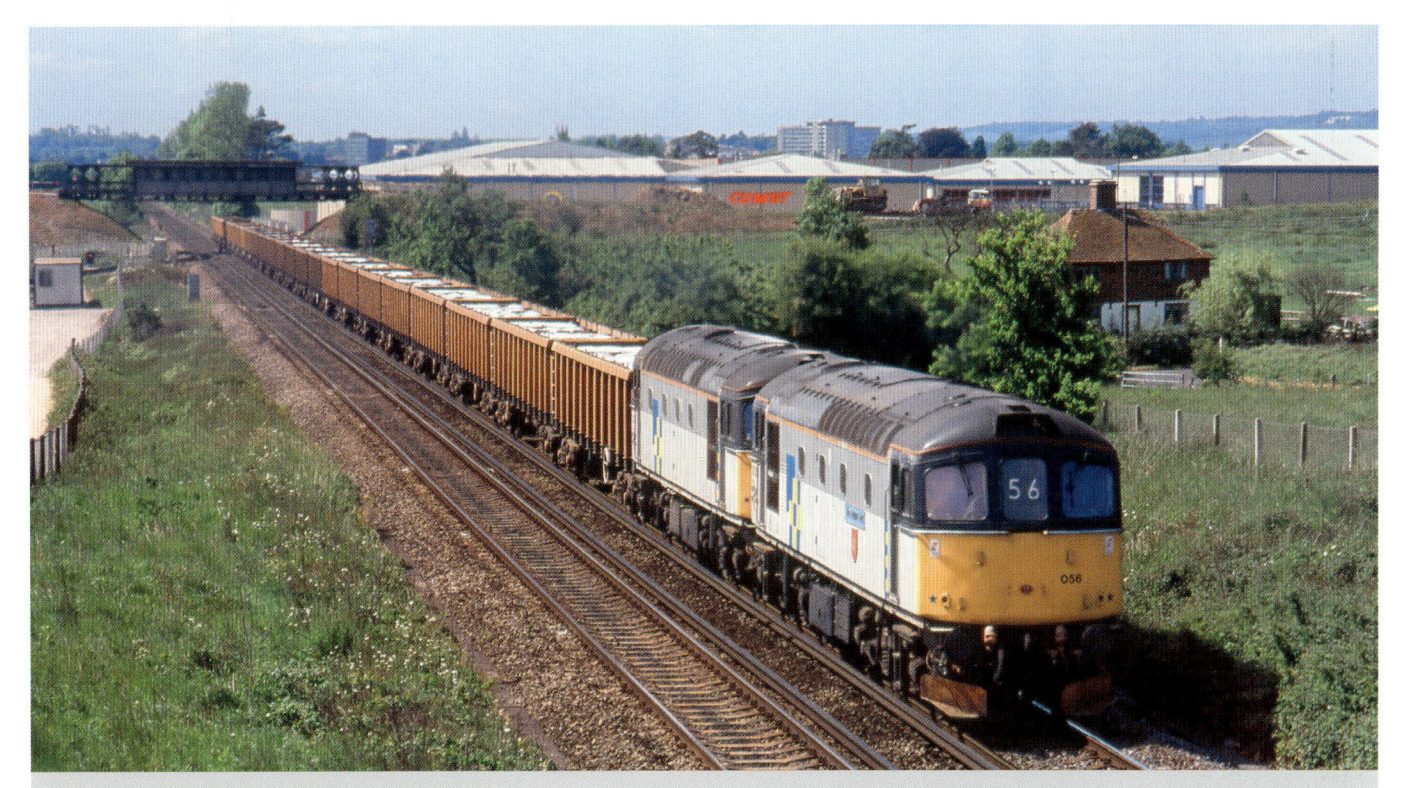

ABOVE: The classic look of the Channel Tunnel concrete lining segment trains is provided by 33056 *The Burma Star* and 33021 atop the 6C56 11.23 Grain to Shakespeare Cliff at Sevington on June 2, 1989. These heavy trains were taxing work for the Class 33s and were usually double-headed, although single 'Cromptons' were not unknown with resultant performance issues. With a long string of PXA boxes in tow, some of these wagons remain in use today on scrap and aggregates flows, now coded KEA and with the attractive golden yellow livery largely obscured beneath three decades of grime. No ready-to-run models exist in any scale, but kit suppliers include S-Kits in 4mm and Impressionist Models in 7mm. Martin Loader

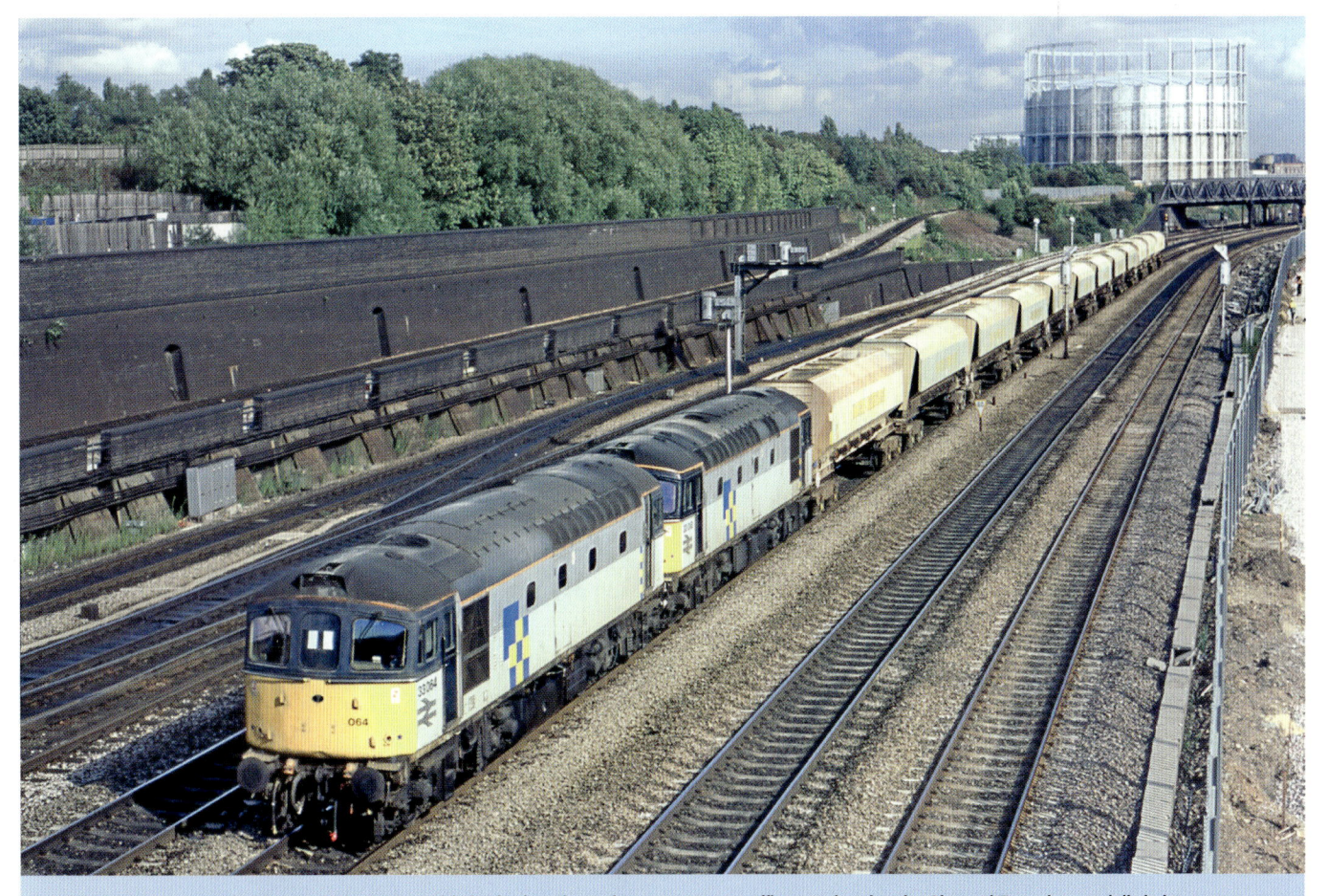

ABOVE: The Construction-allocated Class 33s could also be found on other aggregates traffic not related to the Channel Tunnel, especially in later years when traffic for the latter tailed off. Operating deep in West London, 33064 and 33063 approach Old Oak Common on October 4, 1991, with empty Marcon JHA bogie hoppers returning from the distribution terminal outside Paddington to Angerstein Wharf, near Greenwich. No models exist of these wagons in any scale while the fate of the locos would be very different, 33063 entering preservation in 1997 while 33064 was written off following a collision in April 1994. Dave Cobbe/Rail Photoprints

A legacy continued

Southerners on the move

By the start of the 1990s, the long association of the Class 09s with the Southern Region was under threat as some of the shunters began to be redeployed to new operating areas. A new batch of conversions also appeared to bolster the fleet. Simon Bendall **details the history of the locos in this period while** Alex Carpenter **models two examples using the OO gauge Hornby model.**

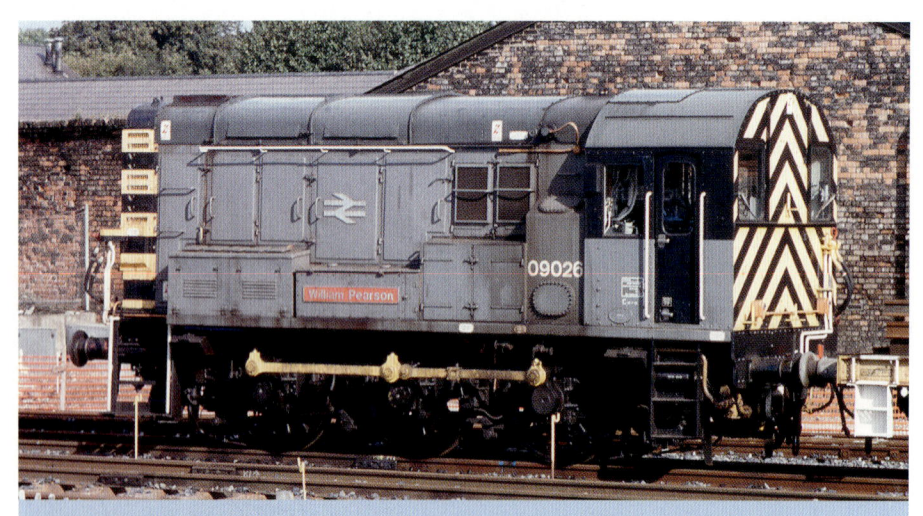

ABOVE: Eastleigh-based 09026 *William Pearson* was the first Class 08/09 to be painted in Departmental grey in February 1989, its home depot applying a non-standard version without any black on the cab and with white numbers and BR arrows squeezed onto the cabsides. When recorded at Salisbury on September 10, 1992, the shunter had passed through Crewe Works for overhaul 14 months earlier, receiving a fresh coat of grey and the full black upper cabsides and doors. The application was still slightly non-standard though with the cast BR arrows relocated to the bonnet doors due to the nameplates. Simon Bendall Collection

The exodus of the original 27mph-capable Class 09/0 sub-class from the Southern Region was already in progress as 1990 began. The first to leave was 09017 back in July 1987 for dedicated use with the Severn Tunnel emergency train, which saw it become 97806 for over a decade. More conventional transfers for use with Railfreight came in 1989 with 09001 and 09015 moving to Cardiff for use on steel traffic while 09008 and 09013 headed to South Yorkshire for similar duties, being based at Tinsley.

Both of the latter along with 09015 would receive Departmental grey in 1991/92, 09008 having carried an embellished BR blue livery for the best part of a year prior to this, Tinsley adding depot plaques, a grey solebar stripe and cab roof, and *Sheffield Childrens Hospital* (sic) nameplates.

Next to leave in 1991 were 09005 and 09014, both heading for Knottingley and overhauls that saw them also go grey in the spring of 1992. The interpretation of the painting instructions for Departmental grey on the shunters varied between different works. RFS Industries at Kilnhurst, where 09005/08/13/14 were overhauled, limited the cabside black to just a rectangle around the window frame.

In contrast, Crewe Works was far more liberal, the black encompassing the whole of the upper cabside, all of the cab door and wrapping around to the small front window above the fuel tank on each side. This is how 09015 was finished and matched the still Southern-based 09009/12/26 which had been painted in 1990/91. This variation held true for all of the other Class 09s that received the grey livery, 09011 and 09019 sporting the extra black after visiting Crewe in 1991 and 09010, 09016 and 09024 getting the Kilnhurst economy style in 1992.

During September 1993, 09008 and 09013 both transferred southwards from Tinsley to Cardiff Canton. These were the last transfers ahead of the splintering of the fleet as the privatisation process began in the spring of 1994. This saw ownership divided between what would become Mainline Freight (09003/06/07/09/10/12/16/18-20/23/24), Loadhaul (09005/14) and Transrail (09001/08/13/15, 97806) while Railfreight Distribution received an allocation for the first time (09011/21/22). These were nominally based at Tinsley and then Allerton but could be found out-based at the likes of Wembley Yard. Completing the carve up were 09004, 09025 and 09026 which were assigned to the South Central train operating unit while 09002 had been withdrawn in September 1992.

Additional conversions

During 1992/93, a programme to create further Class 09s was undertaken at RFS, Kilnhurst, a dozen Class 08s being re-geared to operate at the higher maximum speed. These were renumbered as 09101-07 and 09201-05, the two series differentiating whether they had 110 volt or 90 volt electrical systems, respectively. As the conversions were all done at Kilnhurst, all but one sported the reduced amount of black on the cabsides. The exception was 09107 which, as 08845, was admitted into the modification programme already carrying the Crewe Works version of Departmental grey with the extra black. As it was not repainted again by RFS, it remained in this version of the livery until an EWS repaint in 2008.

Once the allocations had settled down, 09101 and 09102 were part of the Railfreight Distribution fleet based at Reading, one often working at Didcot Yard, while the remainder were assigned to general freight duties. This found 09103, 09202 and 09205 based at Motherwell with one usually out-based at Aberdeen, 09104 and 09201 at Toton with a Knottingley out-base, 09105. 09107 and 09203 at Canton for the Newport trips and 09106 and 09204 at Thornaby.

These allocations were largely maintained from the spring of 1994, the future Mainline Freight transferring 09101 and 09102 to Old Oak Common and also retaining 09201 at Toton. Transrail took the trios based at Cardiff and Motherwell and added 09104 at Bescot while Loadhaul kept the Thornaby pair.

BELOW: Now based at Knottingley, 09014 shows the Kilnhurst version of the Departmental grey livery with the black amounting to a rectangle around the cabside window. Seen on February 18, 1993, the reduced number of black chevrons on the side of the radiator compared to 09026 was another trademark of the RFS repaints. Simon Bendall Collection

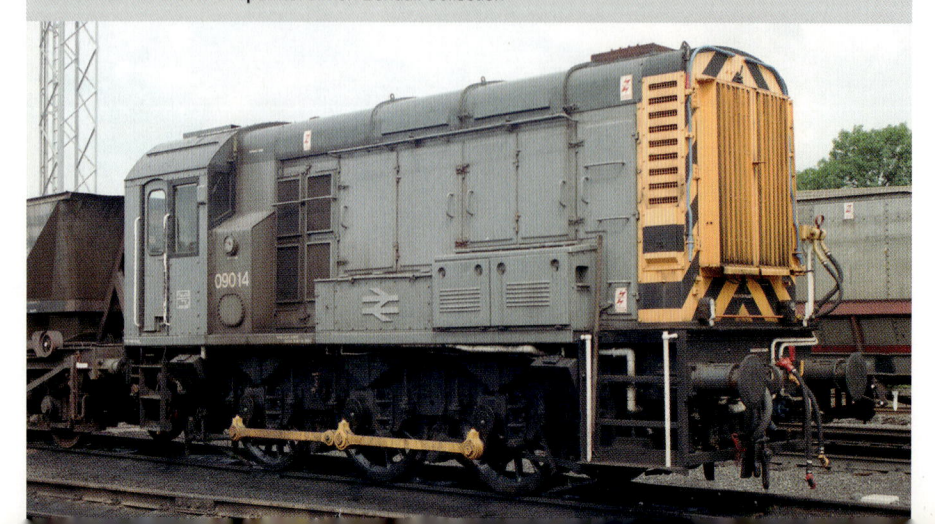

20 www.keymodelworld.com

A legacy continued

Go faster 'Gronks'

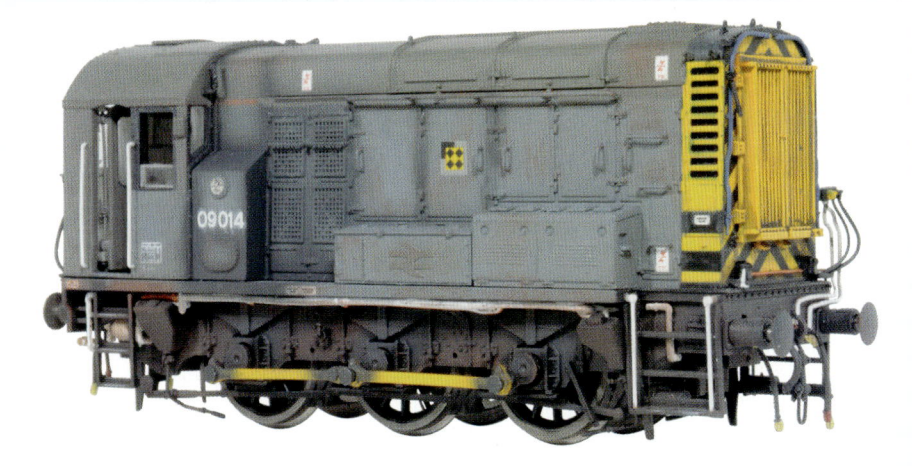

LEFT: **The Hornby Class 08/09 is undeniably the best of the OO gauge options, having a considerable amount of fine detail and a better representation of the pressed bonnet doors. The model of 09014 retains the base factory paintjob, just enhanced with some relatively minor alterations and careful weathering.**

The high-specification Hornby model is undoubtedly the best rendition of the Class 08/09 shunters currently available in ready-to-run form in OO gauge, it boasts an impressive array of detail. However, the manufacturer has failed to capitalise somewhat on the tooling and livery options that could be produced. One example of this is locos fitted with the Southern Region's high-level brake pipes, for which the tooling exists but is rarely used.

Equally frustrating is the lack of some key sector-era liveries, such as Departmental grey, which was produced in the very first batch of releases as 09012 *Dick Hardy* in 2005 but has not been repeated since. Both of the locos featured here use this model as their basis.

The first to be tackled was 09014, which is depicted following its transfer to Knottingley in 1991 for tripping coal hoppers from and to Milford Sidings for repair. Firstly, the printed numbers and nameplates were removed using a blunt scalpel and T-cut applied with a cotton bud. The connecting rods and bufferbeams were the correct colour, so all I had to do to the chassis was add the bufferbeam detail from the accessory pack.

Livery wise, there were two areas that needed attention. Firstly, the removal of the upper black chevrons on the radiator sides, leaving the bottom two in situ; these being simply painted out yellow by hand.

Secondly, most of the black around the cabsides required removal, leaving only the black window frames. Again, this was done by simply painting out with Railfreight grey, which is a very good match to the existing Hornby colour. Some of the lamp brackets were removed as per prototype photos while the HAA-sized Railfreight Coal sub-sector logos were duly added to the bonnet doors along with numbers and data panels as required, before finishing with a coat of satin varnish.

Mixed metals
The second model of 09013 also utilised Hornby's 09012 as its basis, this again requiring the removal of some of the black chevrons from the sides of the radiator along with the black surrounds to the cabside windows and doors. However, as the orange cantrail stripe also needed to come off, it was easier in this case to carry out a partial repaint.

With the model taken apart, the yellow and black chevrons were carefully masked off and the body and cab sprayed with grey primer. Railmatch Railfreight grey was then applied followed by Executive dark grey for the roof. Once the masking was removed, the three uppermost black chevrons were painted out with yellow where they wrap around the sides of the radiator. The only other black on 09013 was around the cabside window frames and also the radiator top, which were picked out by hand.

As this was one of the Class 09s based around Newport for trip workings in the mid-late 1990s, the loco had Metals sub-sector repeaters on its cabsides, these coming from Fox along with the numbers and overhead warning flashes. The fuel gauge was a great little transfer from Precision Decals as was the 'Main tank' lettering below it. The white data panels and depot stickers were from Replica with the etched BR arrows and Canton depot plaques from Shawplan.

The weathering of both models essentially involved only three colours: sleeper grime, roof dirt and dark rust. The sleeper grime was sprayed on, wiped off and sprayed on again lightly, working it into all the areas of the underframe in varying tones. The body itself is mainly a darker shade of grime, so I used roof dirt. Again, sprayed on and wiped off in varying degrees, you can really build up the dirt with the airbrush. Particular areas are around the fuel tanks and where the air intakes meet the solebars, while it was also sprayed around the bodyside doors and roof panels, with emphasis to the lower edges. This helps to give a faded effect too.

Roof dirt was used on the underframe and connecting rods to give the effect of built-up grime and grease. Finally, rust was very finely blown onto some of the bodyside door hinges, parts of the underframe and the exhaust. The model of 09013 was then completed with a Legomanbiffo 8-pin DCC sound chip.

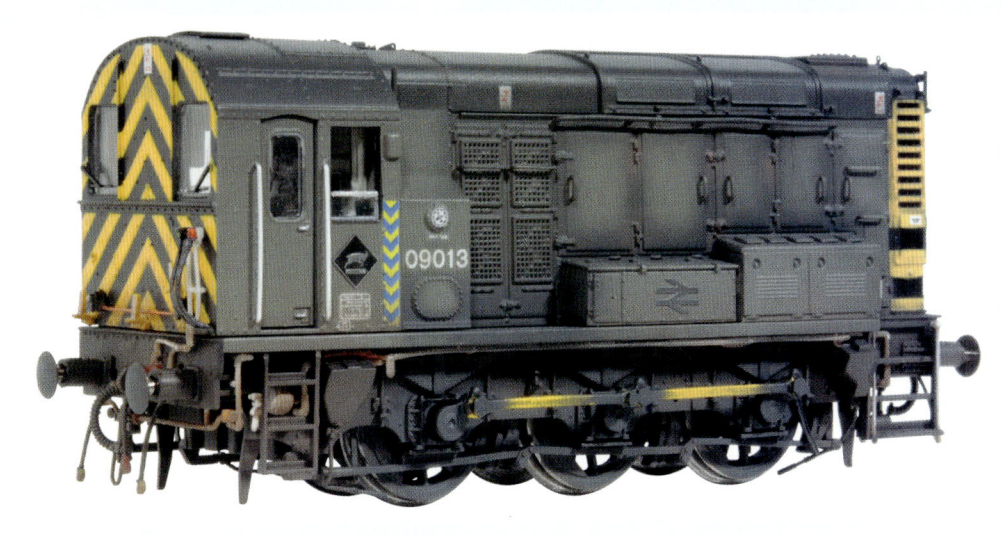

LEFT: **The Class 09s that were allocated to trip workings around Newport in the 1990s looking particularly striking with the Metals repeater stripes and cast Canton depot plaques serving to enhance the livery. 09013 is a more extensive repaint compared to its sister due to the need to remove the cantrail stripe in addition to the black elements on the cabsides.**

A legacy continued

The Long Rangers

The Class 47s equipped with long range fuel tanks were a key part of cross-country passenger operations throughout the 1990s, during which time they were predominately finished in InterCity Swallow colours. Simon Bendall **recounts the creation of the fleet while** Mark Lambert **repaints a Bachmann OO gauge model.**

Although the Class 47s in the 47801-54 number series are near universally referred to as '47/8s' by enthusiasts and modellers, this is actually something of a fallacy as they have always been, and continue to be for those that still survive, officially Class 47/4s. They are denoted as such on the TOPS computer system by their design codes which detail certain characteristics for each loco.

While fictitious, the '47/8' designation is a useful shorthand when talking about the batch of Type 4s that were created in 1989/90 and largely dedicated to InterCity services, all featuring extended range fuel tank modifications. This was the defining characteristic of the 47801-54 series and saw the standard 720 gallon internal fuel tank supplemented by an additional 575 gallon underslung tank, greatly increasing the locos' range, and making their diagramming on passenger trains easier.

The origins of the fleet had come in 1986/87 when the last 16 examples of the class selected to be upgraded from freight-only specification to feature electric train supply (ETS) equipment were completed, becoming 47650-65. Initially allocated to Gateshead and then Eastfield, all received long range fuel tanks as part of the same overhaul, a modification that had previously been applied only to ScotRail's push-pull Class 47/7s. All then migrated to Bristol Bath Road in May 1988, still as part of the InterCity fleet and with most assigned to cross-country workings.

The start of 1989 brought authorisation for further Class 47s to be fitted with additional fuel tanks and also the decision to renumber them into the 478xx series to make the modified locos easier to identify for operational purposes. The already completed 47650-65 were renumbered in sequence as 47805-20 during the course of the year while as other locos were completed, they too gained new identities to fill the 47801-04 gap and upwards from 47821. The last examples were not converted until the early months of 1990, this bringing the appearance of 47842-44 and 47848-53. The last of the series, 47854, was a later addition in 1995 as a replacement for collision damaged 47850, although a few others were also prematurely lost to accident or fire damage in the early 1990s.

Mixed liveries

In some cases, fitting the extra tanks coincided with works overhauls, which resulted in 47834/36-44 emerging in InterCity Swallow livery at the same time as they gained their new identities. Many others were simply renumbered in the livery they were already carrying though, so 47801/02/04-13/15-17/19/20 were initially in BR large logo blue with the usual large numbers and arrows. Other liveries carried upon renumbering included 47803/35 in InterCity Executive, 47826 in the ScotRail-branded InterCity Executive colours, 47847 in BR blue, and 47818/21/23-25/27/29/31-33/49/53 in variations of the InterCity Mainline scheme.

Of the remainder, these all retained large logo blue colours but 47822/28/30/45/46/48/50-52 were given standard sized black numbers on the cabsides while 47814 got small white numbers on the bodysides. 47845/46/48/50-52 were also stripped of their large arrows upon renumbering, InterCity preferring not to display the BR logo on its traction by this time.

Ultimately, 47802/04-23/25-33/35/45-51/53 would all join 47834/36-44 in carrying Swallow by the spring of 1995, some as they cycled through their next works overhaul while others were painted early on at depot level, the Bristol duo of Bath Road and St. Philip's Marsh being particularly involved. Latecomer 47854 was also so painted upon its conversion in December 1995 for consistency despite InterCity being all but obsolete by this time. Of the exceptions, 47801 and 47824 transferred away to other sectors before they could be painted, 47803 was relegated to infrastructure use and 47852 was condemned after incurring damage from rolling into the Old Oak Common turntable pit!

Life extensions

The other major development affecting the long range machines as the 1990s progressed was the decision to give those members of the class with a decent life expectancy a series of upgrades. For the likes of the Railfreight Distribution fleet, this included the wider roll-out of the extra fuel tank but the main element as far as the InterCity machines were concerned was the removal of the cast bufferbeam cowls and cutting back the bodywork in the same area to tackle corrosion. Cab improvements were also implemented to improve the crew environment. These modifications were normally done at main workshops, so it was not a quick programme with 47853 not done until early 1995 for example.

By the time the fleet was divided up in preparation for privatisation in 1994, it was somewhat reduced in number. Some locos had been lost to Rail Express Systems initially insatiable appetite for Class 47s along with that sector taking ownership of the Royal pair of 47834 and 47835. Others were assigned to the Great Western operation, leaving Virgin CrossCountry to inherit 47805-07/10/12/14/17/18/22/25-29/31/39-41/43-45/47-49/51/53/54.

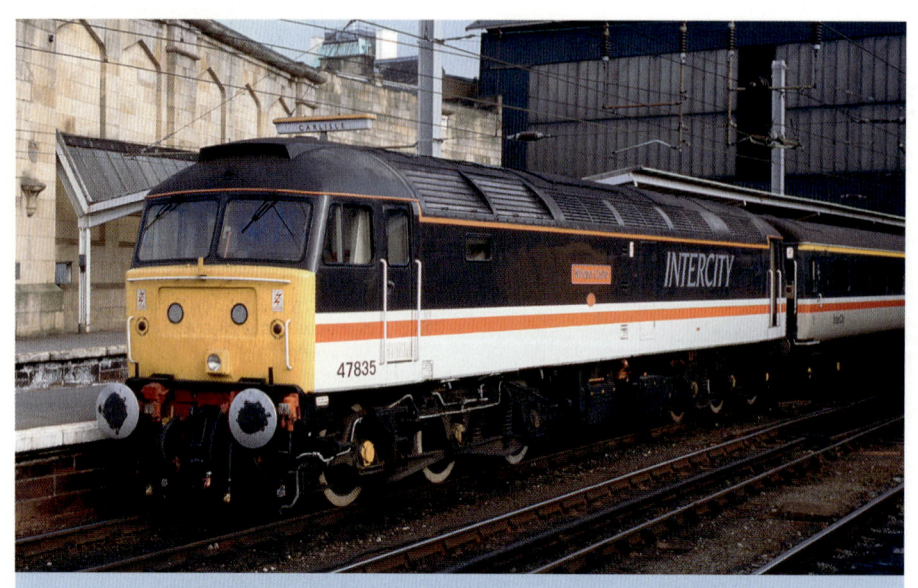

ABOVE: Royal train favourite 47835 *Windsor Castle* was on regular passenger duties when recorded at Carlisle on March 17, 1990, four months after it was repainted in Swallow; its many livery enhancements now requiring something of a clean before its next prestigious engagement. Surprisingly, the loco escaped the removal of its bufferbeam cowlings, which are still retained today in preservation, while its nameplates would be painted black a few months later. Simon Bendall Collection

A legacy continued

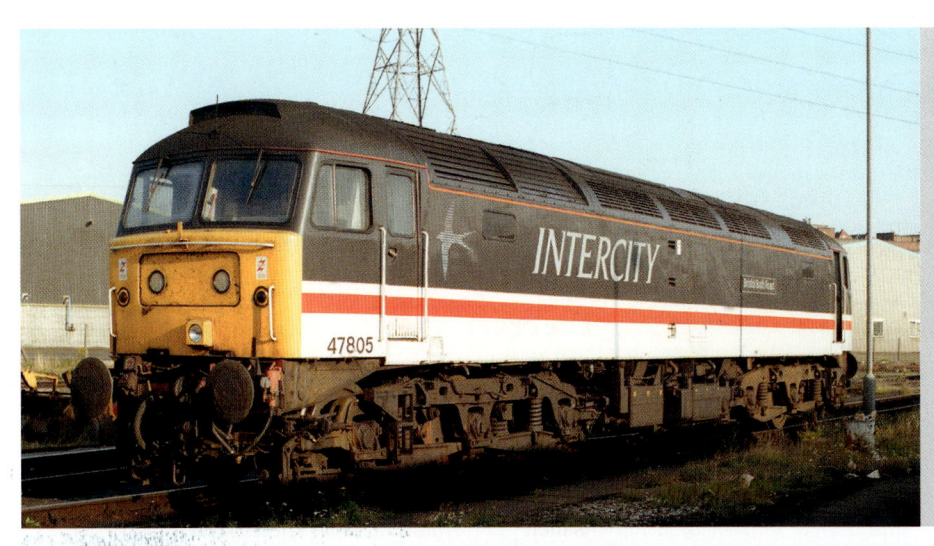

LEFT: Recorded at Saltley depot on August 30, 1993, 47805 *Bristol Bath Road* shows the full suite of life-extension modifications that became so familiar during the decade. Most obvious is the removal of the cast bufferbeam cowling at each end that was a cause of corrosion underneath, this creating the distinctive step in the lower cabside edge in front of the cab doors. This modification also revealed pipework and cabling for the ETS jumpers, giving a further detail to model. Another alteration of the life extension programme was the partial plating over of the cab roof vents, this leaving only the centre section open. The loco would lose its vacuum brake equipment and corresponding bufferbeam pipes the following year and its nameplates in early 1995 prior to transfer away from its namesake depot to Crewe Diesel. Simon Bendall Collection

Model availability

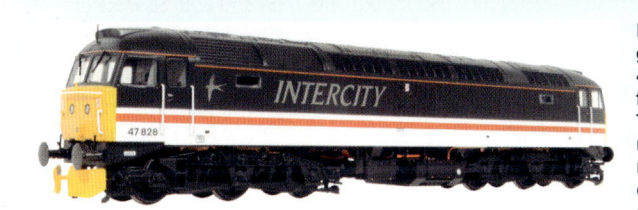

LEFT: Bachmann's new generation of OO gauge Class 47s is represented by 47828 in full InterCity Swallow regalia. This delivers detail and features not previously seen on a RTR model of the class, including enhanced underframe detail and a tooling suite that covers almost all possibilities.

Sometimes it seems there have been almost as many OO gauge models of Class 47s as there were of the real things, the miniature versions dating back to Hornby's model of the mid-1970s. This was largely usurped by Lima's effort from a decade later, which ironically now resides in the range of the Margate-based manufacturer and appears quite regularly in a variety of colours.

The first modern day rendering came from Heljan at the start of this century and helped drive the development in standards and detail that the market enjoys today. While suffering from excess girth, it nonetheless covered a range of variants, an even greater spread of liveries and remains relatively easy to source even today.

Later in the decade, Bachmann released its first iteration of the Brush Type 4s and when this eventually reached variants relevant to the 1980s and 1990s, it had developed into a presentable model that appeared in numerous colours relevant to this special. The 2000s also saw the appearance of Lima's spiritual successor, ViTrains' UK range burning brightly but briefly. The Italian company delivered a Class 47 that was too self-assembly for some tastes with all the detail parts that required adding but yet released a considerable number of liveries in a short space of time.

Much like the Class 20, the summer of 2021 saw Bachmann unveil an all new Class 47 in 4mm scale to replace its previous model, this not only correcting the faults of the original but also delivering the most detailed RTR representation of the Brush machines to date. Initially covering three versions, many more have been tooled and are set to keep the company busy for some years. Competition is on the way though with Heljan's all new and slimmed down Class 47 which is due, at the time of writing, in late 2022.

The Danish manufacturer is also on the second version of the class in O gauge with a greatly expanded range of liveries released in 2021 while the Graham Farish range is additionally enjoying a new generation model, Bachmann having released a number of variants in recent years that eclipse the original N gauge recreation dating from the 1980s.

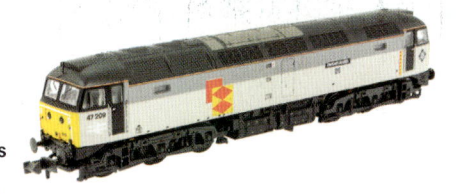

LEFT: While the improved 2021 tooling has now superseded Bachmann's original model of the Brush machines, the numerous releases are far from obsolete this being 47745 *Royal London Society for the Blind* in Rail Express Systems. The Railnet Class 47/7 sub-class is covered in more detail on pages 36-43.

RIGHT: ViTrains' time in the UK market was unfortunately short-lived, the Italians leaving behind a decent Class 47 and a less fondly remembered Class 37. One of its final releases was an extremely limited model of NSE-shod 47587 *Ruskin College Oxford*.

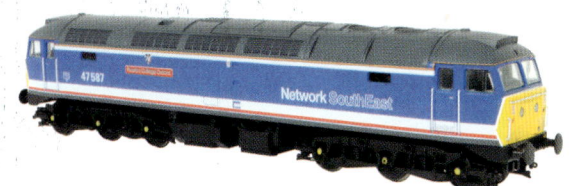

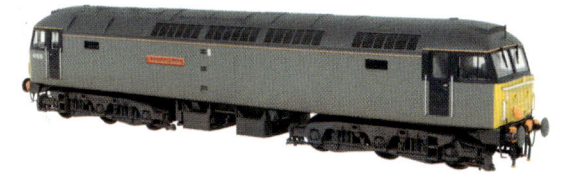

LEFT: Derided by many, valued by others, the original Heljan Class 47 is the epitome of a 'Marmite' model. Still, some effort will elevate it towards its more recent rivals as shown by a detailed 47976 *Aviemore Centre*.

ABOVE: In the 'intermediate' condition of the late 1980s and early 1990s, this Graham Farish release portrays 47209 *Herbert Austin* from the Railfreight Distribution fleet. Image courtesy Kernow Model Rail Centre

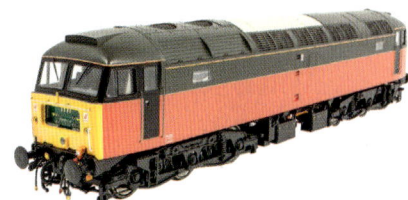

ABOVE: Heljan's revised O gauge Class 47 not only allows for a choice of decals but also headcode panels, this being the Parcels-liveried release. Image courtesy Kernow Model Rail Centre

Modelling BR Locomotives of the 1990s 23

A legacy continued

Creating a royal reserve

This model started life as a Railfreight sub-sector liveried loco, 47190, from the closing down sale at my nearest Modelzone store. Not particularly wanting a Petroleum-badged loco, I started researching other Class 47s with flush fronts at both ends with a view to just renumbering it and changing the sector logos. However, after some hours looking through books and websites such as class47.co.uk, I concluded my best option was to completely repaint it. I chose back-up Royal train loco 47823 *SS Great Britain*.

Disassembly was a lengthy process but eventually I had a bodyshell with no more removable parts that I could dunk in paint stripper. After a good wash and scrub, the first job was to get an even coat of white all around the lower half of the model. I used Games Workshop 'skull white' primer; this never covered very well which is why it was replaced with 'Corax white', so it took a few passes (and at least one re-strip) to build a thin, even coat of white.

I masked the bottom of the body up to where the top of the InterCity stripes would be and sprayed the cab ends with Railmatch post-1984 warning panel yellow. Again, this has a fairly low pigment density and it needed more than one coat, even over white, to give a solid colour. Once this had dried, I masked the cab fronts and sprayed the rest of the model with Railmatch Falcon grey. After everything was touch dry, the layers of masking tape were carefully peeled off to reveal a clean demarcation between all the colours and a small step at the joint between the white undercoat and the grey.

Tackling the stripes

It is almost impossible to avoid steps between layers of paint when spraying, so my cunning plan was to use a transfer for the InterCity red and white stripes to help mask this. I prepared the model for the transfers with a coat of gloss varnish and then applied the stripes (from the Fox range) using some decal softener to get them around details. Amazingly, this worked pretty well, the only downside being the slightly 'off' proportions of the stripes I used. The red/white proportion should be near 60:40 but these ones appeared to be more 50:50.

The italic InterCity lettering and swallow logos were also from Fox. The use of a gloss varnish under and over the transfers before a finishing coat of matt varnish over the whole model completely conceals the small lines of carrier film that join the top and bottom of the letters together, which is a technique I picked up from aircraft modelling. The loco number was made up from Replica rub-down numbers. Getting these straight was tricky but I managed it first time, something I don't think I have done before or since!

The overhead warning flashes were waterslide transfers from Replica with the data panel coming from Fox once more and the etched nameplates from Shawplan. With the body reunited with all its component parts, I added an RCH jumper cable to the right-hand cab front using an A1 etch and fuse wire. This was an early 1990s fitment to locos frequently used on the Royal train to give communication between the driver and train manager.

The original battery box-only underframe moulding was replaced with the correct long range fuel tank assembly from Heljan, the latter being modified to clear Bachmann's light switches and then superglued in place. I added ETS jumpers and Vi-Trains footsteps from the spares box to the now red-painted bufferbeams alongside all the supplied detail parts before re-assembly. The final job was to weather all the underframe parts with a coat of Army Painter 'Hardened Carapace' to give a clean but in-service appearance.

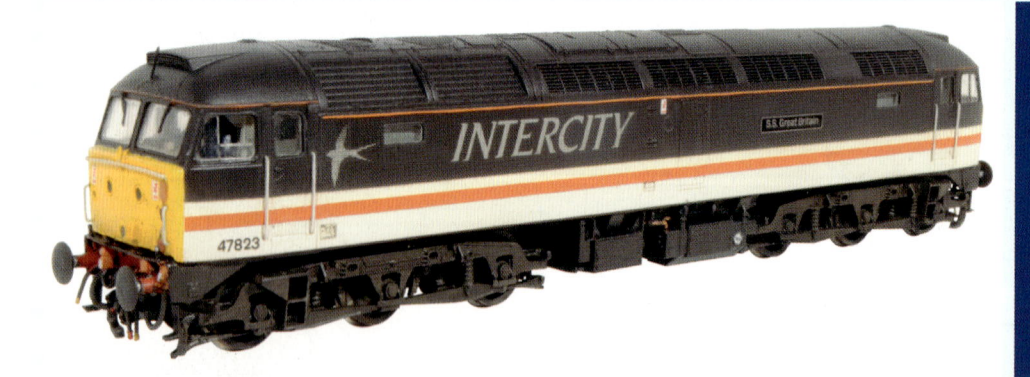

LEFT: Although maintained as a reserve Royal train loco, 47823 was still regularly employed on InterCity duties, be it service trains or charters. Its life extension overhaul did not arrive until 1994 when it became 47787 with Rail Express Systems so retained its bufferbeam cowls while operating with InterCity. One of the main issues with the original Bachmann Class 47 was the rather open nature of the bogie sideframes around the springs, something that the replacement model corrects.

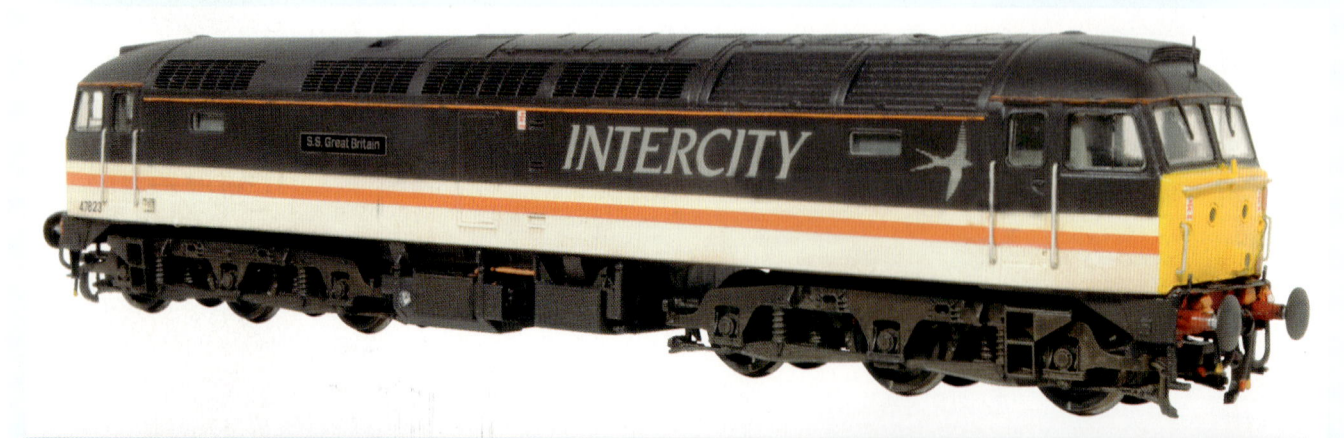

ABOVE: Numerous Class 47s had their former headcode panel recesses plated over at one or both ends during their careers, the marker lights being mounted flush with the ends in these cases. During British Rail ownership, this was invariably due to repairs to collision damage but in more recent times, it has sometimes been done for corrosion reasons, such as with some DRS Class 47s. It is one of a number of physical alterations that can make matching a model to a suitable prototype an interesting challenge!

A legacy continued

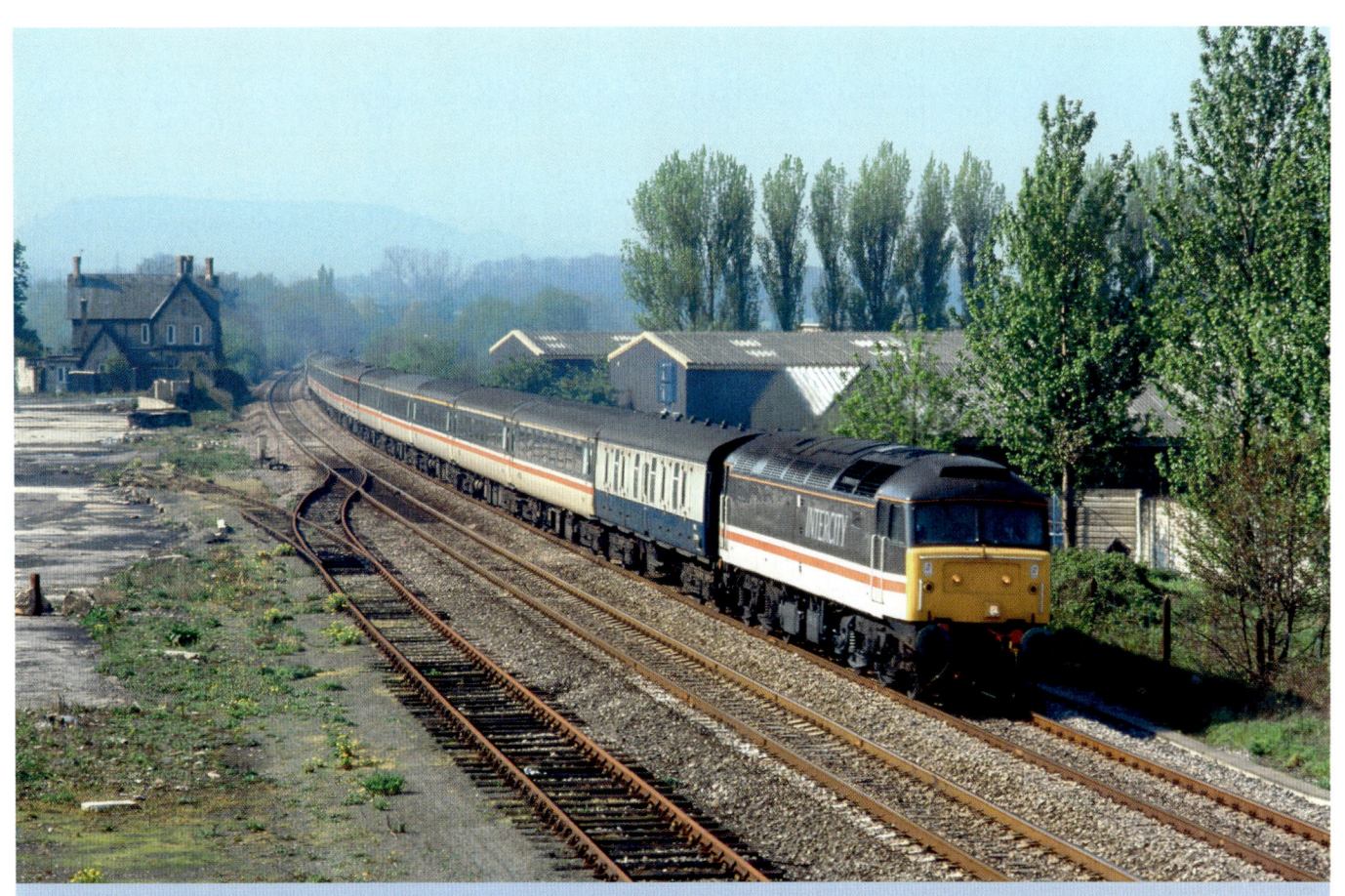

ABOVE: One of the earlier recipients of InterCity Swallow, and cut back bufferbeams, was 47807, which is seen powering past the site of Stonehouse (Bristol Road) station on April 25, 1990. Still spotless following its repaint at Landore the previous month, the Type 4 was in charge of the 1S85 07.07 Plymouth to Aberdeen 'Devon Scot' with at least 12 coaches in tow. At a time when train lengths matched demand, the passenger accommodation for both first and standard is the expected mix of Mk.2d/e/f air-conditioned stock with a Mk.1 BG the only vehicle spoiling the uniform set. A Mk.1 Restaurant Buffet (RBR) is positioned mid-train with the entire formation modellable in 2mm or 4mm using Farish or Bachmann/Hornby products. Martin Loader

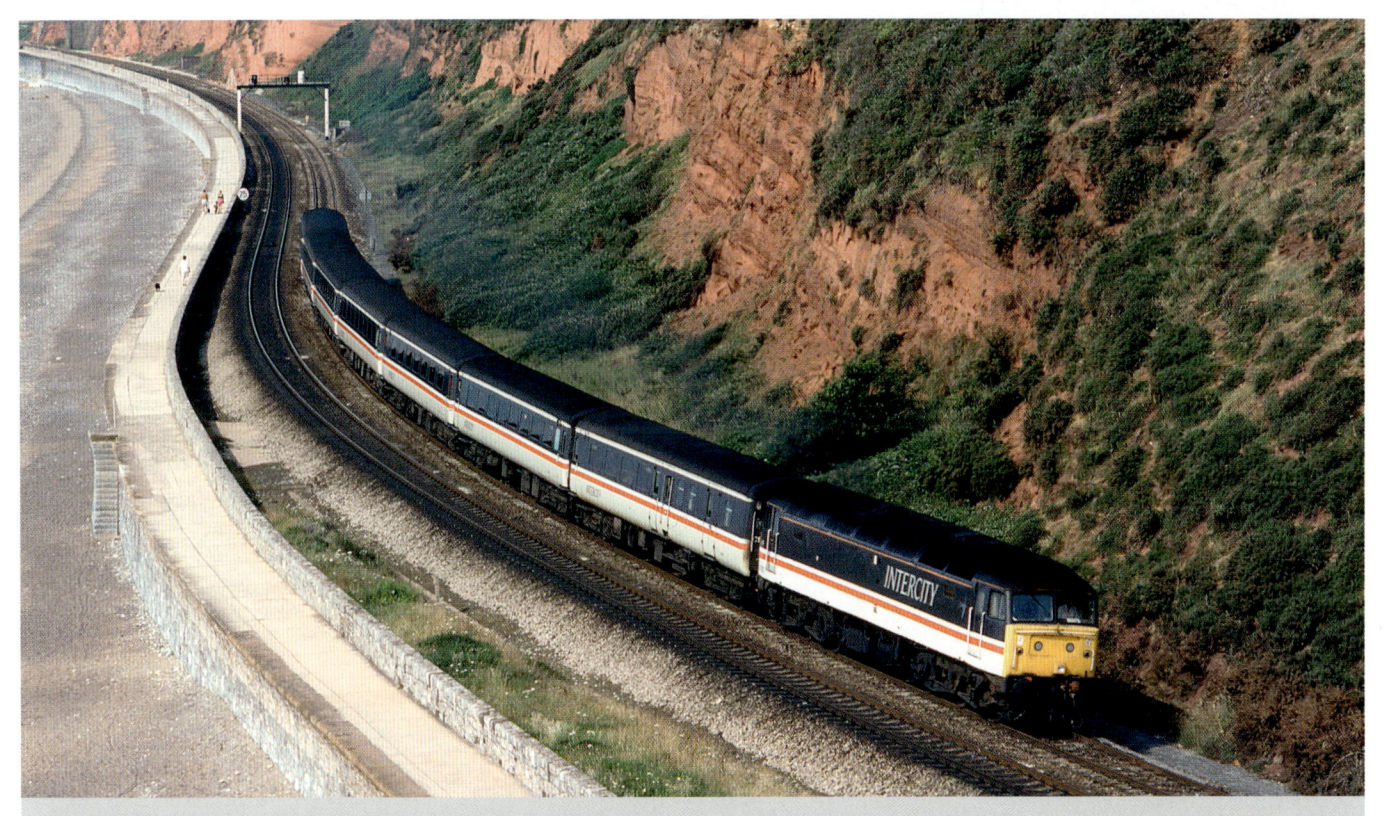

ABOVE: By 1992, the standard InterCity cross-country loco-hauled formation was becoming established but still some way from being dominant, this consisting of a Mk.2d/e/f Brake Standard Open (BSO), five Mk.2d/e/f Tourist Standard Opens (TSO) and a Mk.2f Restaurant First Buffet (RFB), the latter being on the rear in this view as 47812 passes Langstone Rock with a service from Plymouth on June 27, 1992. The loco had received its Swallow livery in August 1990 during overhaul at Doncaster Works, but it would then be another five years before the cut-back bufferbeam modification took place at its next classified attention. This whole train is available from the Bachmann or Farish ranges. Simon Bendall Collection

Modelling BR Locomotives of the 1990s 25

A legacy continued

British Rail's grey days

First unveiled in 1989, the Departmental grey livery was designed to help reduce the number of colour schemes in use on the locomotive fleet. However, it was so widely derided that it soon morphed into 'Dutch' for the numerous Civil Engineers locos. However, this was not the case for those belonging to the Mechanical and Electrical Engineers as Simon Bendall **explains, while** Alex Carpenter **models one of the department's Class 31s.**

Departmental grey, or General grey as it is sometimes referred to, was unveiled by British Rail in February 1989 as part of BBC Television's *'Railwatch'* week of programmes. The event was part of a wider launch of BR's four 'new' standard liveries, the others being InterCity Swallow, Railfreight sub-sector triple grey and the InterCity-derived Mainline scheme. The stated intention at the time was that by 1993, only these four liveries would be in use in order to present a quality, uniform image to both customers and staff.

Departmental grey was intended for use on the 'workhorse' classes, this encompassing those locos allocated to engineers' duties and other non-revenue earning roles, so application to Classes 08, 09, 20, 26, 31, 33, 37/0 and some non-ETS Class 47s was envisaged. In the event, while the list of recipient classes was mostly adhered to, the standard liveries plan was reduced to tatters within a year while Departmental grey would go down in railway history as one of the most criticised liveries ever.

The first loco to receive the new livery was 31453 during classified attention at Doncaster Works, it being released to traffic in February 1989. However, the shade of grey used was deemed to be too light so the next to be done, 31412, emerged in a distinctly darker colour. This found favour with the loco being despatched to Bounds Green for the 'Railwatch' launch. However, with workshops unsure of exactly what shade of grey to use and which locos to apply it to, repaints ground to a halt with newly overhauled locos instead returning to traffic in trusty BR blue!

With clarification eventually received, the application of the grey resumed in June 1989. Focussing solely on the Class 31s, Doncaster Works would be responsible for all but two of the repaints on the class, outshopping a further 16 examples over the next 12 months. This included Class 31/1s 31113, 31166 and 31308 but the remainder were all members of the electric train supply-equipped Class 31/4 fleet, the list being 31417/19/24/31/51/54/55/57/61/62/65/66/68. These were all repainted following overhauls with the exception of 31431, which was re-liveried after receiving repairs to fire damage.

Heating off
From May 1990, a new Class 31/5 sub-class was created, this being for Class 31/4s assigned to the engineers' fleet that had their ETS equipment isolated, which not only reduced maintenance costs but also made them less attractive to Provincial for purloining when the sector was short of motive power. As a result, nine of the Departmental grey examples all gained new numbers, becoming 31512/19/24/31/51/53-55/68. The last of the class to gain the livery were renumbered at the same time as they were done, 31530 emerging from Stratford Diesel Repairs Shops in June 1990 after collision damage repairs while 31511 was painted the same month at Bescot.

Almost as soon as Departmental grey appeared, it started to draw criticism from many quarters including from within BR itself, the main complaint being that it was too drab, especially when dirty. However, it was not until June 1990 that efforts were made to improve it, the aforementioned 31511 being used in livery experiments, receiving both a yellow waistband and a yellow solebar for evaluation. Neither found favour so the loco was returned to traffic in plain grey.

Following further trials at Immingham on 31541, the grey and yellow 'Dutch' scheme was created for use on locos owned by the Civil Engineers, this soon seeing application across the fleet, which included modifying 31113/166/308 and 31512/19/24/30/31/51/53-55/68 along with 31465 which became 31565 at the same time.

However, this did not bring a total end to Departmental grey as 'Dutch' was purely for use on locos belonging to the Civil Engineers with the Department for Mechanical & Electric Engineers (DM&EE) opting not to follow the same route. The latter had also chosen not to implement the policy of ETS isolation so its Class 31/4s remained unaltered and, as a result, were regularly seen on passenger duties in the first years of the 1990s. Instead, the DM&EE favoured the Mainline livery for most of its classes and this was implemented when further '31/4s' were repainted.

Those Class 31/4s belonging to the department that were already in Departmental grey were allowed to retain it, 31417/57/61/62 duly carrying the scheme to withdrawal. Two oddities were 31511 which, despite being a Civil Engineers loco, never got the yellow band and would also be withdrawn in plain grey, having reverted to 31411 in May 1992. The other was the M&EE's 31466, which would eventually get the 'Dutch' treatment but only after the 1992 reorganisation of the engineering departments to put them under sector control, when it became part of the InterCity infrastructure fleet.

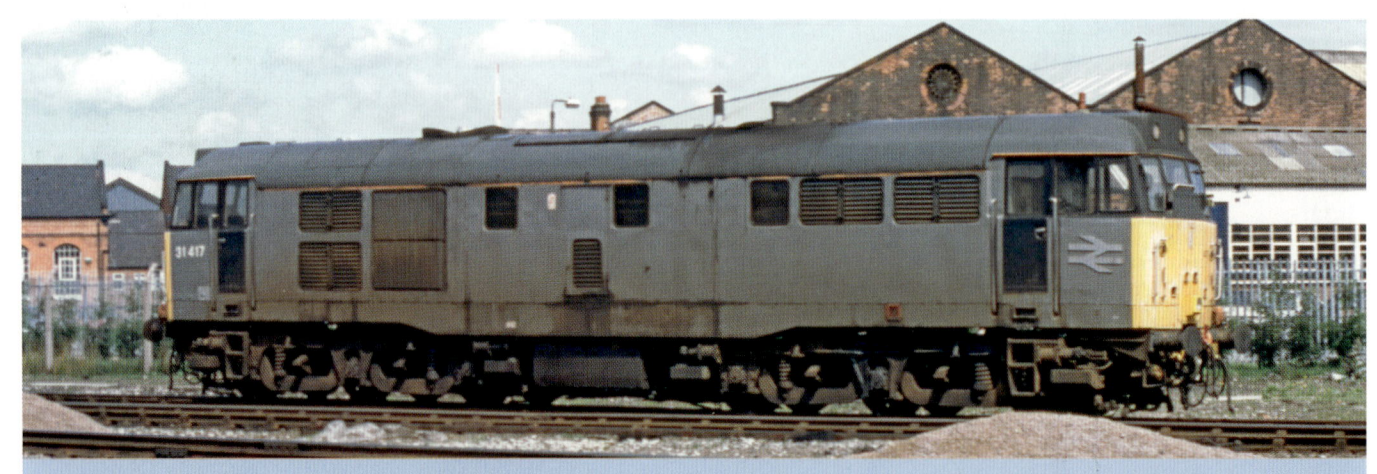

ABOVE: From the Mechanical and Electrical Engineers' fleet, 31417 arrives at Derby in August 1992 and was likely bound for the BREL workshops at Litchurch Lane to collect overhauled coaching stock for return to the assigned depot. The loco was stored in July 1995 by Transrail but disposal was a further 11 years away after passing through the ownership of EWS and Fragonset. 53A Models of Hull Collection/M Smith

A legacy continued

Making drab exciting

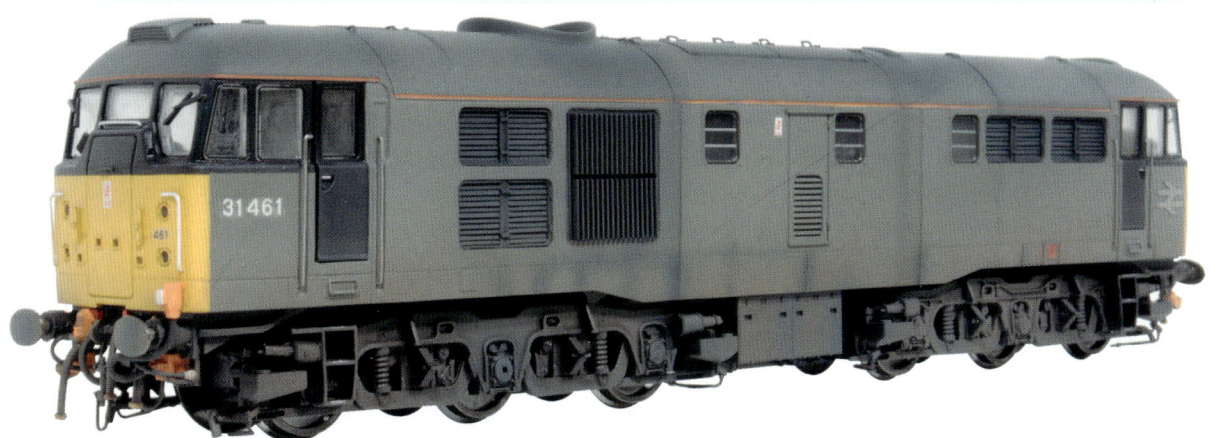

ABOVE: **The 1980s saw several Class 31s receive modifications to their radiators, gaining new side grilles with vertical slats and a cowling around the roof fan. Amongst the ETS-equipped Class 31/4s, just four had cab roof vents instead of headcode boxes, 31461 joining 31418/44/50.**

This OO gauge model started life as Hornby's first 'Skinhead' release in the form of 'Dutch'-liveried 31110. While stripping the model down, it became apparent that a full repaint would not be necessary, just the removal of the yellow bodyside band. This is perhaps easier said than done but I went about it by sanding down the joint between the yellow and grey with wet and dry paper used wet, carefully wearing through the yellow printing wherever possible and taking great care not to damage any moulded detail in the process. The main area to concentrate on was the actual join of the two colours, as this would potentially show through the new paint.

The other handy thing about the Hornby model is that the bodyside grilles are all separate fittings, making preparation for painting a lot easier as they simply push out with a little persuasion. This was useful for this particular model as they were already black so did not require repainting. They can be glued back in place after spraying the bodysides.

Once I was happy that the join between the two colours has been smoothed off, the body was masked to leave just the Railfreight grey to repaint. Firstly, a light coat of Halfords grey primer was applied to show up any blemishes. Next, the Railmatch Railfreight grey was added and allowed to dry. Hopefully upon removing the masking, there will not be much touching up to do; in this case only some black around the inner edge of the cab doors which was difficult to mask. Transfers were from Fox and Replica while bufferbeam detail was a mix of Heljan pipework and ETH sockets, Hornby multiple working fittings and Craftsman ETS cables bent to the desired shape.

Class 31s always attracted dirt with the radiator area descending into something of an oily mess. This was a nice challenge for weathering and delivers good results with a bit of effort. Thoroughly satin varnishing the whole model helps by dulling down and slightly fading the colours ready for weathering. After applying the bodyside 'sleeper grime' washes, I sprayed black around the various panel gaps and left it 'as is', giving a nice effect of built up grime and leaking oil. The lower panel gap is actually the engine room floor so oil and grime seeps out along the join, giving the effect seen here.

I used Railmatch 'roof dirt' for the roof and underframe oil staining, applied using pictures as a guide. Dark grey roofs are quite hard to weather effectively and to get the grime to show up against the dark colour. I used the same method of spraying along the panel gaps on the roof but not covering the whole area as the dirt would be far less visible.

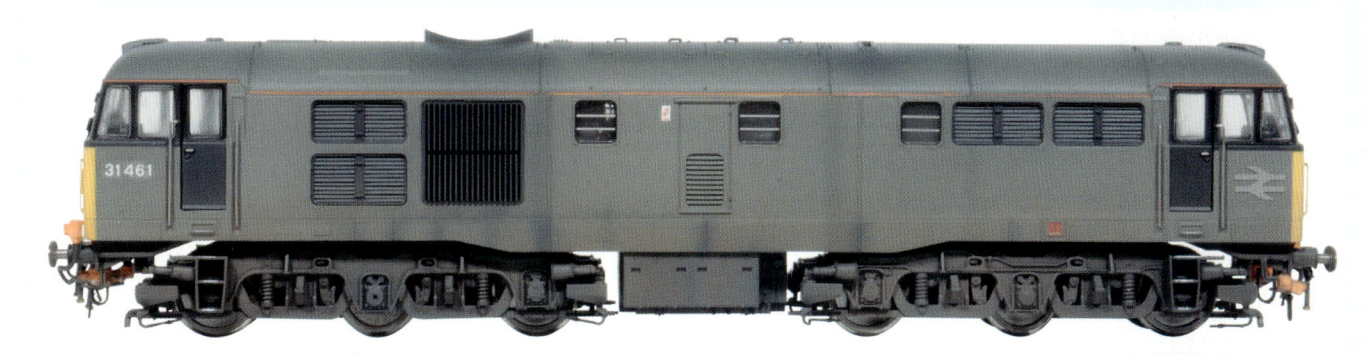

ABOVE: **Although the Departmental grey livery was widely derided for being drab, it actually brought a bit of variety once 'Dutch' became widespread and the Class 31s that retained the livery long enough to get well-weathered are interesting modelling propositions.**

RIGHT: **The fitting of the cast BR arrows was part of the livery's specification, although the use of depot plaques was not, the latter not appearing until 'Dutch' was introduced. The application of black around the cab windows and on the cab doors also brought some relief, the idea again being borrowed from the Railfreight triple grey scheme.**

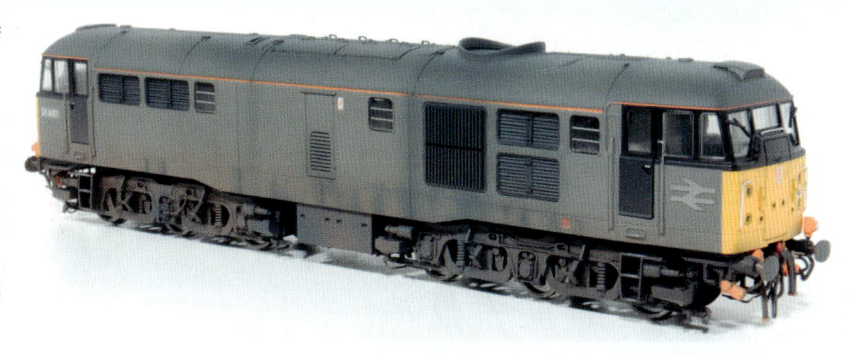

A legacy continued

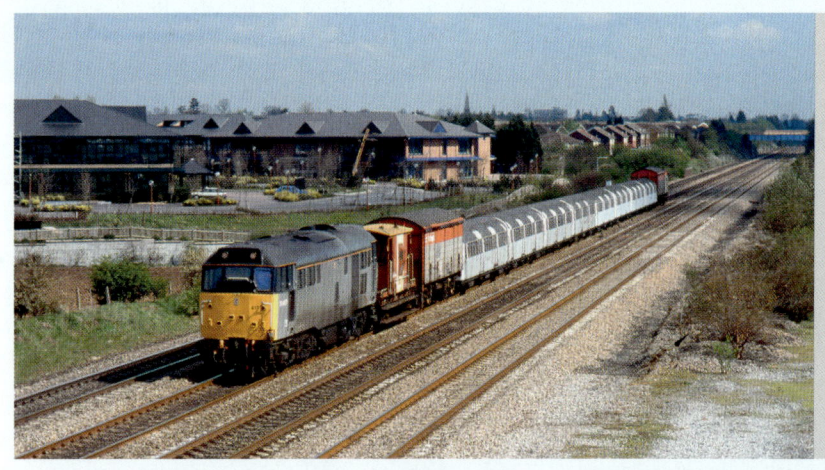

LEFT: The Class 31s assigned to the Mechanical and Electrical Engineers were often found on stock transfers along with passenger work. On April 8, 1990, 31417 ambles along at White Waltham, near Maidenhead, with the 9X03 West Ruislip to Crewe Works transfer of London Underground stock. This would recess overnight at Didcot Yard and was taking Central Line 1962 Stock for attention. This has previously been produced in OO gauge in un-motorised form by EFE and presumably will follow the 1938 Stock in reappearing in re-engineered and powered condition under the Bachmann-controlled EFE Rail brand in due course. A BR brake van coded CAP or CAR is provided at each end along with a REA barrier, the latter being modified VDA vans fitted with compatible couplings. Bachmann produces the VDA in 4mm with it and Hornby both offering the brake van. *Martin Loader*

Model availability

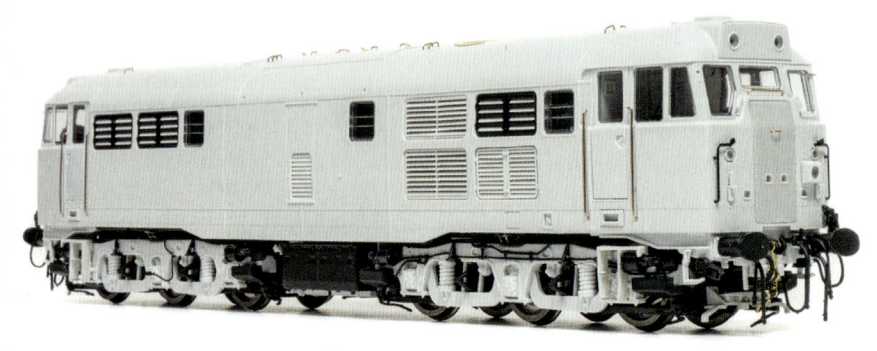

Much like the Class 20s, the Brush Type 2s have been the subject of several models over the decades, especially in OO gauge. Putting aside the vintage Tri-ang model, Lima's recreation from the late 1980s was a good effort and still has fans today thanks to the overall finesse of the bodyshell and shape of the cabs. The latter area is one of the main criticisms of Hornby's current highly-detailed Class 31, which has appeared in various forms and liveries over the past 18 years, albeit with some key ones missing, particularly from the sectorisation era. This has left the market open to a new Class 31 and this is on the way from Accurascale in many different variants with release due in 2023.

In N gauge, modellers have enjoyed a high quality Class 31 in the Graham Farish range since 2015, the initial green and blue incarnations having been followed more recently by refurbished versions appropriate to the 1990s. This tooling replaced the original and rather crude model that was produced by the company in its original incarnation when based on the south coast. Inevitably, Heljan has the 7mm market corned and added refurbished examples to its range last year, these going alongside the long-standing original versions.

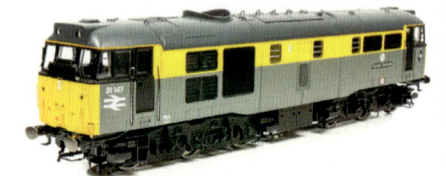

ABOVE: Accurascale's OO gauge Class 31 is due for release next year, this being an engineering prototype of the headcode box version in 1990s and beyond condition. Defining features include an offset headlight on the cab fronts and radio roof pods.

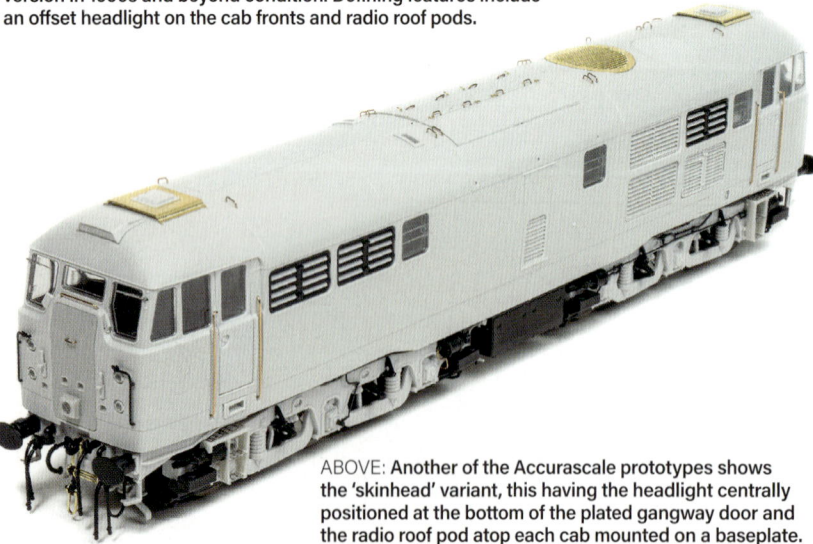

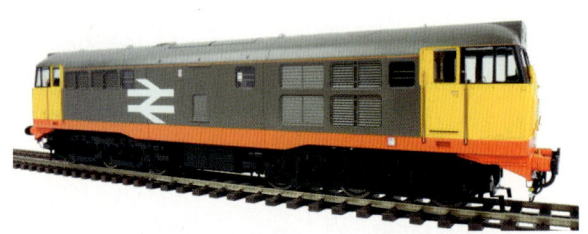

ABOVE: Another of the Accurascale prototypes shows the 'skinhead' variant, this having the headlight centrally positioned at the bottom of the plated gangway door and the radio roof pod atop each cab mounted on a baseplate.

ABOVE: Heljan's 7mm Class 31 has now appeared in numerous liveries, including Railfreight Red Stripe, the un-numbered loco allowing for easy customisation.

RIGHT: The current Graham Farish tooling can cater for a number of detail variations, Railfreight Petroleum 31319 displaying the modified radiator grille and roof cowl along with headlights and roof pods. *Image courtesy Kernow Model Rail Centre*

ABOVE: One of the most recent OO gauge Hornby releases was a headcode box example in the Civil Engineers 'Dutch' scheme, this depicting Bescot-based 31147 *Floreat Salopia*. *Image courtesy Kernow Model Rail Centre*

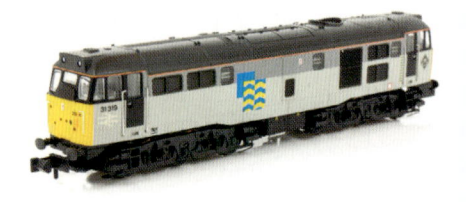

LOCOMOTION MODELS

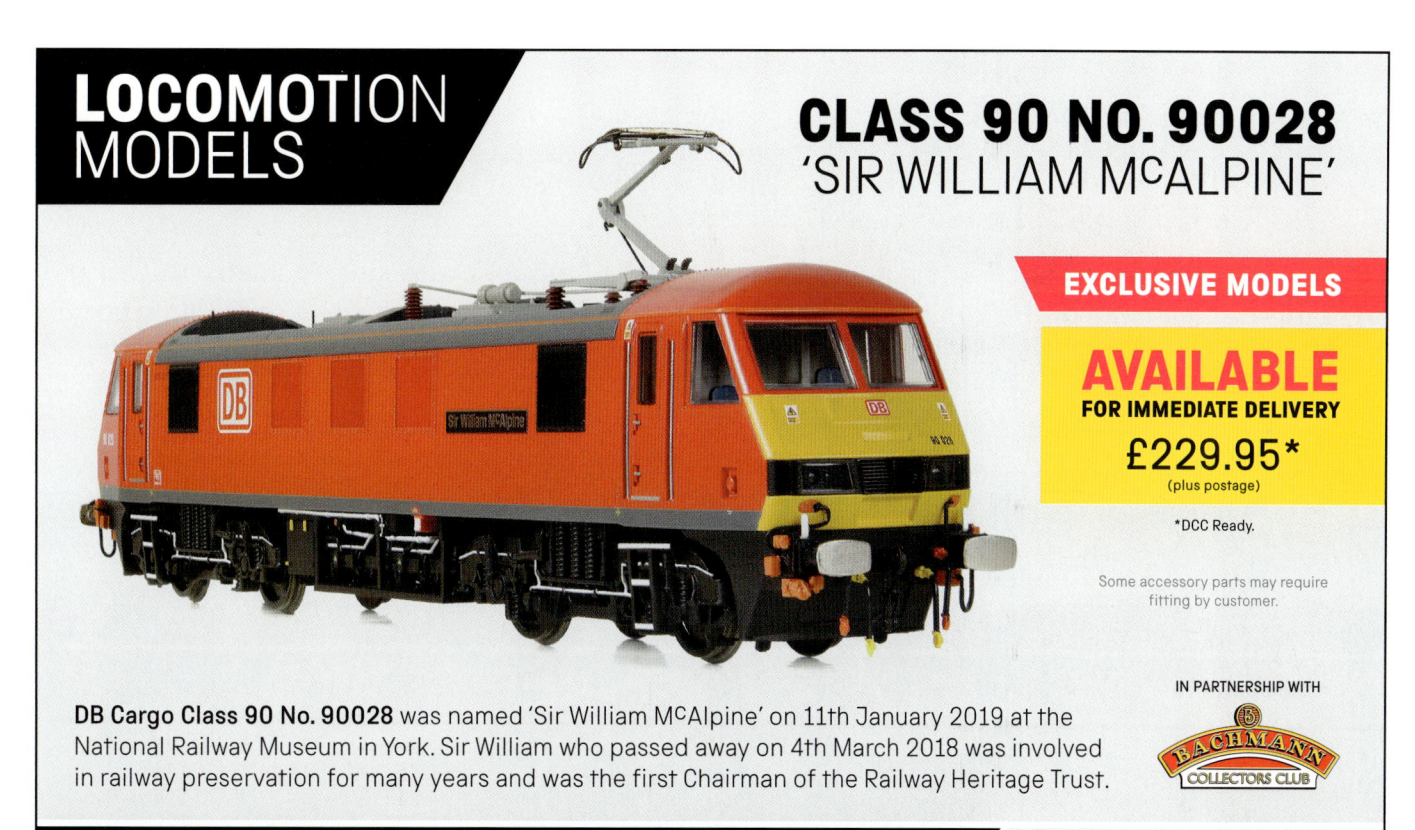

CLASS 90 NO. 90028
'SIR WILLIAM McALPINE'

EXCLUSIVE MODELS

AVAILABLE FOR IMMEDIATE DELIVERY

£229.95*
(plus postage)

*DCC Ready.

Some accessory parts may require fitting by customer.

IN PARTNERSHIP WITH Bachmann Collectors Club

DB Cargo Class 90 No. 90028 was named 'Sir William McAlpine' on 11th January 2019 at the National Railway Museum in York. Sir William who passed away on 4th March 2018 was involved in railway preservation for many years and was the first Chairman of the Railway Heritage Trust.

VISIT LOCOMOTIONMODELS.COM FOR FURTHER DETAILS

MODELS FEATURED ARE **00 GAUGE / 1:76 SCALE**

FIND US ON:

The National Collection in Miniature

Visit the Locomotion Museum Shop for: dapol, Graham Farish, Bachmann Branch-Line, Hornby, Oxford, Woodland Scenics

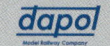

All prices and offers are subject to change without notice

Write for Key!

Having established itself as a leading publisher of railway books, Key Books is now looking for authors to join its international team of contributors. We are looking for existing authors and new ones, who really know their subject, especially if they have a great picture collection that could become an illustrated book.

- BR: FROM GREEN TO BLUE
- CANADIAN PACIFIC IN THE ROCKIES
- CLASS 37s — MARK V PIKE
- CZECH AND SLOVAK RAILWAYS — THREE DECADES OF CHANGE, 1990-2020s — KEITH FENDER
- HIGHLAND RAILWAYS — MIKE WEDGEWOOD

Key Books

To propose an idea or find out more, simply email
books@keypublishing.com

We look forward to hearing from you!

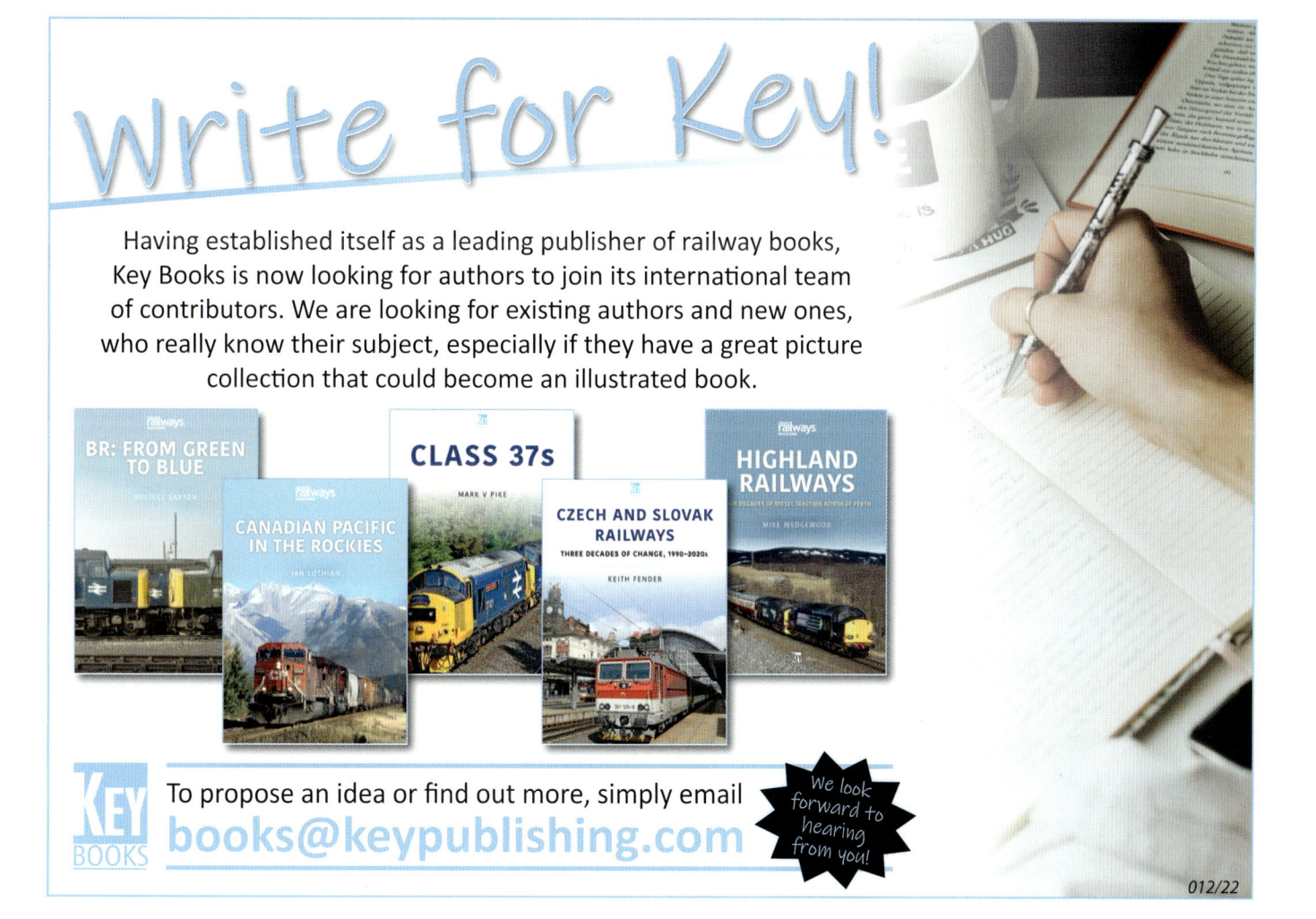

012/22

A legacy continued

The last flights of *Avocet*

By 1990, time had all but run out for the unique Brush Class 89 prototype as the first Class 91s were in service ahead of the commencement of the full electric timetable to Leeds. Now largely limited to charter work, it would not last the year. Simon Bendall **looks at its history while** Alex Carpenter **builds the resin Silver Fox kit in OO gauge.**

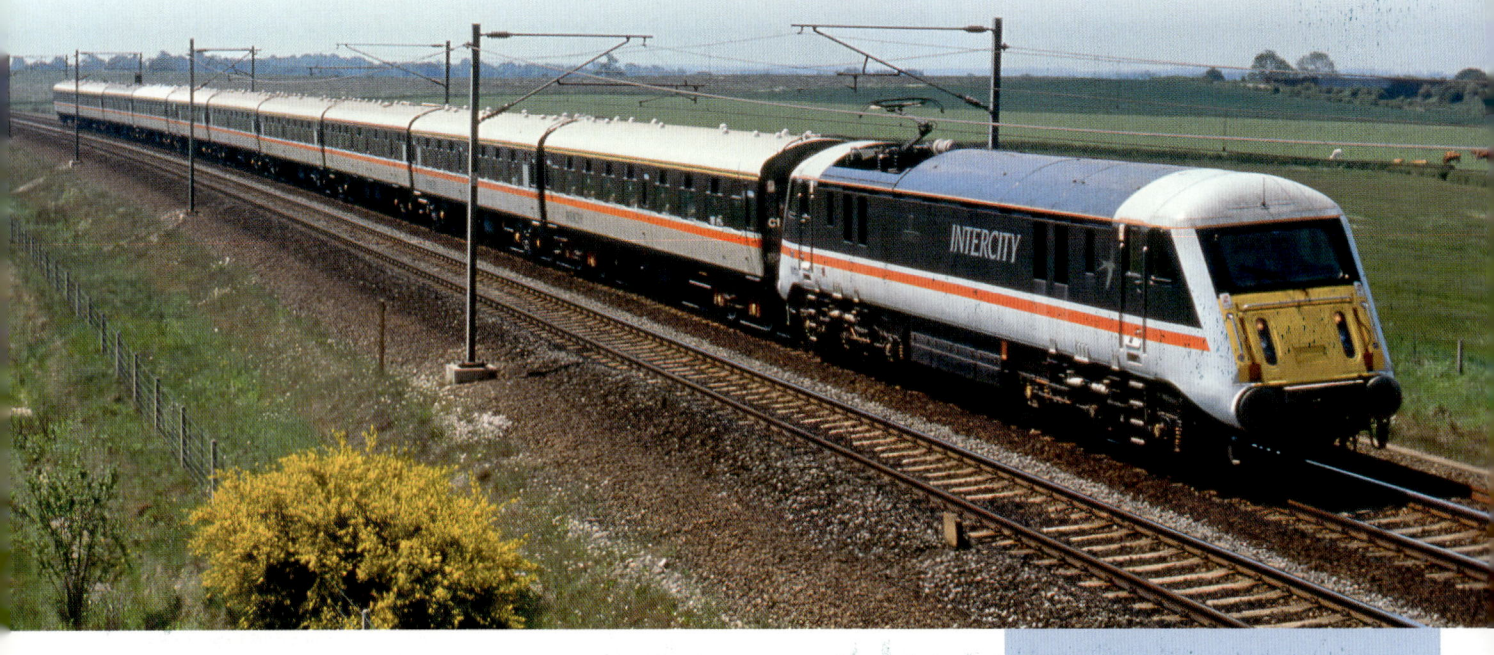

During the early 1980s, British Rail was granted permission by the government to conduct electrification of the East Coast Main Line from King's Cross to Edinburgh. With engineers deeming that a four-axle loco design would not be capable of producing the required performance, the spring of 1982 saw a tender issued for the construction of a prototype Co-Co electric loco. To be capable of 125mph, it was also to feature thyristor control and rheostatic braking. Brush Traction was awarded the contract in June 1983, which sub-contracted its manufacture to BREL at Crewe Works.

However, construction took somewhat longer than planned, it not emerging from Crewe until October 2, 1986, when it was hauled to Derby Litchurch Lane by 25191 for onward road movement to Brush at Loughborough for final finishing and initial testing. Owned outright by BR, 89001 was finished in InterCity Executive livery.

By this time, BR had already opted to revise the specification for the East Coast's new generation of motive power, deciding that a Bo-Bo electric would after all be the best choice and with a revised maximum speed of 140mph. Tender documents for the Class 91s had been issued as long ago as the summer of 1985 with GEC subsequently winning the order. Against this backdrop, the Class 89 project survived cancellation, even though the loco no longer had a purpose nor any real prospect of a follow on production order.

Testing begins

Returned to Derby from Loughborough on February 4, 1987, 89001 headed to Crewe Electric five days later behind 20209. It made its first outings on BR metals around Crewe the same day before light engine runs to Hartford Junction later in the month. Taken back to Derby by 25912 on February 27 for bogie tests at the Railway Technical Centre, the electric was at Old Dalby by April for pantograph testing. Throughout the remainder of the year, trials were conducted on the West Coast Main Line, particularly the Crewe-Carlisle section, hauling some of the BREL International Mk.3 coaches as well as Test Car 10 and Lab 6.

Having proved successful, 89001 was transferred to the East Coast Main Line in December 1987 to begin the driver training programme on electric traction in advance of the arrival of the first Class 91s. This was interrupted between April and June 1988 to allow the loco to visit the IVA transport exhibition in Hamburg, it being accompanied by 90008, 91003 and Sprinter 150263 on the trip to Germany.

Its debut on a passenger train finally came on July 3 when it hauled the 50th anniversary *Mallard* charter from King's Cross to Doncaster where the famous A4 'Pacific' took over. Put into regular traffic on the Peterborough commuter services, it debuted on July 15 before hauling the first revenue-earning electric service from London to Leeds on August 10.

The start of 1989 brought a repaint into InterCity Swallow at Bounds Green in preparation for its naming ceremony at King's Cross on January 16, when the Prime Minster, Margaret Thatcher, named 89001 *Avocet* after the symbol of the RSPB. However, with the Class 91s taking over the Peterborough services from the spring, the use of 89001 began to diminish with only sporadic periods in traffic due to maintenance and failures.

This pattern continued throughout the rest of 1989 and into 1990, by when its use was largely confined to occasional sorties on the white-roofed InterCity charter stock. A choke failure in September 1990 saw it side-lined for good. Formally transferred to store at Bounds Green in July 1991, official withdrawal took place a year later on July 30, 1992. It was then sold almost immediately into preservation to a group of Brush employees, arriving at the Midland Railway Centre that December. Reactivation and a second main line career with GNER would follow between the spring of 1997 and the start of 2001 but this included several lengthy spells out of traffic due to a lack of spares for the unique machine.

ABOVE: With only four months to go before failure ended its BR career, 89001 hustles the Hertfordshire Railtours 'Modern Railways 500' charter along the ECML at Colton Junction on May 27, 1990. Carrying Swallow livery and its *Avocet* nameplates, it worked the tour from King's Cross to York before giving way to green Class 25 D7672/25912 *Tamworth Castle*, as pictured on page seven. The train is formed of InterCity Charter Unit white-roofed Mk.1s, which encompasses seven First Open (FO), two buffets (RBR) and a Brake Composite Corridor (BCK). Hornby has produced the latter in these exact colours but has yet to follow up with the other types, although it has the correct tooling in its OO gauge range.
Martin Loader

A legacy continued

Building the 'Badger'

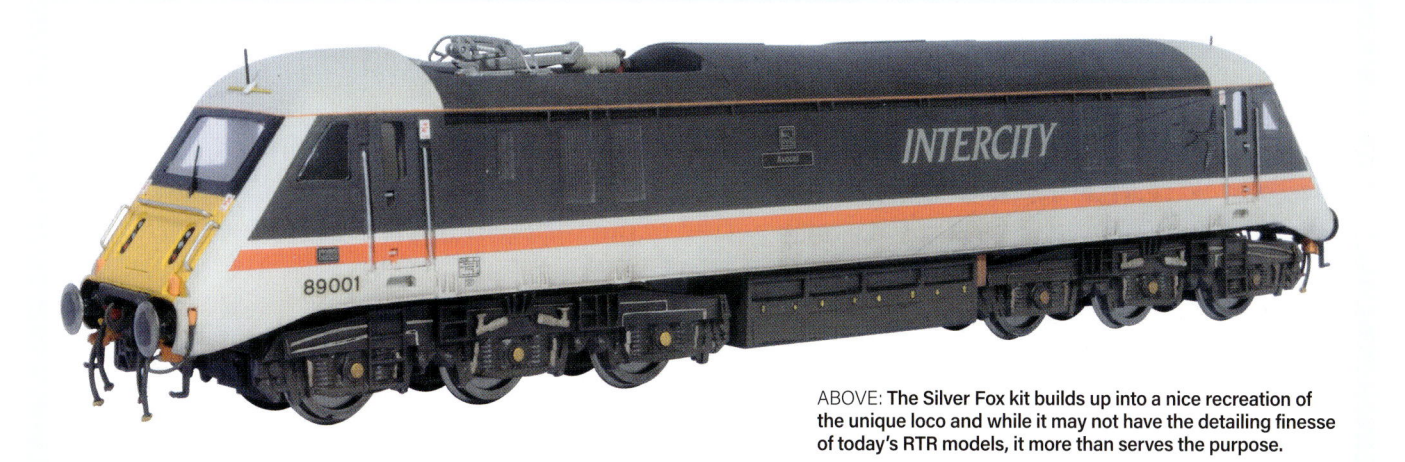

ABOVE: The Silver Fox kit builds up into a nice recreation of the unique loco and while it may not have the detailing finesse of today's RTR models, it more than serves the purpose.

While Rails of Sheffield floated the possibility of a ready-to-run Class 89 in OO gauge in conjunction with Accurascale in 2020, this project has developed little since, at least publicly. Therefore, the resin kit from Silver Fox Models remains a viable route to producing the much-liked AC electric.

Silver Fox supplies a one-piece bodyshell, bogie sideframes and a few other details in the kit (priced £47.50) with the purchaser required to source a chassis, pantograph, paint, and transfers to complete. The recommended chassis is the Hornby (ex-Lima) Class 47, although the company can also supply fully-finished and motorised models in all three of the loco's liveries at £175 each.

The resin parts do benefit from careful cleaning up, particular care being taken along the bottom edge of the body as it is not always easy to tell where the flash ends and the body starts, but time taken here to level it out nicely will pay dividends with the finished model. The windows were initially cleaned up using a scalpel, and then filed out and squared up where needed.

The parts were given a thorough wash in hot soapy water and allowed to dry fully. The key to a good paint finish is primer, so all of the parts were given a coat of etch primer and left for a week to cure. Any blemishes can then be corrected at this stage and lightly re-primed.

Painting
I prefer to use Railmatch acrylics when possible as I get on well with them. First, an all over coat of Falcon grey was applied and left to dry for 24 hours. I always like to leave a day or more in-between masking off different colours, which gives the paint time to 'key'. Next up was the silver-grey, masked off at the bottom of where the white stripe will be. This lets you mark out the positions of the red and white stripes in relation to each other. It is the hardest part of masking the livery, but it is essential to get it right otherwise it will ruin the model. Fox makes the stripes as transfers, but I prefer to paint them as it is more durable.

Once the stripes were painted and dry, the final colour was yellow with the cab fronts being masked off and sprayed. This may need several coats as it has to build up to the right density. Finally, black was applied by hand around the cab windscreens. Once fully dry, overall gloss varnish was applied before adding the transfers, which were sealed in with another coat of gloss, and finally satin varnish. This should render the transfer film invisible. Detail painting of the bogies and underframe was then undertaken as was fitting the etched nameplates, swallow emblems and Brush builder's plates. The model was then given a light weathering.

Motorising
To power the model, I chose to use a Hornby (ex-Lima) Class 66 motor bogie. To mount the new motor bogie, a simple cradle made from three pieces of thick plasticard was glued to the chassis before drilling a central hole in the top, into which the bogie simply clips. The supplied resin sideframes can then be attached. The trailing bogie mounts in the existing chassis hole and is also fitted with the resin sideframes. Weight was added using liquid lead in the underframe tanks.

The three cab front handrails were added from 0.7mm wire, the original mouldings having been carved off before painting. I chose to keep the moulded cabside ones. The supplied buffers were fitted after the buffer shanks were moved downwards by 1.5mm as they sat a little high. Smiths coupling hooks were added as well as dummy drop-head buckeyes from the spares box, these being modified from Hornby HST power cars.

Shawplan air pipes were pre-painted and added, also ETS jumpers and receptacles, these being modified Heljan Class 47 spares. The thin jumper cable ends on the lower cabside corners were made from shortened Bachmann Class 20 items, drilled to take 0.5mm wire, while the glazing was clear plastic sheet, cut and filed to a 'push fit' and secured in place with PVA glue. Shawplan windscreen wipers were added as were the cab to shore radio roof-mounted aerials, the base of which were finished in yellow to match the real loco. Finally, a Hornby Brecknell Willis pantograph was fitted to the roof.

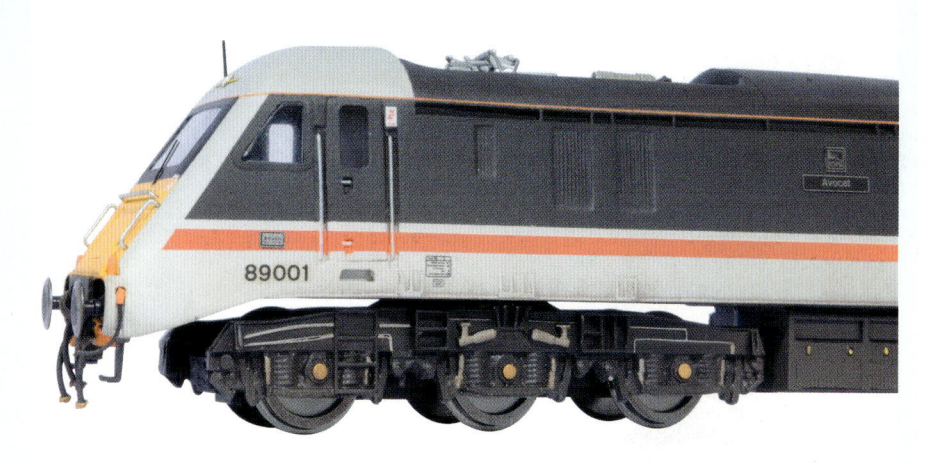

ABOVE: The loco's nameplates, builder's plates and swallow emblems are all from the Shawplan range as are several of the detailing parts. Other separate items serve to enhance the body, particularly around the cab fronts.

A legacy continued

Electras go live

The beginning of the 1990s saw the electrification of the East Coast Main Line completed through to Edinburgh, allowing the Class 91s to enter squadron service atop the Mk.4 coaches. Simon Bendall looks at this early period of operation along with the new Hornby OO gauge model.

Deliveries of the Class 91s from Crewe Works had begun in February 1988 with the emergence of 91001 for initial testing on the West Coast Main Line and then at Old Dalby before spending the remainder of the year undergoing trials and training runs off Bounds Green. Subsequently, 91002-10 were all outshopped between March 1988 and April 1989 before a pause in construction took place while evaluations and modifications were carried out to resolve the type's numerous early teething troubles. It was not until February 1990 that 91011 was released with deliveries then continuing until 91031 was ready 12 months later.

It was already known that the Class 91s would arrive well ahead of their accompanying Mk.4 coaches, the ordering of the latter having been held up, partly due to delays in selecting the bogie type to be used. As a result, BR had already decided to pair the new locos with Mk.3 trailer sets and a HST power car on the other end. The latter would provide train power as the Class 91s were incompatible with the 415V three-phase system of the Mk.3 coaches.

To enable the two to work together, the chosen power cars were equipped with the Time Division Multiplex (TDM) push-pull equipment, effectively making them stand-in Driving Van Trailers (DVTs). It was also deemed prudent to fit a conventional bufferbeam to the power cars to enable easier recovery in the event of failure or the need for conventional haulage. An initial two Class 43s, 43014 and 43123, were converted in late 1987 with a production batch of 43013/65/67/68/80/84 following in 1988/89.

Passenger debut

It was not until early March 1989 that the Class 91s were deemed sufficiently reliable to enter passenger service, initially on the King's Cross to Peterborough and Grantham commuter services but with Leeds workings following soon afterwards, the electrics each being paired with a Mk.3 set and surrogate DVT. Initially, the plan was to have the power cars' Valenta engine running just above idling to provide train power only, not traction. This caused several issues though, not least a build-up of unburnt fuel deposits in the exhausts that resulted in at least one substantial fire.

As a result, authorisation was given to use the Class 43 for traction in addition to the Class 91, the TDM system allowing the driver to control both. The combined horsepower was quite unlike anything seen before on the East Coast with the acceleration possible allowing numerous timing records to be set between stations! Meanwhile, the May 1989 timetable change brought an increase in workings with seven of the eight modified power cars required in service at any one time to partner the Class 91s. However, TDM faults and mechanical issues meant this was not always achieved.

July 1989 saw the first Mk.4 coaches commence testing on the ECML, having emerged from Metro-Cammell's Washwood Heath plant during the previous month. By October, the first Mk.4 set was ready to commence passenger service with the following months progressively seeing further sets brought into traffic. From March 1990, sufficient Mk.4s were in use to allow the surrogate DVTs to be relegated to reserve status and returned to normal service along with the Mk.3 sets.

The InterCity 225 fleet was launched into full service during the summer of 1991, enabling a large number of HSTs to be released to other routes, which included the transfer of the eight bufferbeam-fitted power cars to cross-country duties. From this time, the Class 91s became entirely dedicated to the ECML workings, there no longer being any slack in the fleet to allow them to work InterCity charter trains as they had done on occasions in previous years.

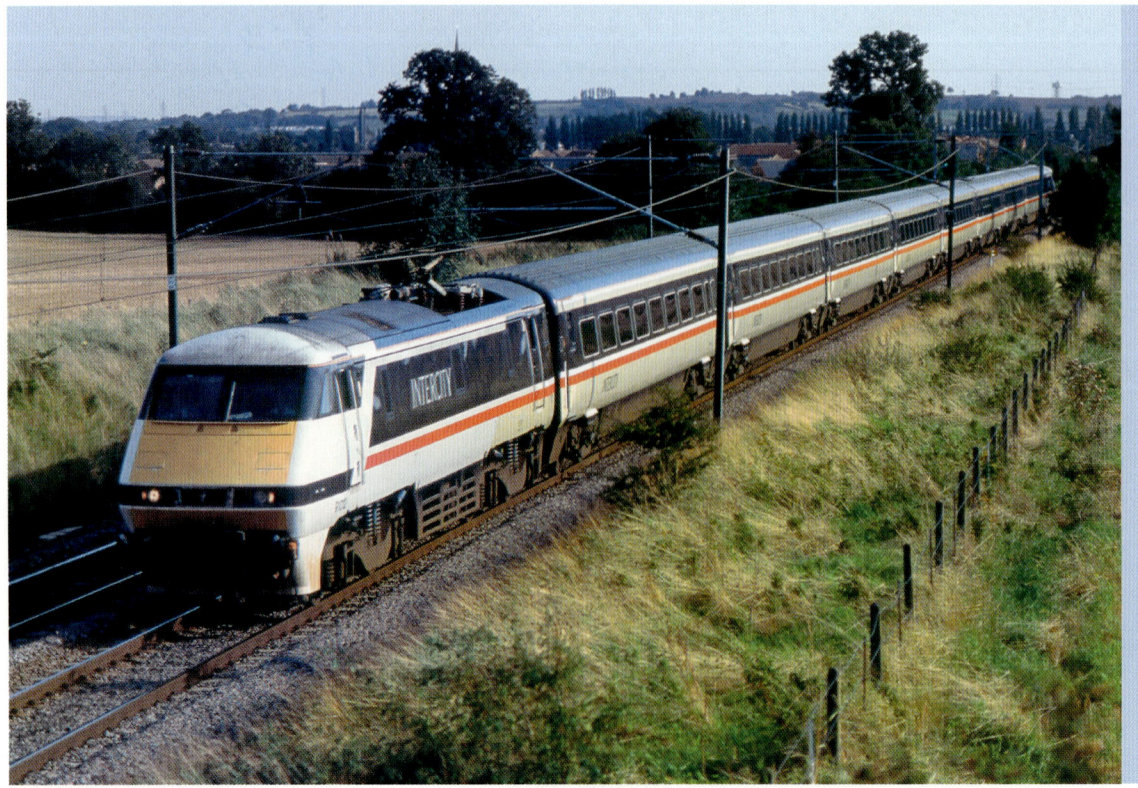

LEFT: For a time, the Class 91s were the flagships of British Rail and InterCity, their stylish lines being eminently marketable alongside the service improvements brought to the East Coast Main Line. On August 18, 1992, 91012 enjoys the early evening sun as it heads north near Peascliffe Tunnel with the 16.25 King's Cross to Leeds. The Mk.4 formation is typical for the time with five standard class vehicles, the buffet and two first class coaches with the DVT on the rear. With Hornby having already released its Class 91, all new accompanying Mk.4s are due later this year. Martin Loader

32 www.keymodelworld.com

A legacy continued

RIGHT: It is perhaps strange seeing Class 91s on other types of coaches after so many years of dedication to the Mk.4s, but this was commonly the case in 1988-90 when the fleet was not fully utilised. On July 24, 1990, 91005 stands at King's Cross while awaiting departure with one of the commuter services to Peterborough. These were formed of Mk.2 air-conditioned stock, including some of the Mk.2f TSOs fitted with high density seating and numbered in the 6800-29 series. The Commonwealth-bogied Mk.1 BG makes for an interesting comparison with the new generation AC electric! Simon Bendall Collection

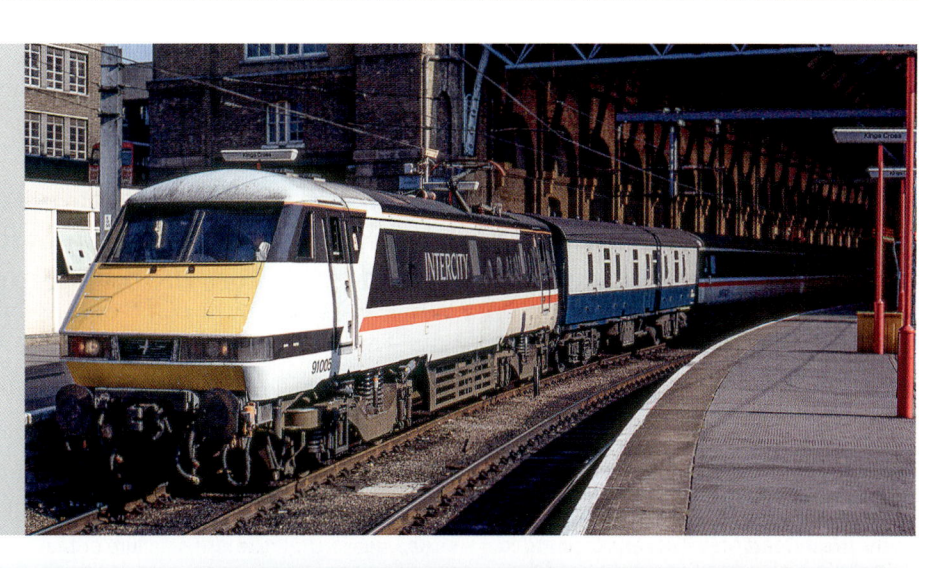

Hornby goes electric, again

As a young enthusiast and modeller in 1991, the cover of that year's Hornby catalogue was inspirational, featuring the manufacturer's Class 91 rushing through a townscape beneath overhead wires and with a set of Mk.4s in tow. This was the British Rail I wanted to model, even if the dreams rather outstripped reality!

Now some 31 years later that same sense of style and speed have been evoked by Hornby's all new OO gauge rendering of the Class 91s, especially when it comes in the form of 91002 *Durham Cathedral* in the superbly-designed version of the InterCity Swallow colours. The model arrived while this volume was in production so sadly too late to take it beyond its out of the box condition, but it is included here for completeness, especially as no examination of the 1990s loco fleet would be complete without the one-time BR poster boys.

Welcomely, Hornby has given the class the 'full fat' treatment with a specification that matches today's expectations. It has also invested sufficiently in the tooling to allow the original as-built body to be produced alongside the refurbished Class 91/1 version with its additional ventilation grilles. Arguably, the class is somewhat difficult to give the highly-detailed treatment to as with such an aerodynamic body and components hidden away as a result, there is much less detail to go to town on compared to other types.

Still, highlights include the etched underframe fairings, the slots in these giving a glimpse of the air tanks and other equipment mounted behind. On the roof, the Brecknell Willis single-arm pantograph is sprung and poseable and far removed from the metal fitting that adorned the original model three decades ago, even if it lags behind what Accurascale and Bachmann have achieved with their comparable Class 92 and Class 90, respectively.

The model is up to expectations in other areas as well with pre-fitted ETS components, air pipes and dummy buckeyes in the accessory bag, and switchable day and night lighting.

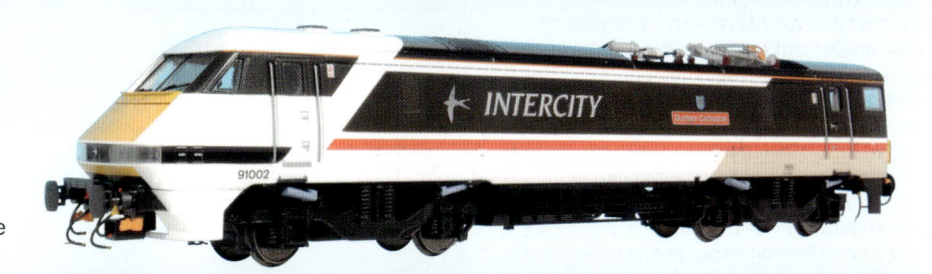

ABOVE: The designers did a superb job on re-styling the InterCity Swallow livery to match the lines of the Class 91s, giving a look that is still modern today. Indeed, with LNER bringing back an amended version of the livery, the class has gone full circle.

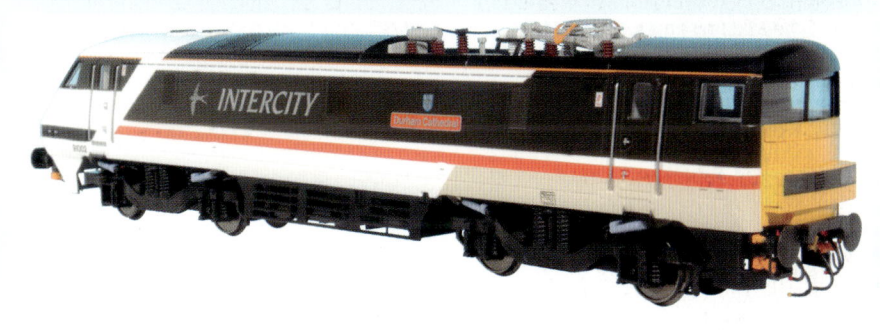

ABOVE: The Class 91s avoided the mistake of the HST power cars by having a full driving cab at the blunt end. While its use may have been occasional, it allowed sets to keep running in the event of TDM failure or similar by running the loco round and attaching to the DVT.

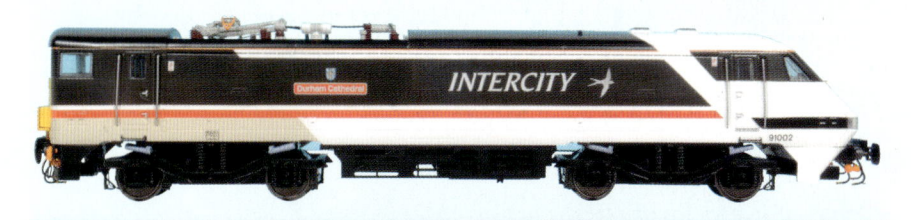

ABOVE: The etched underframe fairings are a highlight of the model, delivering not only the necessary finesse but also a view of the components behind, something which is quite distinctive on the real locos.

Separate nameplates are also included to apply over the printed ones if desired. The deceptively complex InterCity livery is well applied with excellent colours while the printing is good throughout. While that dreamed of ECML layout may never have been built, the Hornby Class 91 rekindles some fond memories of long ago while also giving the type the modern rendering it has long deserved.

New looks for the decade

As the early 1990s progressed, several of British Rail's sectors adopted new names while the locomotive fleets also underwent restructuring in preparation for privatisation. There was also time for further new liveries to emerge before the break-up of the national operator began as Simon Bendall details.

The first of the sectors to adopt a new identity was Provincial, which morphed into Regional Railways from December 1990 with an adapted livery following during 1991, although it was another year before any locos became involved in receiving this. Under this new brand, the sector continued to have responsibility for all passenger services that did not fall under the remit of InterCity and Network SouthEast. Operating on a decentralised basis, five regional centres were created with the aim of providing services attuned to each area while also giving good connections between them. By the spring of 1992, ScotRail, North East, North West, Central and South Wales & West were all in existence and coping reasonably well with the challenges of providing both rural and urban services in an unfavourable economic environment.

The next significant rebrand came in October 1991 when the Parcels sector was put on a more business-orientated footing and given a complete marketing overhaul to become Rail Express Systems. Rather than just clinging to whatever Royal Mail traffic it could, the sector was now charged with trying to secure new flows as private courier firms began to make their presence increasingly felt. Investment allowed the locomotive fleet to be improved, the Class 47s in particular benefitting from a package of modifications, while similar upgrades were also delivered to the parcels van fleet. The rapid spread of the new RES livery was also obvious, transforming previously tired-looking parcels trains into unmistakable adverts for the benefits of corporate identity.

A less obvious change during 1991 was the decision of the four bulk-haul freight sub-sectors to drop the Railfreight name in favour of Trainload to better reflect the nature of their business. While this had no impact on the loco fleet, it was reflected on a few wagons such as the smattering of covered steel wagon prototypes. The decision to now prefix Coal, Construction, Metals and Petroleum with Trainload also affected some depot and yard signage and was very much implemented on marketing material and other official paperwork.

InterCity and Network South East were both content enough with their brands not to make any further significant alterations, although InterCity did briefly contemplate replacing the red stripe on its livery with claret in 1993. This went as far as four HST power cars, 43010/139/140/146, and at least one set of Mk.3 trailers receiving the revised colour for evaluation, but the idea progressed no further and the affected stock was returned to normal.

Engineers disbanded

Some of the most significant changes of the early 1990s centred on the loco fleets of the various engineering departments. The first came in June 1990 when the Civil Engineers successfully campaigned for an alteration to the Departmental grey livery, it won official approval to add an upper yellow band to its locos. The 'Dutch' livery as it became instantly known spread rapidly across a number of classes while, at the same time, the grey and yellow was becoming more prevalent on engineers' wagons thanks to new conversions and overhaul programmes. As a result, matching sets of locos and stock could soon be

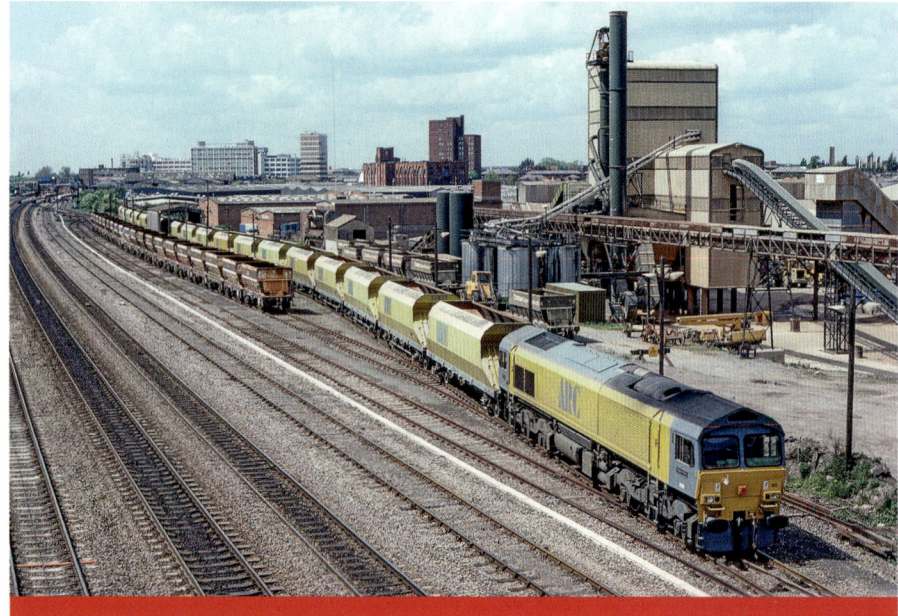

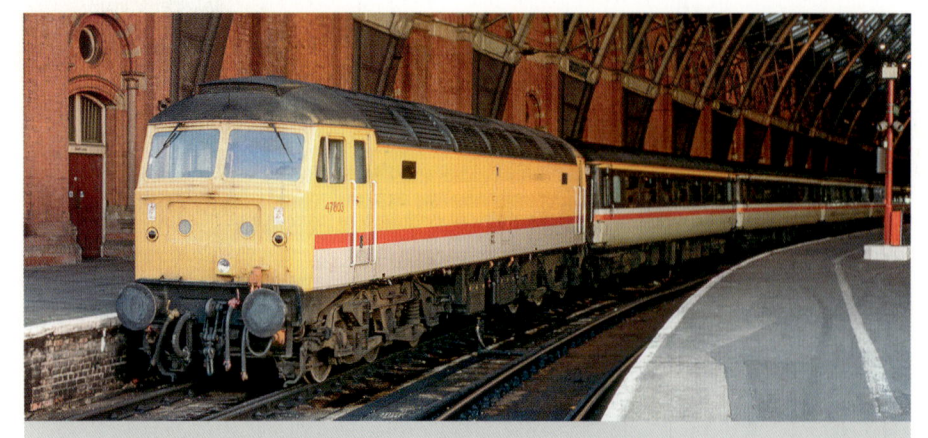

ABOVE: ARC became the second private rail freight operator on the network in October 1990 with the delivery of its four Canadian-built Class 59/1s. Put into traffic from the following month, they revolutionised the company's operation out of Whatley Quarry to distribution terminals across London and the south east. Some 18 months later, 59103 *Village of Mells* draws its rake of JHA bogie hoppers through the discharge shed at Hayes in West London on May 11, 1992. After some three decades of the Lima, now Hornby, Class 59 in OO gauge, a new model should finally arrive from Dapol later this year. More competition is apparent in N gauge where Dapol and Revolution Trains are striving to be the first to get their new offering to market. Simon Bendall Collection

ABOVE: Long range fuel tank example 47803 was officially relegated to the InterCity infrastructure fleet in October 1992, being assigned to the Midland and CrossCountry routes. Six months later, it was repainted into this predominately yellow livery with red 'Infrastructure' lettering emblazoned down the sides, although the latter lasted mere weeks. The relegation of the Type 4 to such mundane work was somewhat questionable as it was still regularly found atop InterCity services across the country, such as in November 1993 when pictured at St. Pancras. Storage by Mainline Freight would come in June 1995, but disposal would not be for another 12 years. Simon Bendall Collection

New looks for the decade

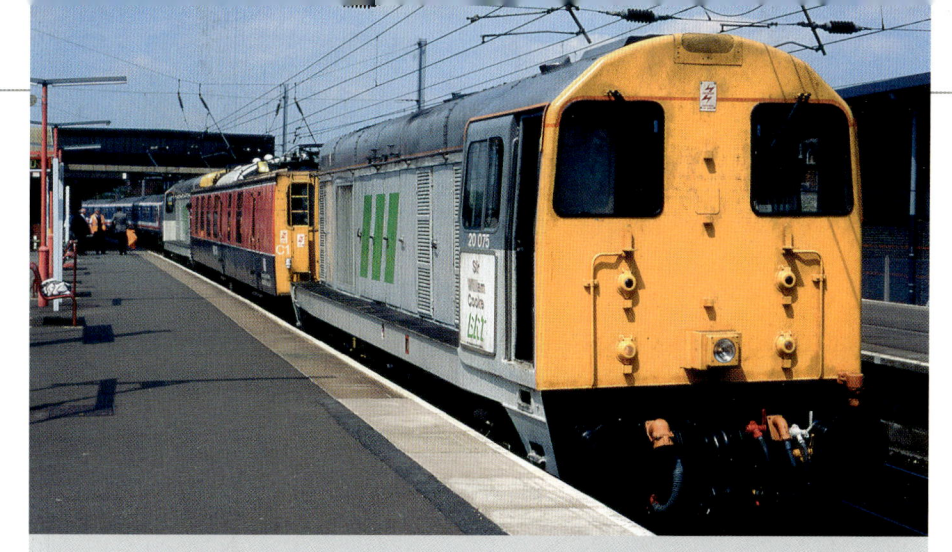

ABOVE: The BRT-liveried duo of 20075 *Sir William Cooke* and 20128 *Guglielmo Marconi* were somewhat unusually employed on May 22, 1995, as they stand at Bedford sandwiching overhead line test coach ADB975091 *Mentor*. The oddball combination would continue south to St Pancras before touring the West Midlands two days later, including visiting Birmingham New Street. At this time, the duo was more usually employed on freight traffic with Transrail and working off Bescot. Simon Bendall Collection

seen across the network, replacing the dreary look of such trains that was common in the 1980s.

A significant organisational change arrived in the spring of 1992 as the various engineering fleets were largely dispersed to the control of the three passenger sectors of Regional Railways, InterCity, and Network SouthEast. This was an early step towards privatisation that ensured all stock, including engineers' wagons, was accountable to a business unit. The locos remained assigned to what were now called infrastructure duties and typically allocated to a geographical area.

For example, NSE fleets were divided up into pools that were either based north or south of the River Thames while the Regional Railways allocation was spread amongst the five regional centres mentioned above. InterCity preferred groupings by main lines so locos were assigned to the East Coast, West Coast and Great Western with a joint fleet covering the central Midland and CrossCountry routes. Several Class 31 were also set aside specifically for duties that had previously fallen under the remit of the Mechanical and Electrical Engineers, such as hauling overhead line maintenance trains. Not that this stopped them from widely wandering onto other duties.

Beyond 'Dutch'

With a host of new locos now on their books, the three passenger sectors indulged in some limited dabbling with additional brandings or full repaints. In the case of Regional Railways, it opted to continue with the 'Dutch' grey and yellow livery for its machines, only 31233 gaining the sector's bodyside lettering for its naming as *Severn Valley Railway*.

Network SouthEast chose to turn out a handful of engineers' pool Class 73s and an additional Class 33, 33035, in its colours before deciding to also continue with 'Dutch'. Sadly, this denied us the sight of Class 37s in red, white, and blue, even though the plan got as far as creating painting diagrams.

Only InterCity opted to experiment with a new predominately yellow Infrastructure livery, turning out 47803 in the startling scheme in April 1993, followed by 31116 in a Union Pacific-inspired version six months later. Reaction to both was negative at best so again 'Dutch' was perpetuated on the sector's fleet.

Centralised locos

Not all motive power could be easily dispersed though with Central Services created in April 1992 to mop up many of the remaining locos. This was a BR headquarters-based body that was responsible for specialist infrastructure functions such as the Civil Link air-braked engineers' network. To power these trains of track materials, it was given a selection of Class 31s based at Bescot and Crewe-allocated Class 47s as well as the soon to be withdrawn pair of 50008 and 50015 at Laira.

Also included under the remit of Central Services was the provision of locos for the test trains predominately based at the Railway Technical Centre in Derby. This gave it control of the six dedicated Class 47s, 47971-76, along with late replacement 47981 and around half a dozen Class 20s.

However, it was not until February 1993 that this new operation really made its mark with the debut of a new maroon and grey livery on 20092 and 20169. These were branded as Technical Services which was, slightly confusingly, a division of Central Services and they were soon joined by 47972 in the same colours. No further locos were repainted although a handful of test coaches were done.

Those locos that lasted in traffic long enough would eventually pass into EWS ownership, the Class 20s and Class 31s along with the Civil Link Class 47s after they were all folded into what would become the Transrail fleet in 1994. The test train Type 4s followed after some allocation 'jiggery pokery' that eventually saw them grouped and sold off with their RES sisters.

Telecoms Choppers

The other new organisation that was created upon the disbandment of the engineers' fleets in the spring of 1992 was British Rail Telecommunications (BRT). This was charged with managing much of the railway's communications network and required locos fitted with slow-speed equipment to power its cable-laying trains. As a result, it acquired a fleet of just over a dozen Class 20s, many coming from what was now Trainload Coal.

In the event, only four would see prolonged use, 20075 and 20128/31/87 initially passing through Doncaster Works for overhaul, from where they emerged in early 1993 carrying fresh coats of BR blue with a discreet green and white BRT logo on the bonnet sides. Inevitably in the image conscious world of railways, a new corporate livery duly arrived in September that year with 20131 receiving an application of two-tone grey with green logos. Its three classmates would duly follow during the course of 1994.

The quartet were initially popular with Regional Railways for use on passenger trains, pairs regularly finding their way to Skegness in the summer of 1993. Two years later, BRT reached agreement with Transrail to maintain the Class 20s and allowed their use on freight traffic around the West Midlands when not needed, an arrangement that continued with EWS. However, 1997 saw the quartet sold to Direct Rail Services after BRT, now owned by Racal, withdrew from rail operations.

Following this reorganisation of the engineers' fleet, the next restructuring would come in the spring of 1994 as the locos were divided between the regional freight companies.

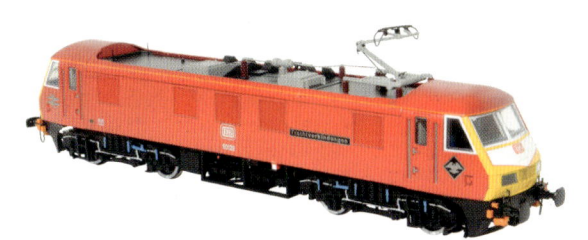

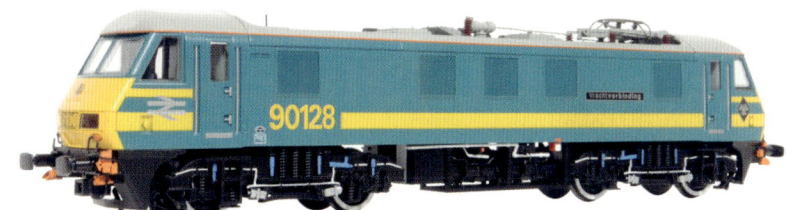

ABOVE: Special liveries, usually of a heritage flavour, continued to sporadically appear in the early 1990s. One of the highlights of 1992 was the repainting of three Railfreight Distribution Class 90s into the colours of the national railway operators of France, Belgium, and Germany, this being designed to promote international freight links ahead of the opening of the Channel Tunnel. With the release of Bachmann's OO gauge Class 90 in 2019, two of this trio have so far made it into model form. Both are portrayed as running soon after repainting with SNCB blue and yellow 90128 being exclusively available from the Bachmann Collectors' Club. Meanwhile, DB red 90129 is a more recent limited edition commissioned by Kernow Model Rail Centre.

Modelling BR Locomotives of the 1990s 35

New looks for the decade

Parcels relaunched

The autumn of 1991 saw the Parcels sector recast as Rail Express Systems, this bringing a much-more business-orientated approach, a debatable new look and investment in the locomotive fleet, particularly the Class 47s. Simon Bendall looks at the modifications that were conducted while James Makin details a number of 4mm Bachmann models.

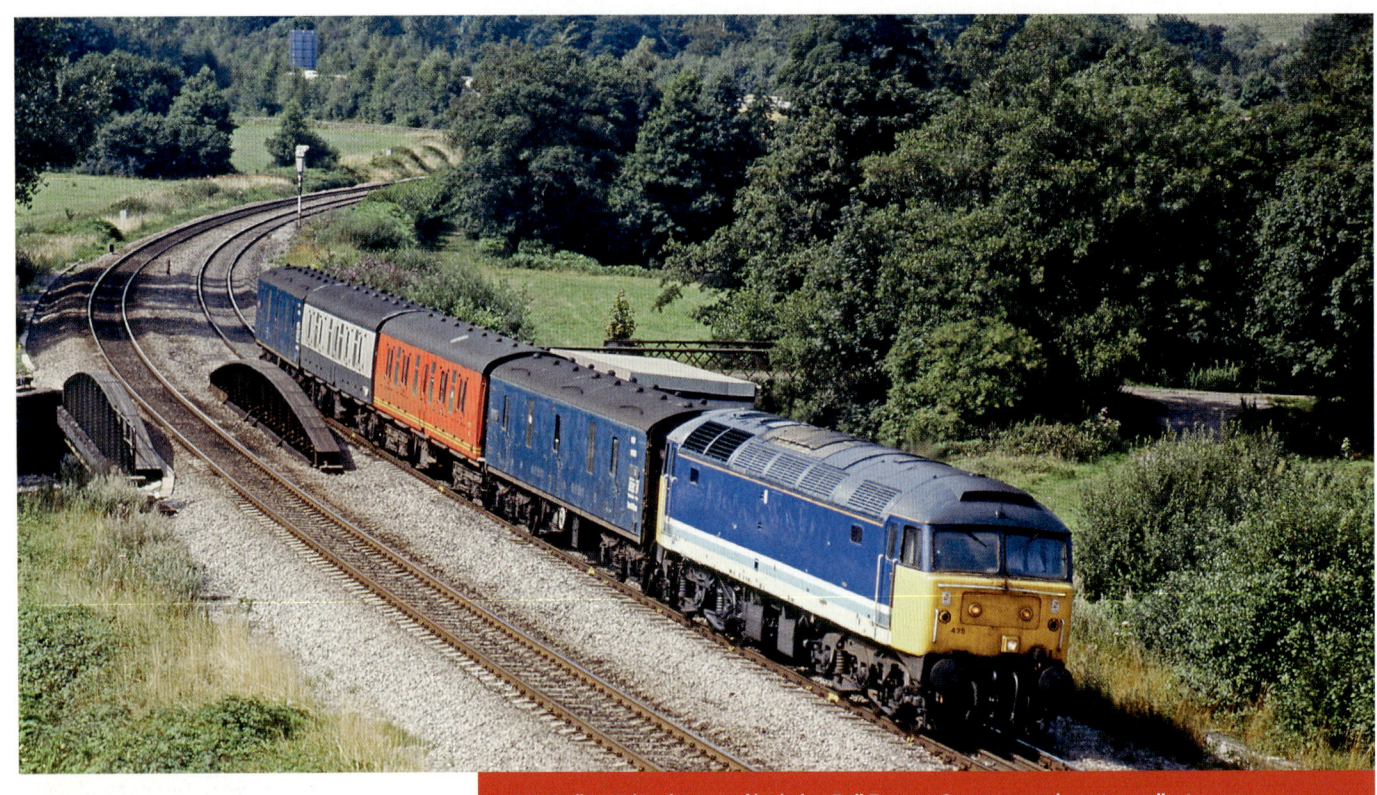

ABOVE: Illustrating the sort of look that Rail Express Systems was keen to eradicate as soon as possible, 47475 crosses the Ely River at Clawdd Coch with the 1A70 Swansea to Swindon Cocklebury postal vans on July 28, 1992. This was the only main line loco to carry Provincial livery, being painted in January 1989 for use on TransPennine services. Within a month of this image, the loco would be in RES colours. The vans encompass two Mk.1 GUVs in original condition flanking two Mk.1 BGs, the Parcels-liveried example riding on B4 bogies and the BR blue/grey on Commonwealth. Brian Robbins/Rail Photoprints

October 1991 saw the launch of another livery that proved to be controversial for British Rail, the Rail Express Systems (RES) red, grey and blue scheme joining Departmental grey in provoking some strong reactions.

Up to this point, the Parcels sector had been the only operating department without its own corporate identity. While the Parcels red/grey livery introduced in 1990 had provided a smart if bland improvement, there was still no 'brand' to use in marketing. Locos and rolling stock still carried an array of liveries, a point made worse by an influx of Class 47s formerly with Network SouthEast and the Railfreight sub-sectors in 1991, with the result that trains could frequently contain stock in a half dozen liveries. This was great for photographers but not for selling an image to customers.

The Roundel Design Group, creator of the Railfreight sub-sector liveries in 1987, was charged with rebranding the Parcels operation, both in name and livery. The name Rail Express Systems was chosen to reflect Rail - the national and international rail network; Express - 100mph trains travelling through the night and Systems - an integrated organisation serving the needs of customers.

The new livery was developed from the existing Parcels red/grey scheme,

BELOW: Illustrating the predecessor to RES, 47582 *County of Norfolk* is seen at Old Oak Common on a late summer's day in September 1991, it had become the penultimate Class 47 to receive Parcels red/grey two months earlier. The work at Doncaster had also included some of the life extension modifications, most obviously removing the bufferbeam cowls, but long range fuel tanks would not be fitted until 1995 when it was overhauled at Crewe, becoming 47733 and receiving RES colours. Simon Bendall Collection

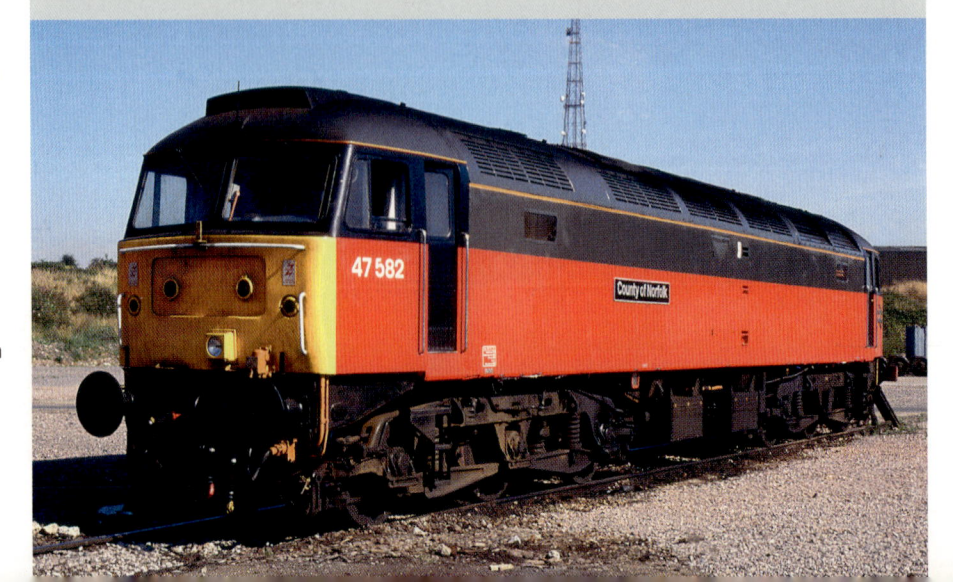

New looks for the decade

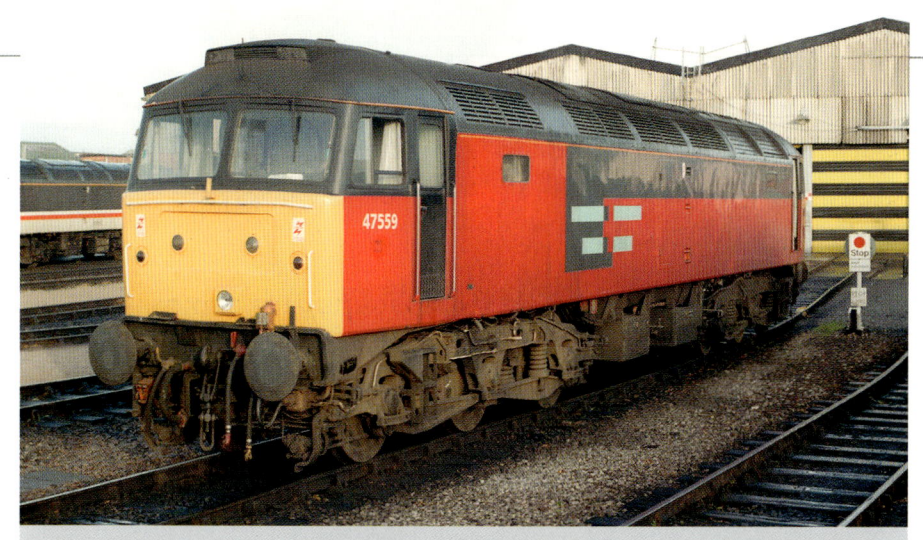

ABOVE: Illustrating a typical Class 47/4 in RES, 47559 stands at Crewe Diesel in the autumn of 1992, having been painted at Glasgow Works that March. The loco has seen the roof vent partially plated up but the bufferbeam cowls remain in place, although they would be removed the following year and the extra fuel tank fitted, both in advance of becoming 47759. *Simon Bendall Collection*

the predominately red base having to be retained to remain compatible with the Royal Mail Travelling Post Offices. Changes made included the replacement of the Executive dark grey with a grey-blue shade known as Express parcels grey, while the long-standing Rail Alphabet gave way to a new font, Frutiger, for numbering and lettering. Cast BR arrows and depot plaques, the latter to a new design, were also included in the specification but were not always applied in practice. It was, however, the blue and grey bodyside graphic that caused the most debate, opinion being divided on whether it worked or not.

An early unveiling

After trials on a Mk.1 GUV, the first loco to be painted was 47594 in July 1991, some three months prior to the official launch, at the unusual location of the Midland Railway Centre. The reason for the early re-livery was so that the Class 47 and a rake of repainted mail vans could take part in a photoshoot at St Pancras that month. The intention was that, following this, the loco would be hidden away at Old Oak Common for over two months to await the formal October launch. However, this was rather undermined as 47594 was seconded on several occasions in August to work, amongst others, Paddington to Birmingham InterCity services.

The RES launch finally arrived on October 11, 1991, with an event at Crewe Diesel depot. Joining 47594 were sister locos 47597 and 47625 along with 90020 and shunter 08633. All five were named during the launch, the trio of Class 47s becoming the first locos to receive the 'Res' themed nameplates, which would come to adorn further classmates as the months progressed.

By this time, RES had opted to concentrate solely on Class 47s for its main line diesel traction, the tired Class 31/4s having been let go back in the spring. The Type 4s were supplemented by small fleets of Class 86 and Class 90 electrics but the Brush machines saw the bulk of the attention and investment. Such was the company's insatiable demand for motive power at this time that several long-stored Class 47/4s were snapped up and resurrected to traffic, while surplus Type 4s from InterCity would also be taken on.

A key goal of the rebrand was that the new colours would be rolled out quickly across both locos and rolling stock. As a result, several depots worked alongside the main workshops to conduct re-liveries at a rapid pace from the start of 1992, with the most inappropriate colours, such as the aforementioned triple grey and NSE, being targeted for early removal. In all, the Class 47/4s painted were 47475/90-92, 47500/03/17/21/24/30-32/35-37/39/41/51/57-59/62/64-68/73/76/78/80/81/83/84/87/88/94/96-99 and 47600/03/05/06/12/15/18/24-28/30/31/36/42/53 along with ex ScotRail push-pull machines 47701/04/05/07/09/14/16.

Core fleet

The end of 1993 had seen RES embark on a renumbering programme for the Class 47s it regarded as long-term machines, a new number series starting from 47721 onwards, and eventually ending at 47793, being decided upon to reflect the implementation of the life-extension modifications such as extended range fuel tanks and cut-back bufferbeam cowlings. It would also come to identify the locos fitted with cab front RCH jumper cables for working with the new Propelling Control Vehicles (PCV) on the recast Railnet mail services, but this was a later alteration and did not drive the application of the new numbers.

However, while the renumbering scheme was still in progress, privatisation overtook events with RES being sold to Wisconsin Central in December 1995 and absorbed into EWS the next year. With the Americans having no love for the venerable Type 4s, the renumbering programme was abandoned before 47565/66/72/74-76/84/96 and 47624/27/28/34/35/40 could become 47723/24/28-31/35/40/48/51-55, respectively.

This also meant that 47572/74/75 and 47634/35/40 were denied the accompanying repaint into RES colours, all remaining in Parcels red/grey as the 'blue flash' livery was duly abandoned from the spring of 1996. However, with so many freshly overhauled locos in RES colours, it was inevitable that the livery would last well into EWS days with many of the Class 47s withdrawn without another repaint.

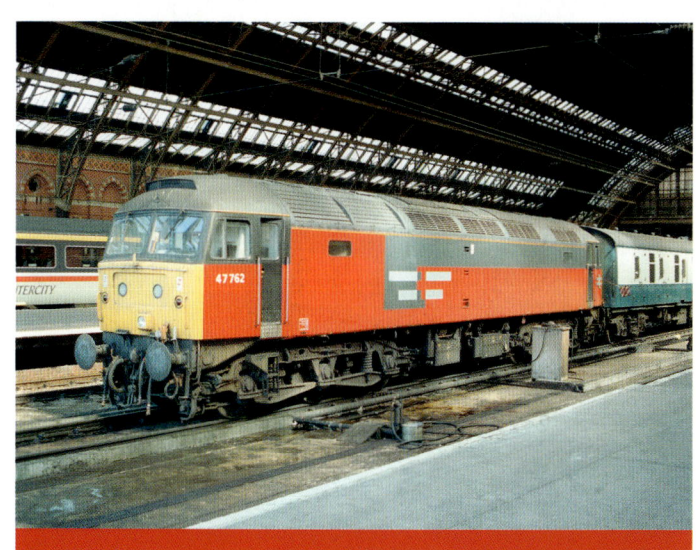

ABOVE: The former 47573 stands under the Barlow train shed at St Pancras during 1994, it had been renumbered as 47762 at the start of the year. The loco has the full set of life extension modifications but has yet to receive the control cables on the cab fronts, which would not appear until the following year. *Simon Bendall Collection*

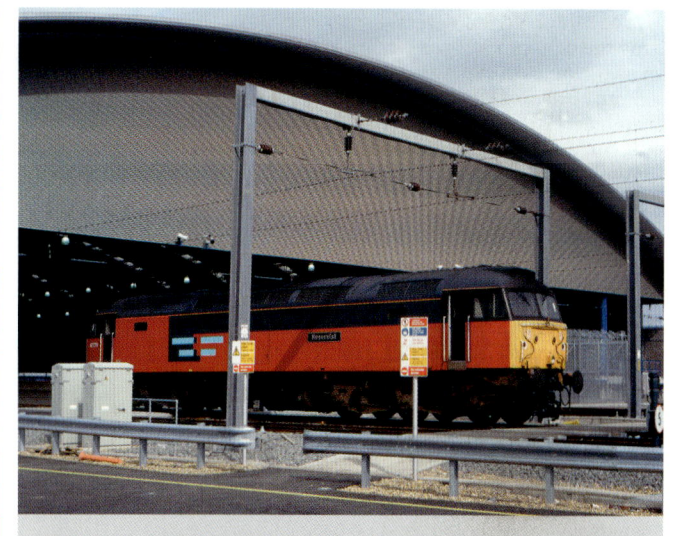

ABOVE: The RES Class 47s in their final form is exemplified by 47773 *Reservist* stabled outside the Royal Mail's Princess Royal Distribution Centre at Willesden in 1997. Now under EWS ownership, the loco has the RCH jumpers in place along with new LED tail lights, these being easily identified thanks to the white surrounds. *Simon Bendall Collection*

Modelling BR Locomotives of the 1990s 37

New looks for the decade

A resplendent fleet

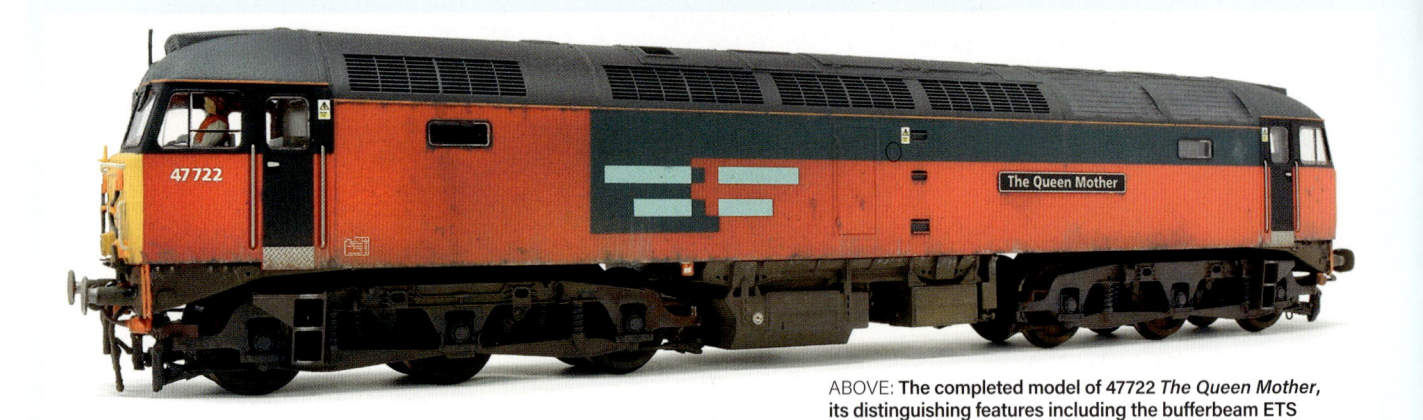

ABOVE: The completed model of 47722 *The Queen Mother*, its distinguishing features including the bufferbeam ETS alterations along with the 'rectangular oval' buffers.

By the late 1990s, the fleet of refurbished Class 47s that once belonged to Rail Express Systems was now under the ownership of EWS, but the locos were still going about their daily routine of hauling mail trains across the country alongside their AC electric counterparts.

Modelling Didcot in Oxfordshire around 1998-2001, I was seeking to create a small batch of Class 47s that were representative of the fleet during this period. These could not only be seen passing through at the head of the many Railnet services but also in frontline passenger service with Virgin CrossCountry, having been hired from EWS to make up for a shortfall in loco availability.

Bachmann's RES Class 47 release of 2013 made for the natural starting point, the model of 47745 being readily available and also substantially discounted at the time, enabling a reasonable fleet to be assembled, especially if buying at the right time. The model already featured most of the right details, including the long range fuel tanks, cut back bufferbeams and RCH jumper cables, while the livery was well applied.

There is still plenty of scope though to take the model from a standard factory release and transform it into something unique while also representing these hard-working machines in the twilight of their careers. The first job was to select the identities of each machine as this affects the minor detail differences that can be seen between them.

A red quartet
First up was 47722 *The Queen Mother* which was renumbered from 47558 in 1995 and inherited the name from 47541, with new plates cast in the RES house style. The loco had standard headcode recesses at each end but with variations to the Bachmann model around the bufferbeam area. This was next joined by 47736 *Cambridge Traction & Rolling Stock Depot*, which was notable in having received a black-painted former headcode panel along with numbers on each end, which was unusual for a Class 47/7.

The third choice was 47787 *Victim Support* which, as 47163, was once part of the famous duo of Stratford Class 47s to wear Union flags to mark The Queen's Silver Jubilee. The loco was involved in a serious accident at Kensal Green in 1977, which led to its rebuilding with flush-fronted cabs at both ends. Finally, there was 47788 *Captain Peter Manisty RN* which had been transferred across from InterCity in 1994 under former identity 47833. It had previously been painted in a dubious representation of BR two-tone green and had a flush front at one end. All four locomotives would outwardly appear very similar but the minor detail differences all make for an interesting fleet.

The Bachmann donor models were dismantled with the glazing left in the bodyshells but masked with Humbrol Maskol and a start made to remove their former identities. The Bachmann printed numbers and names were taken off with a cotton bud dipped in Humbrol enamel thinners. Working away smoothly with a gentle motion, the printing lifts after a few minutes, leaving a glossy red surface underneath.

Body alterations
For the two locos that required flush-fronted ends, the handrails were first removed along with the light lenses. The necessary headcode panel recesses were then filled with Humbrol model filler, cocktail sticks first being placed through the marker light holes. Once dried, the cocktail sticks were removed, having helped to preserve the original positions, and making it easier to ensure that the Bachmann lights would still line up once the model was reassembled.

The model filler was then sanded smooth with some repeat application where required to get a completely smooth finish. After this, Shawplan's headcode panel marker light etches were added on each model, taking care to note the prototype arrangement of whether a sealed beam marker lens or marker light arrangement was required, and the wire handrails reaffixed. Each model

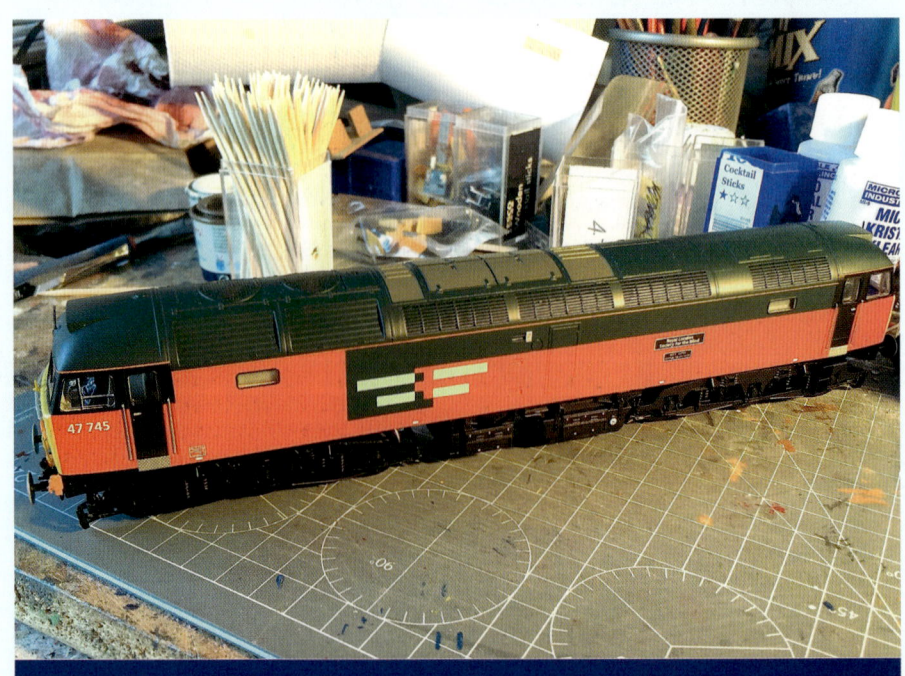

ABOVE: The donor model used for all of the RES Class 47s was Bachmann's 47745 *Royal London Society for the Blind*, which not only gives the appropriate livery but also the correct set of details.

New looks for the decade

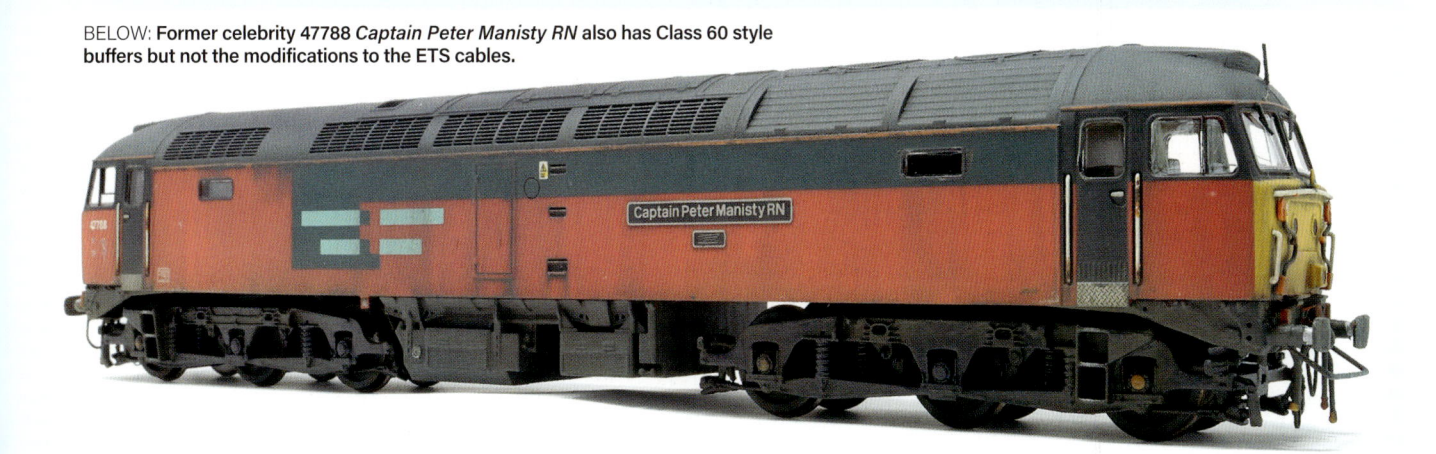

BELOW: **Former celebrity 47788** *Captain Peter Manisty RN* **also has Class 60 style buffers but not the modifications to the ETS cables.**

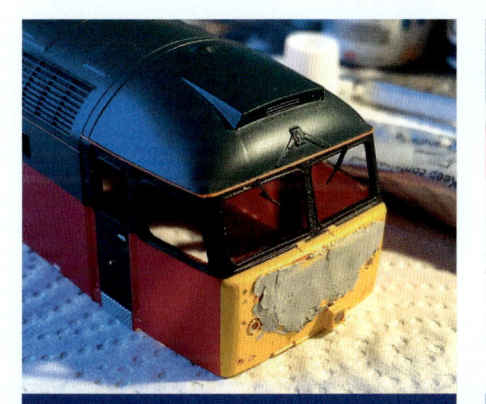

ABOVE: **Work is underway to fill the headcode panel to create a flush-front; the marker light apertures being opened out before the filler dried, which was then later sanded smooth.**

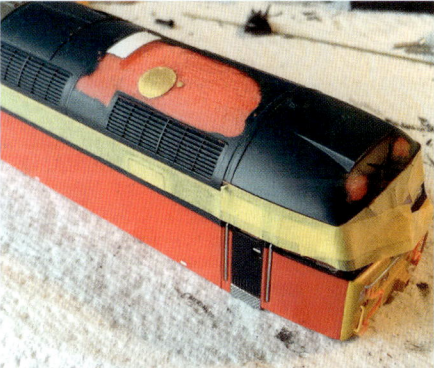

ABOVE: **The mould lines have been filed off the cab roofs and around the cantrail grilles while a blanking plate for the Spanner-type of boiler exhaust has been added from the Shawplan range. The white plasticard rectangle represents the electrical access panel found on certain class members.**

ABOVE: **With the end smoothed up, etched marker lights from Shawplan have been added and the handrails put back in place.**

was masked to allow the new flush ends to be painted, starting with a white undercoat before adding Phoenix Precision's post-1985 warning panel yellow.

While generally well moulded, Bachmann's original Class 47 was let down by prominent vertical mould lines on the cab roofs as well as horizontal lines around the boiler end of the roof, both of which can be gently sanded down to remove them. Next, the different types of plated-over boiler port were represented. The Bachmann model is supplied with the plated rectangular version, however across the chosen prototypes there were a variety of designs to be found. Shawplan's etched brass replacements were used, supplemented by pieces of plasticard where needed to represent the full range of details across the four class members.

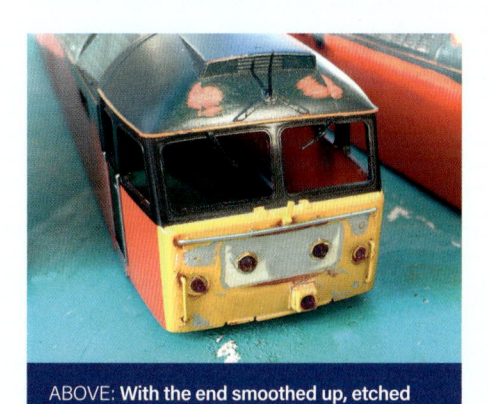

Similarly, the roof fan grilles can be replaced with the Shawplan etched versions, which leaves the roof ready for a coat of dark grey paint. The shade of this need not be that specific as this will change during the weathering phase.

New identities
The bodyshells were given a coat of Railmatch gloss varnish. Supplied in aerosol form, a quick spray gave a glossy finish onto which the transfers were added. Fox Transfers and Railtec both supply useful decals for the livery elements, while etched nameplates can be purchased from the Shawplan and Fox ranges, which between them cover nearly all of the RES Class 47/7s that ever received a name.

The etched nameplates were secured with Railmatch matt varnish, sparingly applied using a cocktail stick. The reason for using varnish as an adhesive is that it gives plenty of time to adjust the plate to ensure it is straight and level. One added benefit of the gloss finish is that any painting touch-ups required at this stage can be made with fine brushes; any slippages can easily be wiped away without affecting the base colours.

Small extra bodyshell details were added at this stage, such as painting the handrails the correct shades, whether that be polished steel, white or yellow. The tail lights on RES locos also received a LED upgrade with a white-painted surround, so this is replicated on the models with a small ring of white added using a fine 5/0 brush.

The bodyshells were then coated with Railmatch matt varnish, again using an aerosol to save valuable time, after which they were left for approximately a month to allow the varnish to fully harden ready for the weathering stages.

Weathering
The weathering was matched to photographs of each loco around the turn of the century. In general, the overall look could be described as in good condition but yet tired in places, evidence that these machines were worked hard by EWS on Royal Mail services right up until the introduction of the new Class 67s.

Much use was made of washes to kickstart the weathering process by watering down neat Humbrol paint with enamel thinners to a consistency of milk, applying the paint to the locomotive body and then wiping it off in a downward vertical motion. To start with, a wash of dark brown (Humbrol No.186) was painted on and wiped off with kitchen towel. The matt varnish layer applied previously acts as a 'key' for the weathering wash to cling to, which can be useful to tint the overall colour of the livery in some cases. In this case, a cleaner appearance was desired, so a cotton bud dipped in neat enamel thinners was rubbed vertically up and down the bodysides to remove much of the grime.

Certain areas can be left dirty to replicate the streaks of dirt brought down from the roof via rainwater capillary action. The process was then repeated again with other colour shades to build up a realistic

Modelling BR Locomotives of the 1990s 39

New looks for the decade

BELOW: All of the RES Class 47/7s had long range fuel tanks fitted, these being installed around one end of the underframe and enveloped two of the battery boxes as shown by 47787 *Victim Support*.

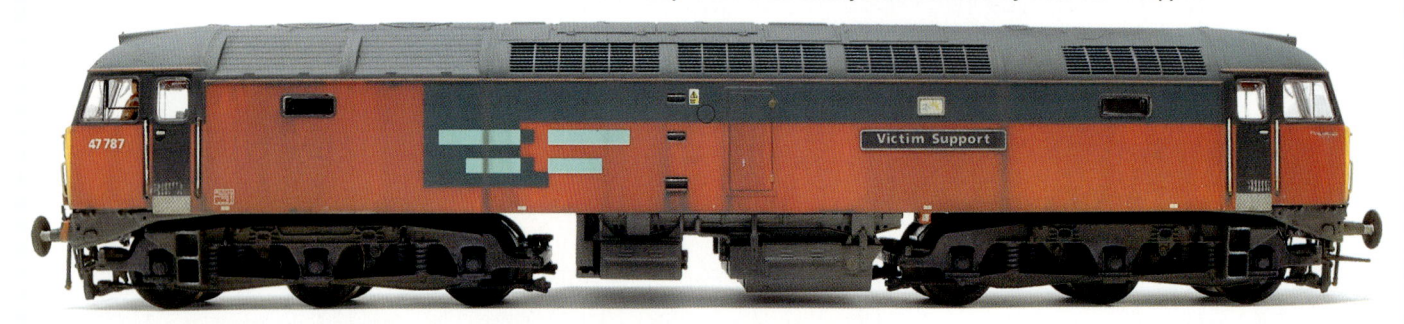

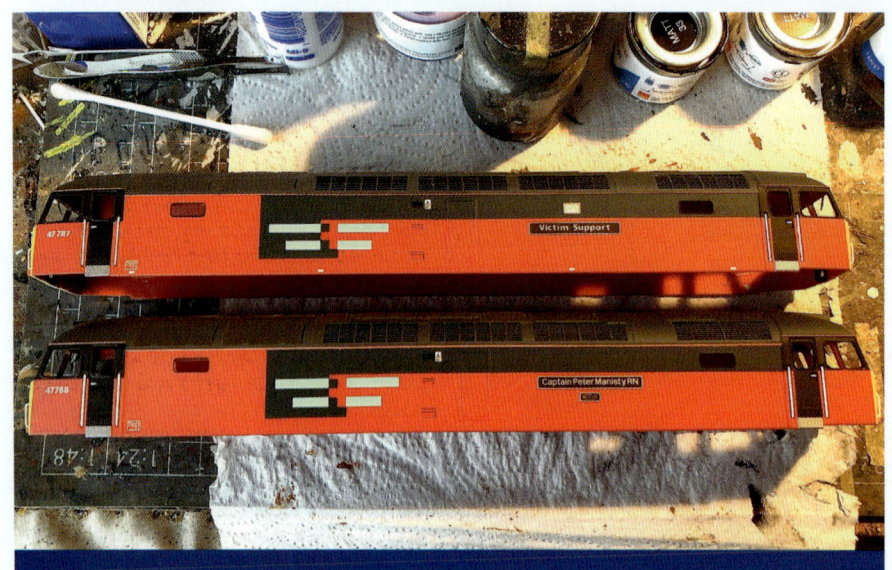

ABOVE: Two of the bodyshells have received their new numbers and etched nameplates as well as detail painting, such as the cab door handrails, and now await varnishing.

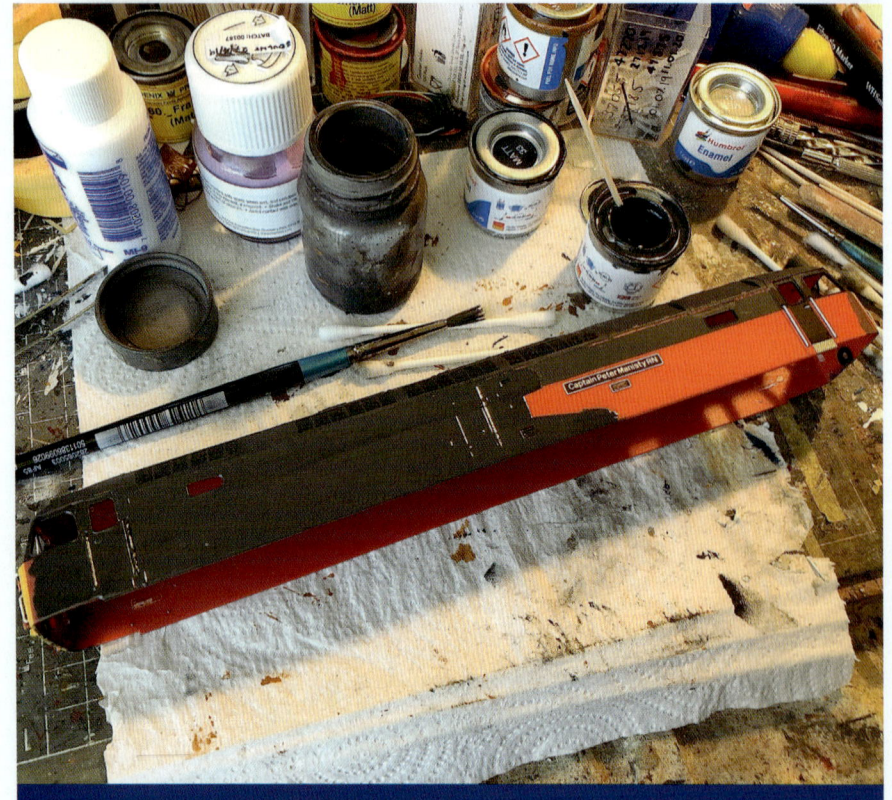

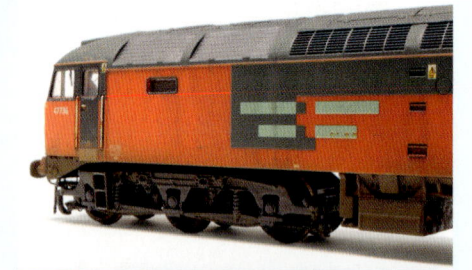

ABOVE: With the bulk of the dirt applied, adding flecks of chipped paint and rust is the next job, this really bringing the models to life. The rust showing through the blush flash is particularly effective.

ABOVE: The first stage of weathering sees a thinned coat of Humbrol dark brown applied. Although looking extreme, much of this would then be wiped off, remembering to work vertically at all times.

finish, including shades of darker browns (Humbrol Nos.133 and 251) and dark grey (Humbrol No.32).

After the washes were applied and removed, the next stage was to add any individual marks, damage, scrapes, and rust patches as applicable. Through careful observation of photographs on Flickr, Google Images or Smugmug for example, you can build up a picture of what is needed on your chosen loco in a specific year. A number of surface rust patches were prevalent on the locos, and these were created by using fine 5/0 brushes to carefully touch in shades of brown, working from light to dark, with the darkest rust at the epicentre of the outbreak. Humbrol shades of Nos.62, 186, 113, 133 and 251 are used in tandem to build up a rust patch.

Meanwhile, there are other patches and damage, or parts of undercoat exposed; these are colour matched to the prototype images and applied with small brushes. When looking for a good weathering brush, go for a 5/0 or a 10/0 and take care when choosing a brush to go for one that ends in a precise pinpoint as this helps in applications like this where precision is key.

Underframe detailing

Alongside the body detailing, it is important to consider any changes that need making to the underframe. Generally, if using Bachmann's 47745 release, any changes will be relatively minor but there is the option to further open out the battery box and fuel tank moulding.

Careful study of photos showed that some Class 47/7s, such as 47722 modelled here, had repositioned ETS cables and additional orange electrical pipe runs going up to the cab. In this case, the Bachmann mouldings

New looks for the decade

BELOW: The black headcode panel of 47736 *Cambridge Traction & Rolling Stock Depot* made it stand out a little more. The driver figure repainted in modern attire is also noticeable as are the rust patches represented on the cab roof.

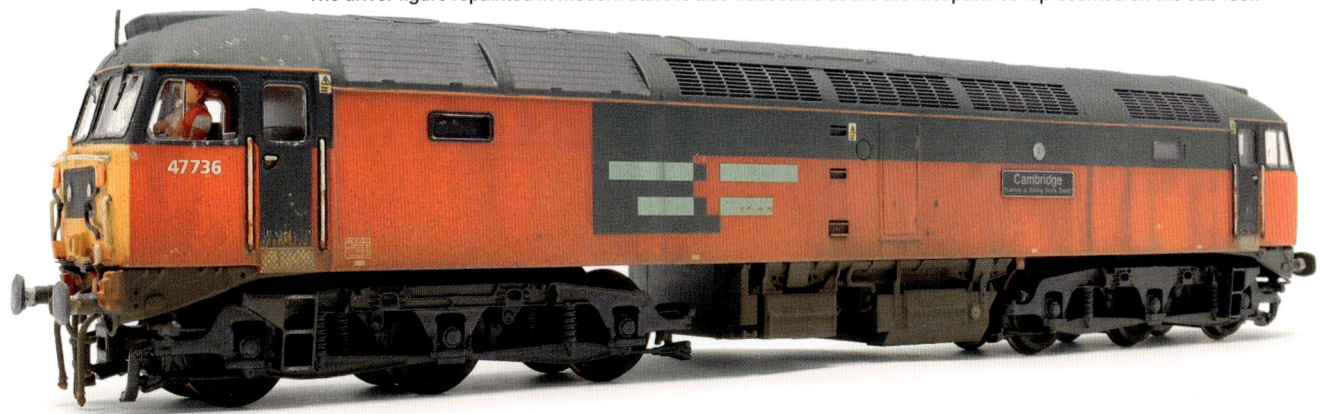

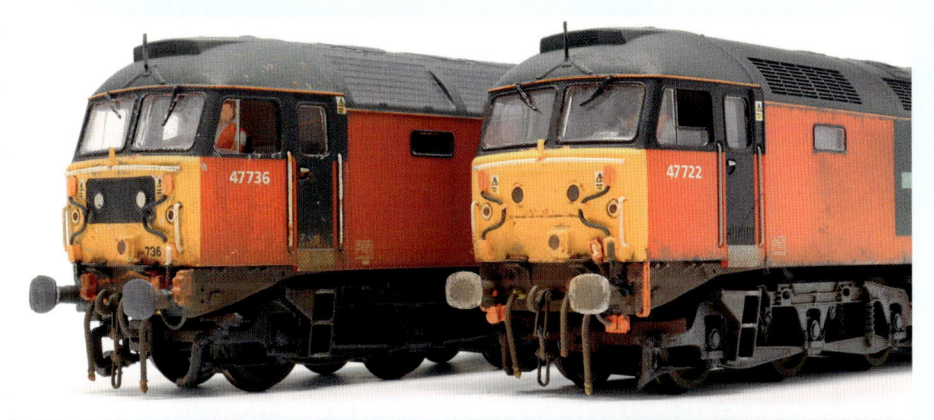

ABOVE: The two styles of ETS bufferbeam fittings are displayed here with 47736 having the as-built style and 47722 the revised layout with additional conduit as found on some locos with cut-back bufferbeams.

were removed and replaced with parts from the spares box while thin brass wire was added on the sides of the bufferbeams and painted orange.

The bufferbeam pipework itself was that supplied by Bachmann with some additional elements scratchbuilt from 0.45mm brass wire and superglued into the bufferbeams. The style of buffers also varied between locos with some receiving the Class 60 'rectangular-oval' type in place of the round Oleos supplied on the model. Once the detailing was completed, the chassis were all given a coating in dark grey (Humbrol No.32) as a basis upon which to add the weathering.

At this point, the moulded cab interiors were dealt with, the floor being painted black to hide the reduced depth. The driver figure also had the moulded BR flat cap removed and was repainted into more modern clothing with a high-visibility jacket as applicable.

A final dusting

With the main weathering completed on the bodyshells and the chassis painted and ready to go, the bodies were reunited with the chassis and any masking tape removed, including Humbrol Maskol from the window glazing. The final stage is to apply an overall airbrush coating of grime to bring together the final look as well as acting to tone down some of the weathering colours used in the previous stages.

Starting with the lower chassis, Phoenix Precision 'brake dust' and 'track dirt' were airbrushed on, taking care not to go over the top and risk ruining the models at such a late stage. Moving upwards, 'roof dirt' and 'dirty black' were sprayed downwards across the roof. Finally, a custom mix of dark grey and blue was mixed and sprayed exclusively around the exhaust port on each loco to give a rich oily sheen to the exhaust deposits seen in this area.

Later, the chassis and cantrail grilles received a dry-brushing with Humbrol Metalcote 'gun metal' (No.27004) to highlight the raised edges while little details such as the buffer shanks were picked out in silver, along with the cab footsteps to highlight wear and tear over time.

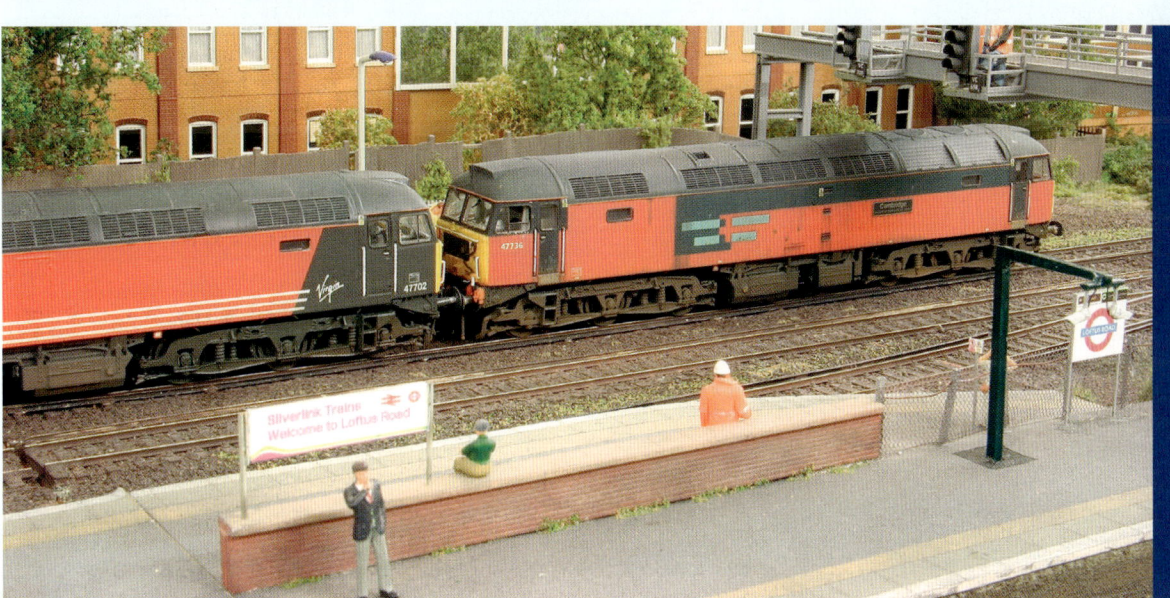

LEFT: RES-liveried Class 47s were common on Virgin CrossCountry services assisting their hard-pressed classmates. Seen on Worthing MRC's Loftus Road layout, 47736 has come to the aid of 47702 on a Brighton-bound working.

Modelling BR Locomotives of the 1990s 41

New looks for the decade

RIGHT: Repainted a month earlier, 47524 passes Aller on April 28, 1994, in charge of the 13.55 Plymouth to Crewe. Even at this date, mail trains could still be seen without RES-liveried vans in them, the formation consisting of seven Mk.1 BGs and a solitary Mk.1 GUV as the penultimate vehicle. By now, virtually all such vans were riding on Commonwealth or B4 bogies, this being another policy of RES to increase operational speeds to 100mph. RTR models of both types are available in the Graham Farish, Bachmann and Heljan ranges in 2mm, 4mm and 7mm, respectively.

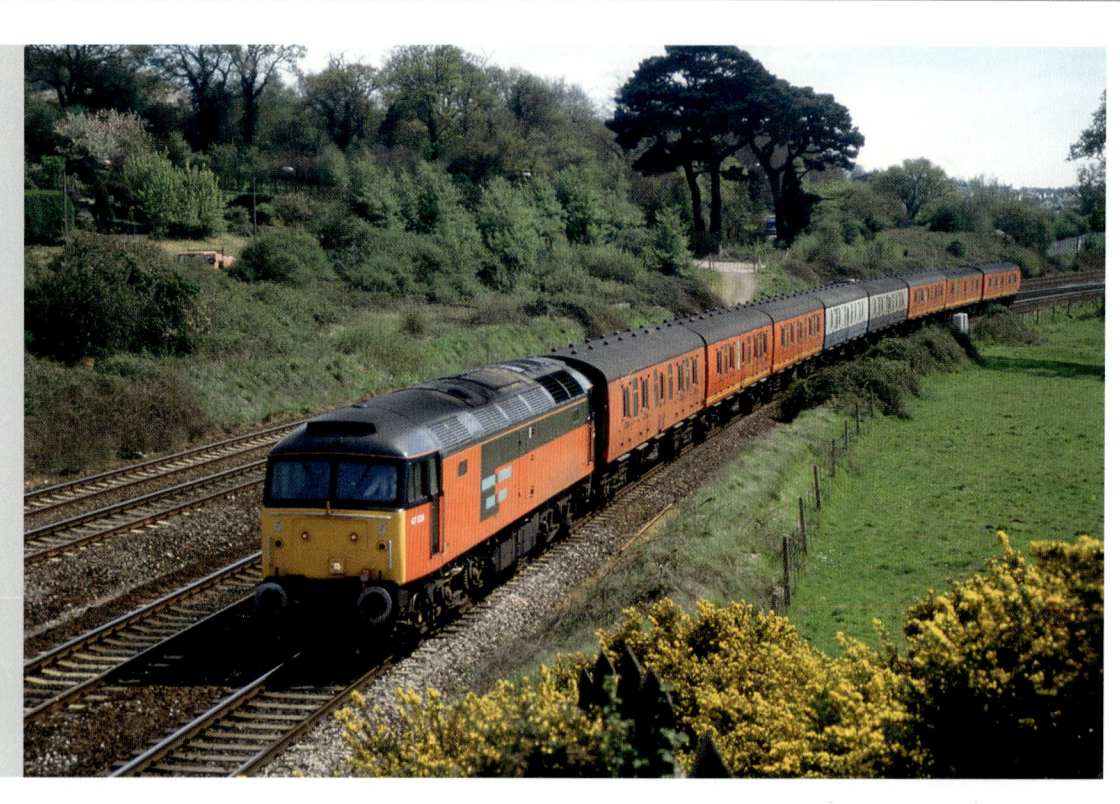

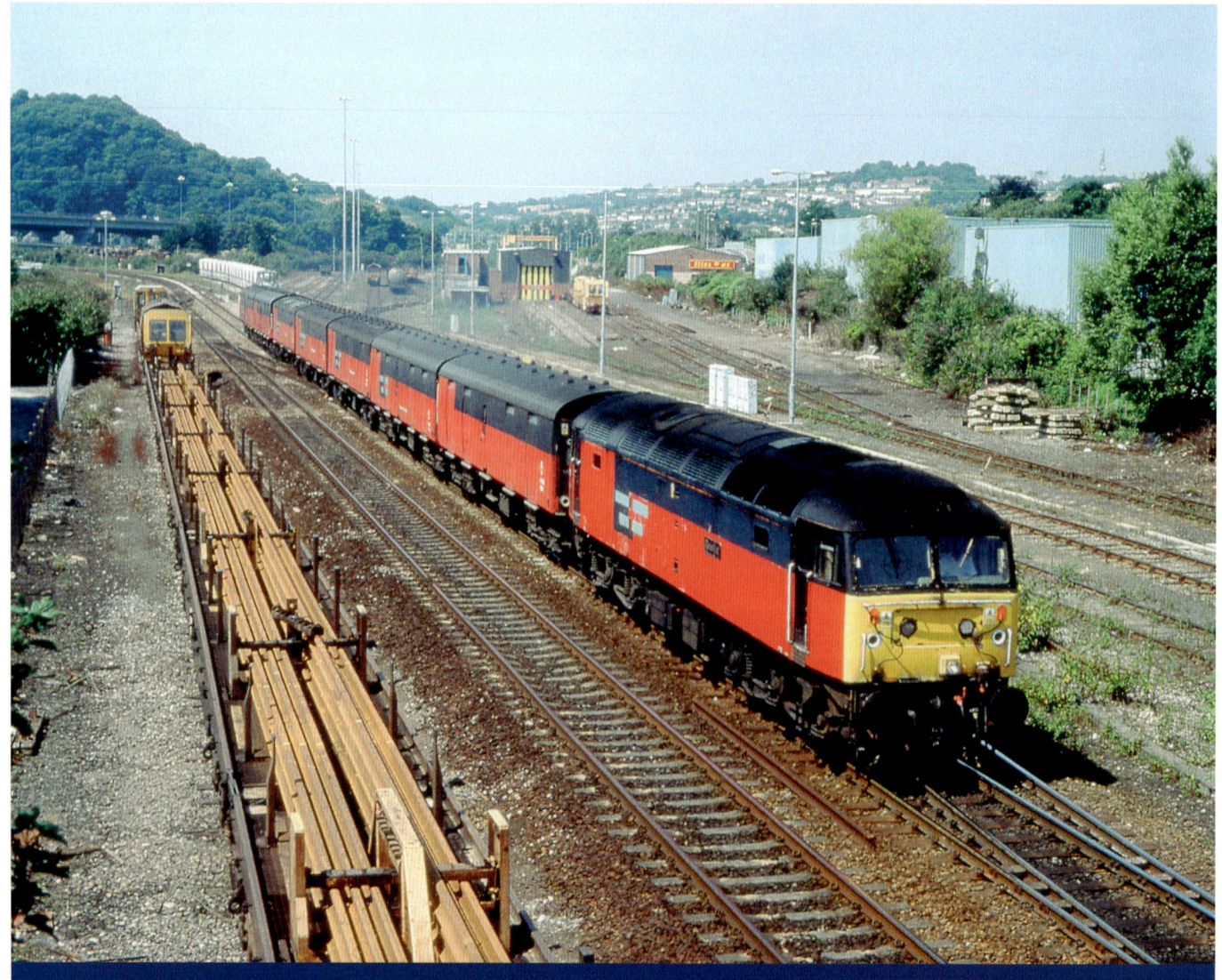

ABOVE: A tatty 47769 *Resolve* accelerates past Tavistock Junction a short way into its journey with the 1S81 12.44 Plymouth to Shieldmuir in June 1999. On the left is a stabled long-welded rail train while the local track machine depot is in the background. The set of roller-door vans features four Super BGs, a pair at each end sandwiching three Super GUVs. Both types are available in OO gauge from Bachmann and Hornby (ex-Lima) respectively but only the Super BG can be found RTR in N gauge in the Farish range.

New looks for the decade

RIGHT: Of the former ScotRail push-pull locos, 47704 was the only one not to spend any great amount of time on hire to Network SouthEast, it failed soon after arriving with the other Parcels examples for West of England duties in July 1991 and was returned to Crewe. It was in better health on February 27, 1993, when hired in to work the Saturdays-only 1O86 09.23 Plymouth-Waterloo as it thrashes up Hemerdon Bank. As the loco-hauled services wound down, NSE had surrendered some of its Mk.2a coaches to Regional Railways, replacing them with a motely assortment of surplus stock in return, including the two blue/grey TSOs in this set. The formation is also only eight coaches with the Mk.2c TSOT missing.

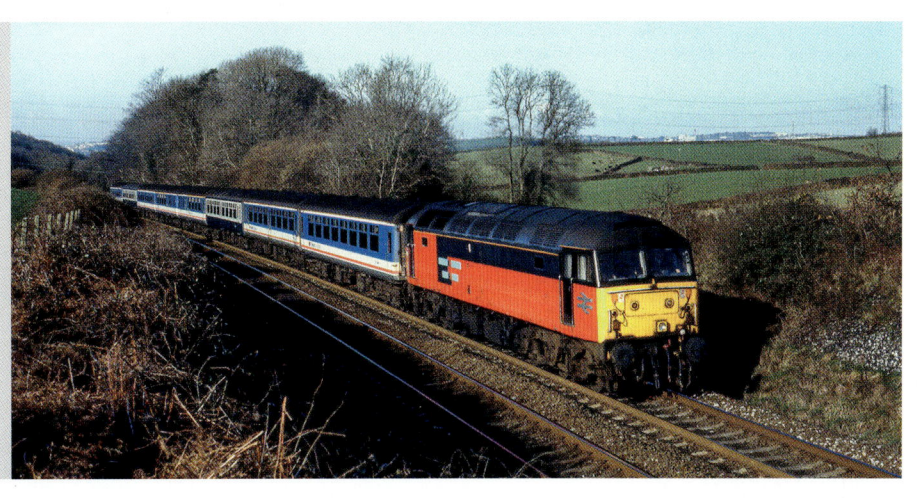

RIGHT: Now an EWS machine, 47739 *Resourceful* is captured at Exeter Riverside on August 8, 1996, having brought the high speed track recording train west from Reading. Class 47s would be regular motive power for such workings in the latter half of the decade as Serco took over their operation. The formation features support coaches DB977338 and DB977337, recording coach DB999550 and push-pull driving trailer DB977335, the latter carrying the short-lived red and grey Technical Services colours.

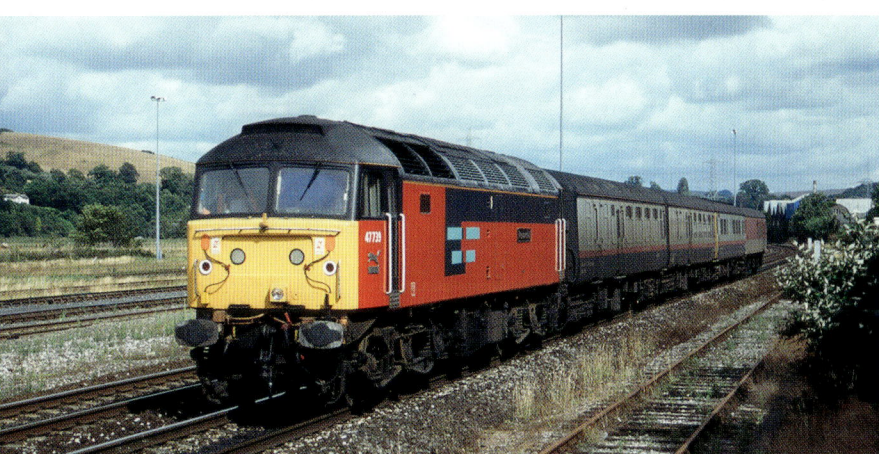

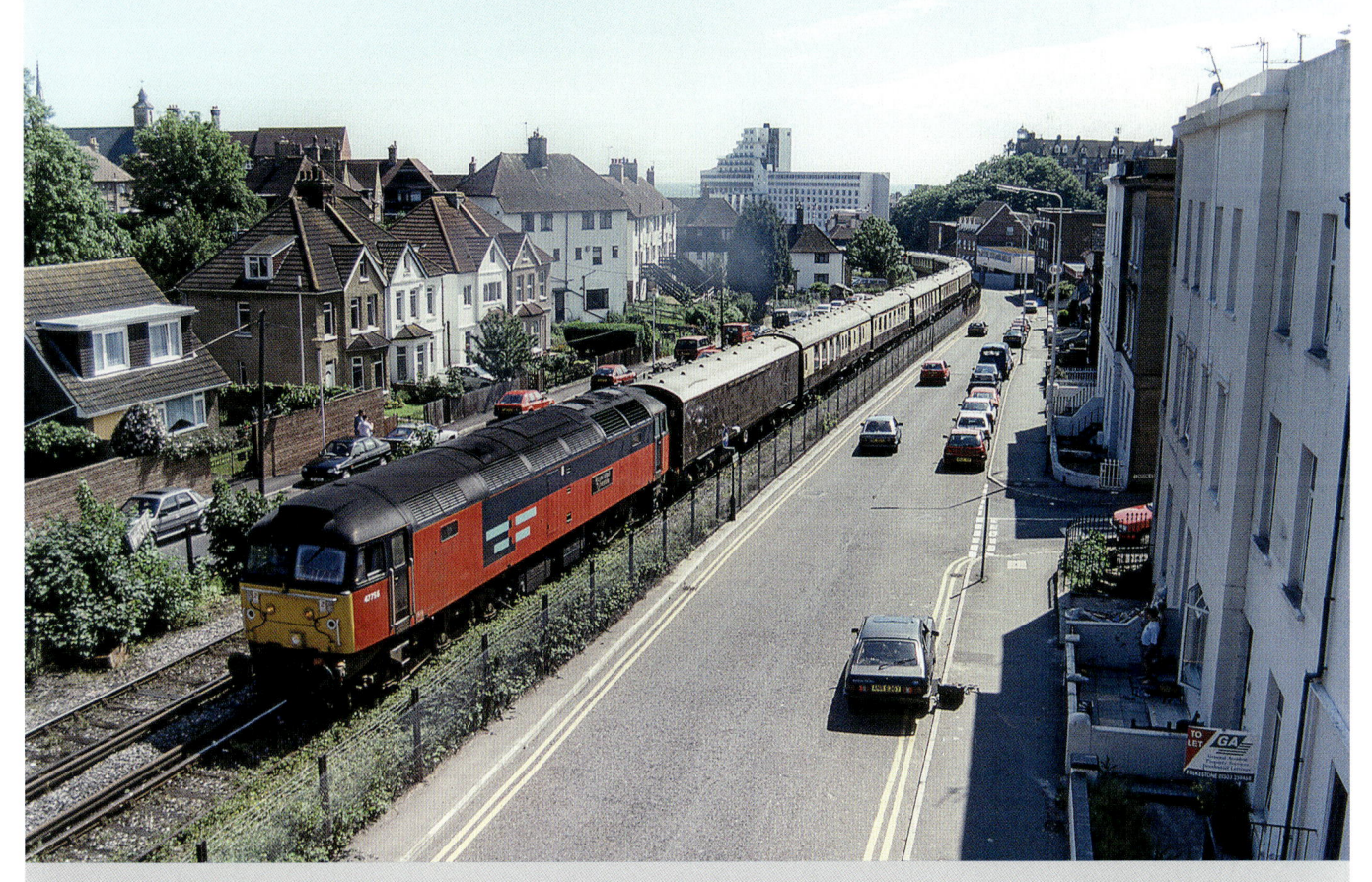

ABOVE: Charter trains were an important part of the duties for the RES Class 47s, both under BR and EWS ownership. On June 7, 1996, 47756 *Royal Mail Tyneside* is working hard as it brings the Pullman stock of the Venice Simplon Orient Express up the steeply-graded Folkestone Harbour branch. As well as working such prestigious stock, they were commonly found atop Mk.1s belonging to the likes of Rail Charter Services and others. The leading vehicle is baggage car 99542, a former ferry scenery van. All photos: Simon Bendall Collection

Modelling BR Locomotives of the 1990s

New looks for the decade

Electro-Diesels go 'Dutch'

The introduction of the additional yellow band on Civil Engineers locos from the summer of 1990 brought a welcome splash of additional colour to the network. **Simon Bendall** examines the introduction of 'Dutch' and its application to the Southern's Class 73s while **Mark Lambert** improves the livery application on the OO gauge Dapol model.

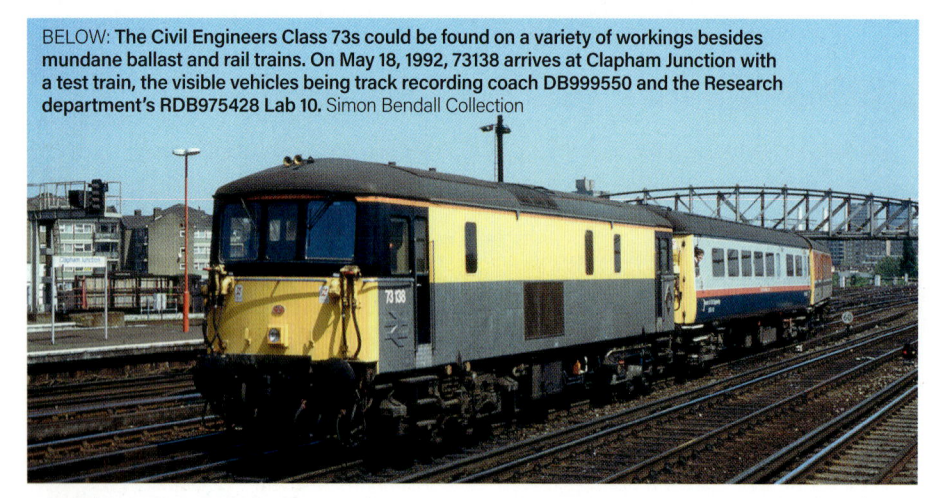

BELOW: The Civil Engineers Class 73s could be found on a variety of workings besides mundane ballast and rail trains. On May 18, 1992, 73138 arrives at Clapham Junction with a test train, the visible vehicles being track recording coach DB999550 and the Research department's RDB975428 Lab 10. *Simon Bendall Collection*

The Civil Engineers' grey and yellow livery, quickly dubbed 'Dutch' on account of its similarity to the corporate colours of the Netherlands Railways, came about principally because of the efforts of one man and the power of the railway press. Quite why the story of its adoption was so convoluted is open to speculation but the obvious move of painting a yellow band on the disliked BR Departmental grey livery even necessitated letters to the Chairman of the BR Board!

Until the mid-1980s, the only locomotives allocated to the Civil Engineering function were a handful of shunting locos. All this was to change as sectorisation spread its wings, with the Director of Civil Engineering (DCE) being made responsible from January 1988 for a fleet of 280 locomotives from eight classes. The resulting mixture of liveries meant there was no clear form of identity or ownership, and it was to resolve this that the plain grey livery was created.

Even before Departmental grey was launched, it was clear that the DCE was less than impressed. There were internal calls for some form of DCE branding to be applied to allow staff to recognise departmental locos without the need to refer to a list. After experiments with bolt-on plates, the simple solution was a yellow and black diagonal-striped sticker, which was to be applied to, typically, the secondman's cabsides of those locos not scheduled for repainting. This also displayed the initials of the loco's assigned region while the concept was additionally borrowed by other engineering departments. For example, red versions for the Research division appeared on 47971 and 47972 in BR large logo blue while multi-coloured 31413 gained a fetching light blue variant for the Mechanical and Electrical Engineers.

A tide of yellow

With numerous locomotives due for repainting in 1990, the DCE's rolling stock manager, Roger Price, took the initiative. The timing was spot on as both internal newspapers as well as national rail magazines could not quite comprehend the idea of painting locomotives in all-over dark grey. This less than complementary media coverage, combined with negative feedback from staff, resulted in the livery trials on two Class 31s detailed on page 26.

The final trial involving an upper yellow band on 31541 met with widespread approval almost immediately. The BR design department was eventually convinced of its merit and the official approval letter went out, copied to the BR Chairman, in early September; this coming after a number of locos had already seen the additional pigment applied!

On the Southern, many Class 33s were quick to receive 'Dutch' colours, aided by the fact that several were already in plain grey as Eastleigh Works was part way through an overhaul programme on the 'Cromptons'. It was a similar story with the region's other stalwarts, Selhurst gradually outshopping grey and yellow Class 73s after overhaul.

Of the dozen locos repainted in 'Dutch', 73133 was the first in September 1990 for its naming as *The Bluebell Railway*. Also completed towards the end of the year were the trio of 73105, 73131 and 73138 with 1991 bringing an additional six repaints on 73107/08/10/19/28/29. Thereafter, the application of grey and yellow largely ceased on the electro-diesels as the engineering departments were divided up amongst the passenger sectors, Network SouthEast largely preferring to use its own livery on the class. There were two more 'Dutch' re-liveries though, 73130 late in 1992 and 73118 in the spring of 1993.

As with other locos overhauled in the early 1990s, the good condition of the paintwork ensured 'Dutch' Class 73s were active throughout the short reign of Mainline Freight and then on into EWS ownership. The last two examples, by now heavily faded, were withdrawn in 2002, these being 73108 and 73110.

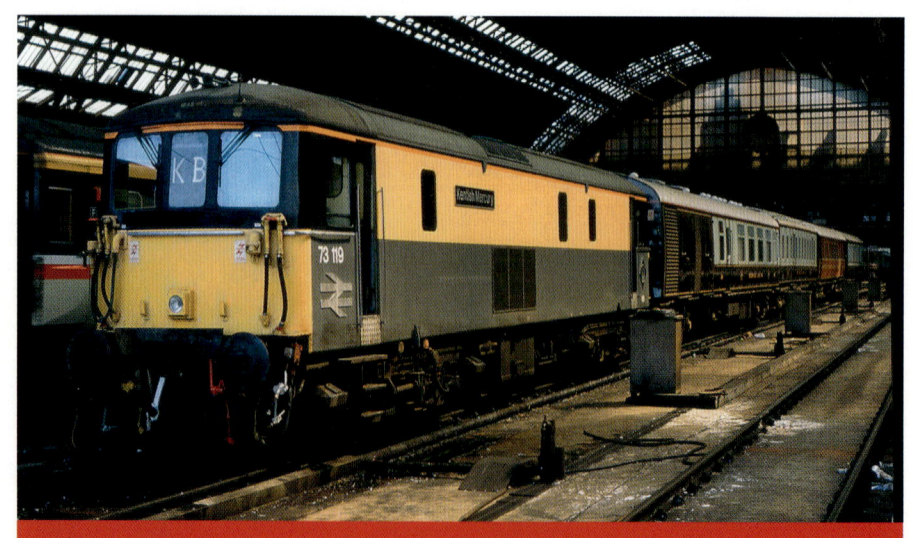

ABOVE: St Pancras was the unlikely location to find 73119 *Kentish Mercury* on August 20, 1995, as it stands in one of the centre roads with the 'Queen of Scots' luxury train. At the time, this set was based in the carriage shed at Clapham Junction and was engaged on a filming contract. The coaches are Mk.1 generator coach 99886 (ex BSK 35407), 1890-built LNWR Restaurant Kitchen 99880, Great Northern teak-bodied saloon 99881 dating from 1912 and 1892-vintage West Coast Joint Stock dining saloon 99052. The set was regularly employed in the 1980s and early 1990s but today is owned by West Coast Railways with only 99052 making the very occasional foray onto the network. *Simon Bendall Collection*

New looks for the decade

A colour-corrected 'ED'

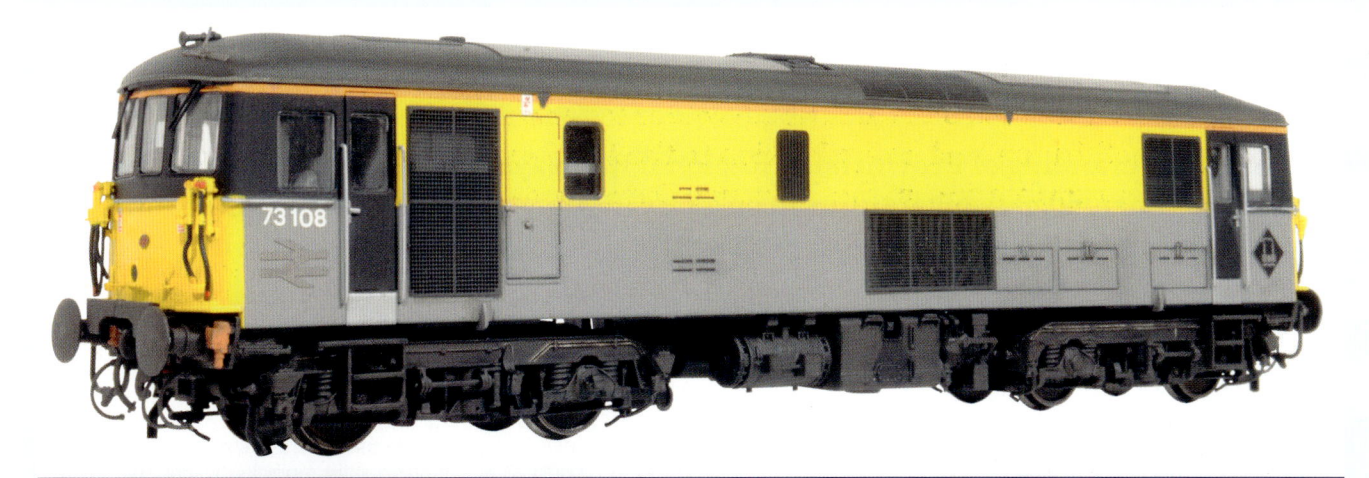

ABOVE: Correcting the colours makes all the difference to the appearance of the Dapol Class 73, giving a finish that matches the quality of the tooling.

Dapol's OO gauge Class 73 is a generally accurate and detailed model with good haulage capability, but it has been spoiled by some bizarre colour choices on many of the releases. I have repainted a couple of 'Dutch'-liveried models and this one is my favourite. Every colour on the model is wrong except for the white used for the numbers and the orange for the cantrail stripe. The yellow is too much of a lemon shade, the body grey too dark and the roof grey is too light. My solution with this model was to accept the yellow and go for a faded look to the other colours to tie in with it.

The key part to this repaint is masking. Having removed the body from the chassis, I masked the yellow stripe (including the orange cantrail), the cab fronts and the black parts including the doors but excluding the grilles. This left me with an exposed roof and lower bodysides. I used Flint grey for the lower bodysides and the glass fibre roof panels as this is a bit lighter than Departmental/Railfreight grey and produces a slightly faded look to the loco.

Once the paint had dried, I masked the lower bodysides and the roof panels and sprayed the remainder of the roof with Executive dark grey. This is the colour it would have been when first repainted but the use of a matt varnish at the end of the process makes it seem a shade or two lighter. Once the roof had dried, I removed all the masking and tidied up any fuzzy edges with a cocktail stick; the hard, semi-gloss factory finish on the yellow makes this a doddle.

More adjustments

After 24 hours, I returned to the model and masked all the areas around the grilles along with the glazing. With a fine needle setting on the airbrush, I carefully sprayed all of the bodyside grilles with Executive dark grey. This is not to fade them but to correct them as Dapol has painted all of the grilles black. Removing the tape around the grilles then allowed the whole model to receive a coat of matt varnish before removing the masking on the glazing.

Once everything had dried fully, I fitted the etched BR arrows and depot plaques, put some rub-down numbers on and added a small 73A shedplate to each cab front just above the headlight. All the etched parts came from Shawplan with the numbers from a Wolf sheet, which were available from Modelmaster at some point. The only detail I needed to fit was the cab-to-shore radio aerials and ground plates, which were made out of plastic strip and brass wire and then fitted above the driver's window at each end. I painted the ground strip a lighter shade of grey, as the real thing seemed to have been.

Before I refitted the body, I gave the whole of the underframe, bufferbeams and bogies a coat of Army Painter 'Hardened Carapace', wiping it off the bogie pipe runs with a damp brush, so the white was still visible and picked out the buffer shanks with silver paint. Once I had got the body back on, the sides lacked a little something, so I picked out all the panel lines round the doors and battery covers, as well as the ventilation slots, using Tamiya Panel Line Accent Colours.

I used dark brown on the yellow parts and a mix of black and light grey on the grey parts. These are super-thin washes which run into panel lines by capillary action and just need to be touched against the detail in one or two places. They are designed to be used with Japanese Gundam models and come with a fine brush built into the lid.

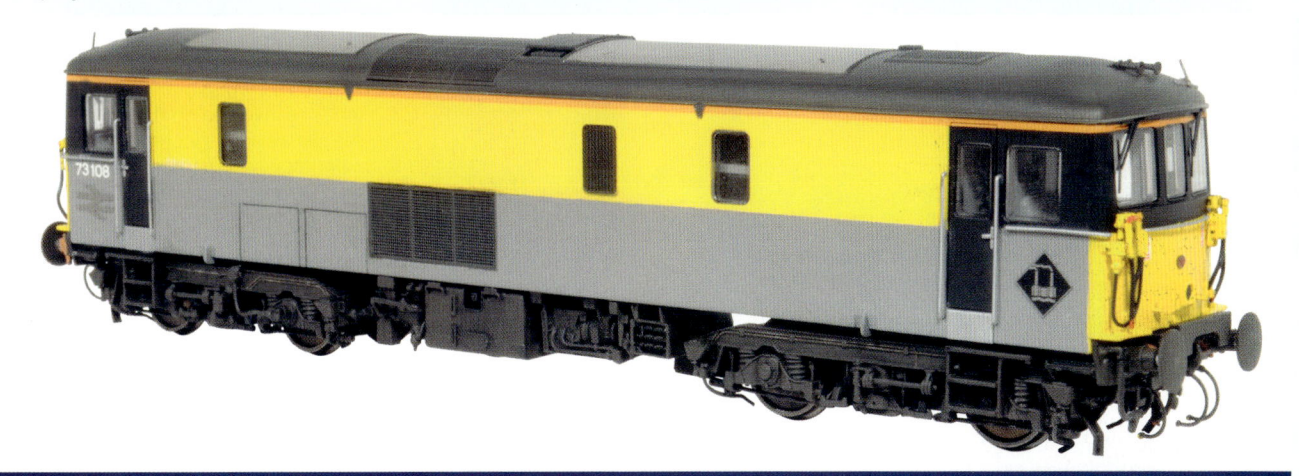

ABOVE: The Dapol model needs very little in the way of additional detailing, just adding the radio roof aerials that became prevalent in the late 1980s and early 1990s. Many Class 73s, and Cromptons as well, carried the shedplates of Stewarts Lane on the ends.

New looks for the decade

Regional recast

Following the rebranding of Provincial as Regional Railways, the sector took a renewed interest in loco-hauled passenger trains in order to overcome a shortage of multiple units. This became most evident on the North Wales coast where Class 37/4s played a large part in workings to Holyhead for eight years as **Simon Bendall** explains, while **Timara Easter** upgrades a 4mm Bachmann model.

The introduction of the Class 158 DMUs at the beginning of the 1990s allowed the renamed Regional Railways to largely move away from loco-hauled services in a number of areas where they were once commonplace. However, this fleet of units and the subsequent redeployment of other DMU types that they triggered was insufficient to cope with passenger numbers in some areas, leading to overcrowding.

By 1992, the sector was obliged to look at retaining some loco-hauled services in the northwest of England due to a shortage of suitable units and to deliver enough capacity. Initially, traction came in the form of Class 31/4s declared surplus by Rail Express Systems and supplemented by a few other examples surrendered by the Civil Engineers. These were partnered with pressure-ventilated Mk.2 coaches, these mostly coming from Network South East in the form of the Mk.2a variant.

The sector opted to largely retain the previous Provincial livery but with some alterations, including adjusting the shade of grey used on the lower bodysides and introducing the 'linking device', this being the marketing name for the three dark blue and two white thin horizontal stripes found on the cabsides. Regional Railways lettering also appeared, this being white on locos and black on the coaches due to the colours it was overlaid on. Just five of the Brush Type 2s were repainted, 31410/21/39/55 in 1992 with 31465 following early in 1993. Others in the pool over time included BR blue examples 31408/32/38/42 and Departmental grey 31411 with the sub-class continuing on North Wales passenger duties into 1995.

Type 3 power
During 1993, Regional Railways acquired a number of Class 37/4s for use on revitalised loco-hauled services along both the North Wales coast and the Highland main line. This gave a second lease of life to the ETS-fitted sub-class, many having been relegated to freight use after finishing in Scotland at the start of the decade.

The initial Crewe allocation, from which the North Wales machines were drawn, was 37407/08/14/18/21/22/25/29 with 37414 the first to gain Regional Railways colours in March 1993. It was soon followed by 37422 and 37429, all three having previously been in Railfreight triple grey with Construction logos. Similarly finished 37418 and 37421 but with Petroleum badges this time were next to be repainted in April 1994 and November 1993, respectively.

Meanwhile, north of the border, Inverness-based 37427 was specially repainted to mark the reintroduction of loco-hauled services to Edinburgh over the Highland Main Line from the start of the 1993 summer timetable. Uniquely, it was given ScotRail lettering on the bodysides instead of the usual Regional Railways legend. Its initial companions on these duties were 37402/04/28 with the first two later replaced by just 37431. Sadly, this last hurrah of Highlands loco-haulage came to an end following the 1994 summer season, which had included workings to Kyle of Lochalsh.

Transrail takes over
In England, Mainline-liveried 37402 had moved to the North Wales pool by the start of 1994 and would join its eight classmates in the ownership of Trainload Freight West, soon to become Transrail, from the spring of that year. This loco would duly gain unbranded Railfreight triple grey while 37407 swapped its Mainline colours for full Transrail garb and 37425 would lose its long obsolete Construction sub-sector scheme for Regional Railways in October 1995.

This was a particularly late use of a BR sector livery but was done so that the loco matched the coaches, which was the same reason that latecomer to the fleet 37420 was similarly painted in April 1996, just as EWS took control. Another late addition to the Holyhead workings around the same time was 37417, also in unbranded triple grey, while throughout this time, celebrity 37408 *Loch Rannoch* continued to carry BR large logo blue.

In an unusual move, Transrail decided to fit ownership plates to some of the Regional Railways liveried locos, these being applied to the driver's cabsides and carried the legend 'This locomotive is the property of Transrail Freight Ltd'. At least 37418/20/22/25/29 are known to have carried these plates for a time.

Under EWS ownership, the number of Class 37/4s involved on the North Wales passenger workings increased yet further, including newly-repainted maroon and gold examples, this diluting the ranks of the Regional Railways-liveried locos with some transferred away to freight duties.

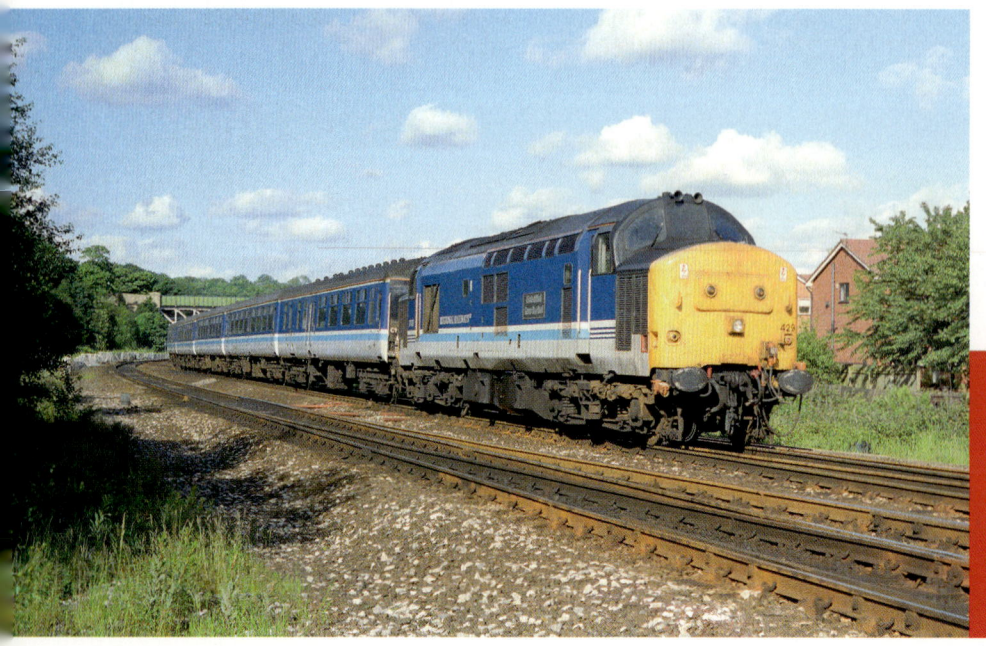

LEFT: The loco modelled opposite, 37429 *Eisteddfod Genedlaethol*, approaches Lostock Junction on June 8, 1994, with the 1F01 17.25 Manchester Victoria to Southport. The loco-hauled workings in the northwest were much shorter-lived than their North Wales counterparts, coming to an end in 1995. The formation is entirely Mk.2a stock with a BSK (a permanently de-classified BFK) and four TSOs, which are available in 2mm from Graham Farish and 4mm from Bachmann. Bill Atkinson

New looks for the decade

A regional respray

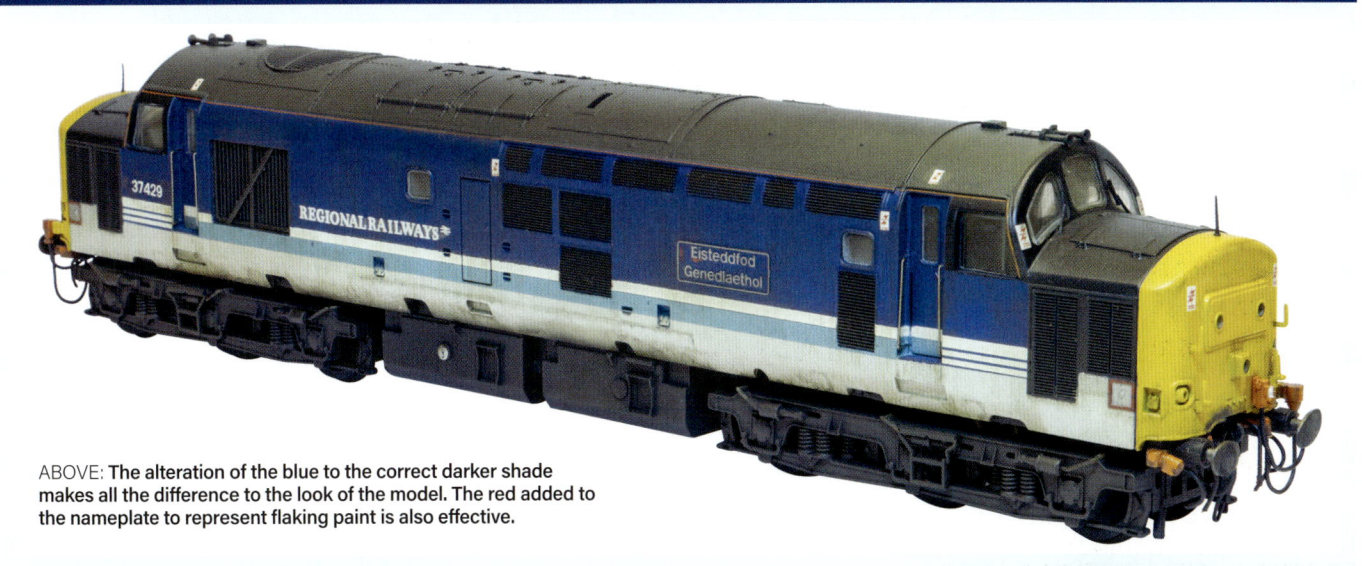

ABOVE: **The alteration of the blue to the correct darker shade makes all the difference to the look of the model. The red added to the nameplate to represent flaking paint is also effective.**

Some years ago, I bought one of the Rails of Sheffield limited edition Bachmann models of 37427 *Highland Enterprise*, on which I intended to modify the incorrect shade of blue. However, modelling plans changed, and it stayed in its box for several years. Not so long ago, I decided to model the last loco I travelled behind on the North Wales coast back in 2000, which was 37429 *Eisteddfod Genedlaethol*. To my shame, it is the only time I have been to Holyhead by rail!

Correcting the shade of blue was a fairly straightforward affair. I masked off the livery elements that were to be retained and removed all the printing that would otherwise show through the paintwork before wafting a layer of grey primer over the bodyshell. This was then followed by Phoenix Precision's Regional Railways dark blue over the top.

During 1996, 37429 received a repaint, which resulted in the bodyside grilles being painted dark grey instead of the bodywork colours. These areas were picked out carefully with a flat brush and Executive dark grey, firmly dating the model to the last years of the loco's life. Etched nameplates came from Shawplan as did the replacement etched roof grille, while the numbering was an HMRS Pressfix sheet and the Regional Railways branding from Railtec Models.

37429 retained the Western Region style of lamp brackets on the noses, having this in common with a few others in the sub-class. The etches available from Shawplan are excellent and each merely needs a 0.45mm hole drilling in the nose before securing in place with a modicum of superglue.

Bufferbeam details

To make the ETS gear, the socket on the secondman's side of the bufferbeam came from Heljan Class 47 spares and that under the driver's side was scratchbuilt from plastic section. The corners of the bufferbeam were carefully trimmed to then accommodate the parts. Further bufferbeam detailing included Hornby Class 31 buffers, Roco main air pipes and Smiths screw couplings with the remainder of the bufferbeam pipework made from thin black coated wire left over from DCC decoder installations.

The outer ends of the air horns were given a bit more of a 3D feel by carefully drilling a hole in the centres with a fine drill bit and then using a 1.5mm drill to open out the fluted shape. The Blue Star multiple working plug and mount on the lower corner of both noses is a little on the clunky side, so it was reduced a little in size by filing and reshaped to better resemble the real thing. A little touch I felt worth doing was where one of the nameplates had started to show the original red paint underneath the blue, which I replicated by dabbing in a couple of tiny spots of paint with a fine brush.

When it came to weathering the model, I chose to portray it as I first saw the real loco back in 1998 at Didcot, by which time it had lost the two Transrail ownership plates, one from each driver's cabside. Using an airbrush, I built up the dirt, starting with the lighter colours first and gradually getting darker. I began with a mix of Humbrol Nos.62 and 186 plus a dash of Metalcote gun metal, which eventually got darker once matt and satin blacks were added to the mix in small amounts.

Most of this was removed after each pass of the airbrush, working downwards with a moistened flat brush (dipped in white spirit) to replicate the effect of rainwater. A final misting over the lower bodysides with a mid-brown mix helped to meld things together.

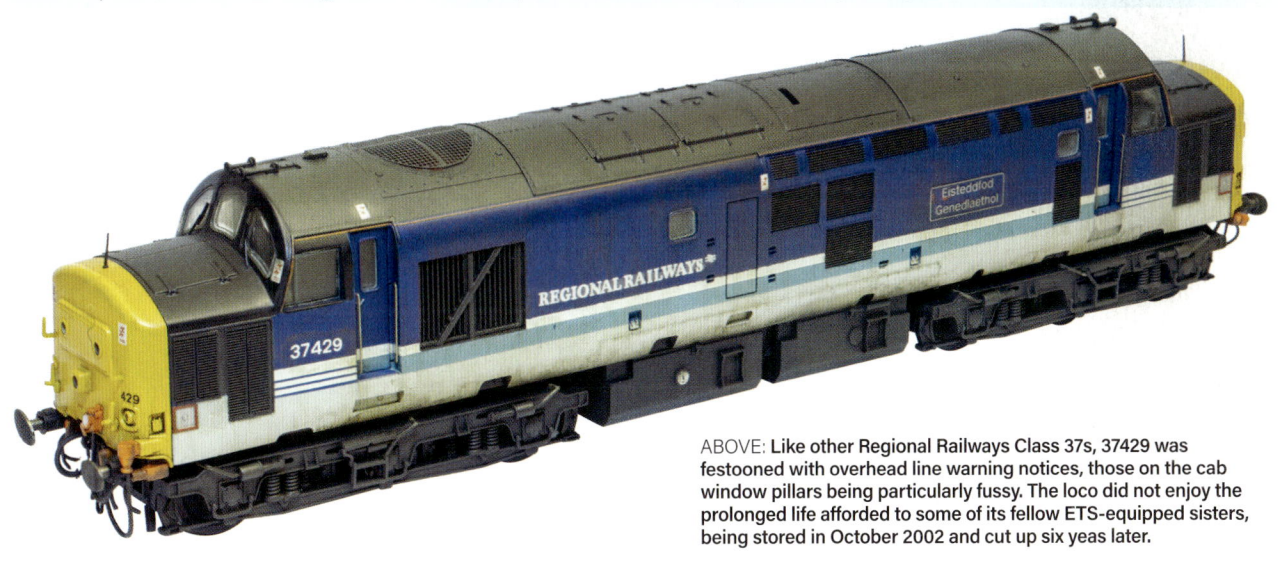

ABOVE: **Like other Regional Railways Class 37s, 37429 was festooned with overhead line warning notices, those on the cab window pillars being particularly fussy. The loco did not enjoy the prolonged life afforded to some of its fellow ETS-equipped sisters, being stored in October 2002 and cut up six yeas later.**

Modelling BR Locomotives of the 1990s **47**

New looks for the decade

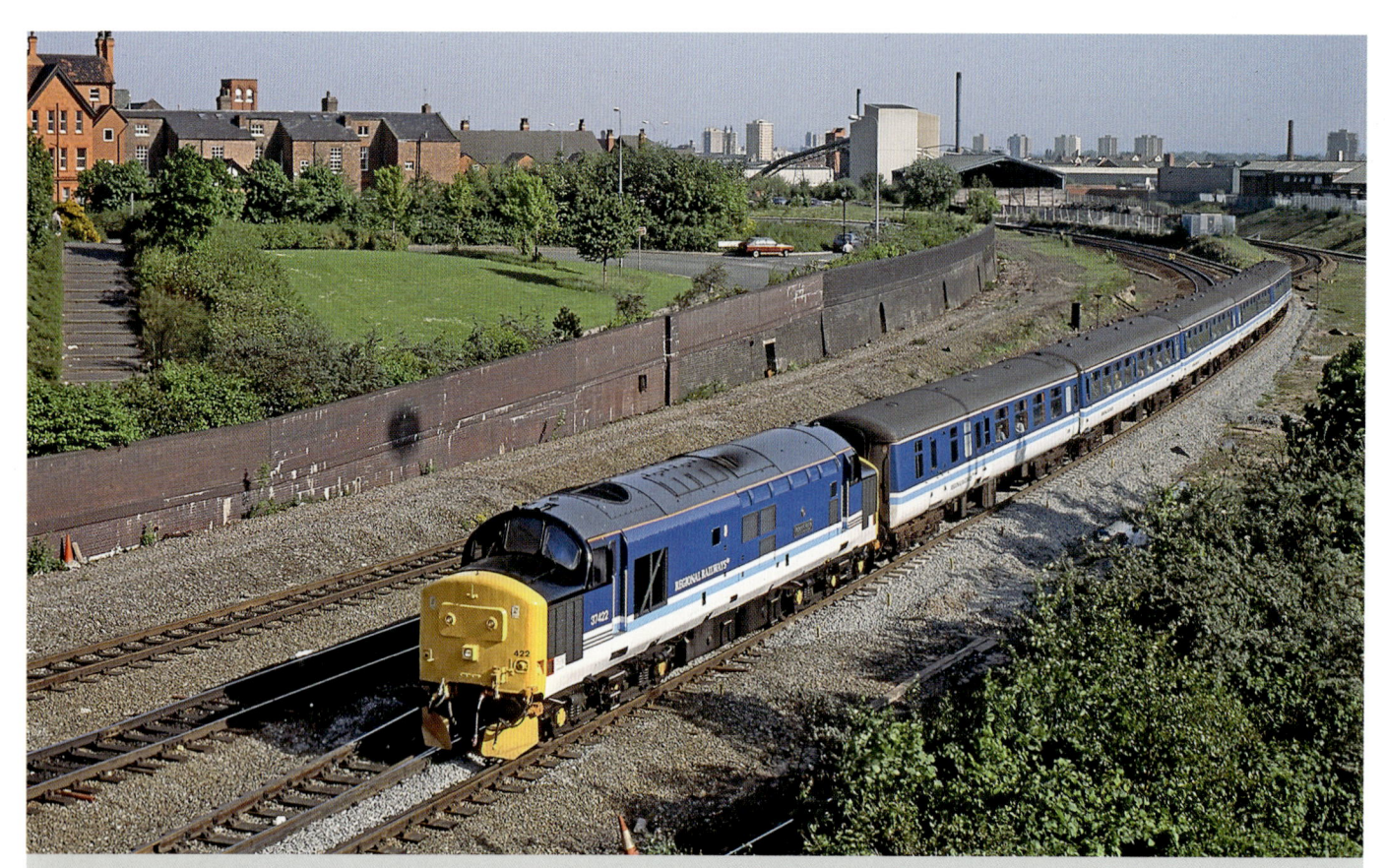

ABOVE: These four images showcase the Crewe-based Class 37/4s in their first year of operation under the Regional Railways banner. On May 11, 1993, a near spotless 37422 *Robert F. Fairlie Locomotive Engineer 1831-1885* had been repainted in Regional Railways colours just a few weeks earlier at Crewe Diesel TMD as it approaches Salford Crescent with the 17.14 Manchester Victoria to Blackpool North. The five coach set of matching pressure-ventilated Mk.2s features a declassified Mk.2c BSK leading three Mk.2a TSOs and then a Mk.2a BSO on the rear. The availability of Mk.2a models was detailed on the previous page while Accurascale has the Mk.2c under development in OO gauge. John Whiteley

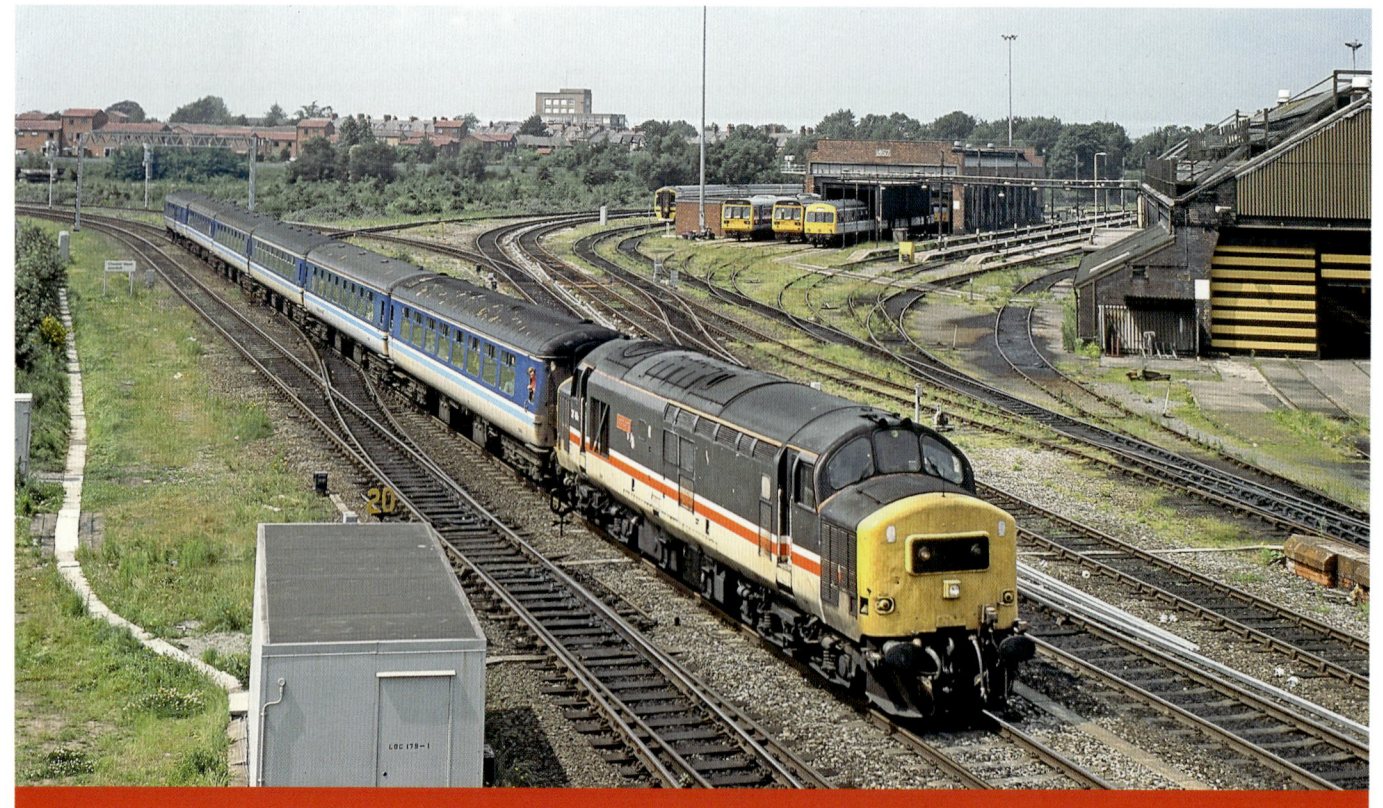

ABOVE: In careworn Mainline livery applied three years earlier, 37407 *Loch Long* approaches Chester and passes the DMU depot with the Sundays-only 12.50 Llandudno to Crewe on June 13, 1993. The six coach formation is interesting in being entirely formed of Mk.2b and Mk.2c vehicles, which were far less common at this time than the ubiquitous and older Mk.2a design. The five TSOs are arranged as two Mk.2c then a 2b, a 2c and another 2b with the brake being rather indistinct but possibly a Mk.2c BSO. Notably the first and third TSOs are refugees from the by then abolished TransPennine loco-hauled services as they still retain Provincial colours. Although subtle, the Executive light grey used on this pair has a beige tint compared to the silver-grey employed on the other coaches while the lack of Regional Railways lettering is a more obvious clue. John Whiteley

New looks for the decade

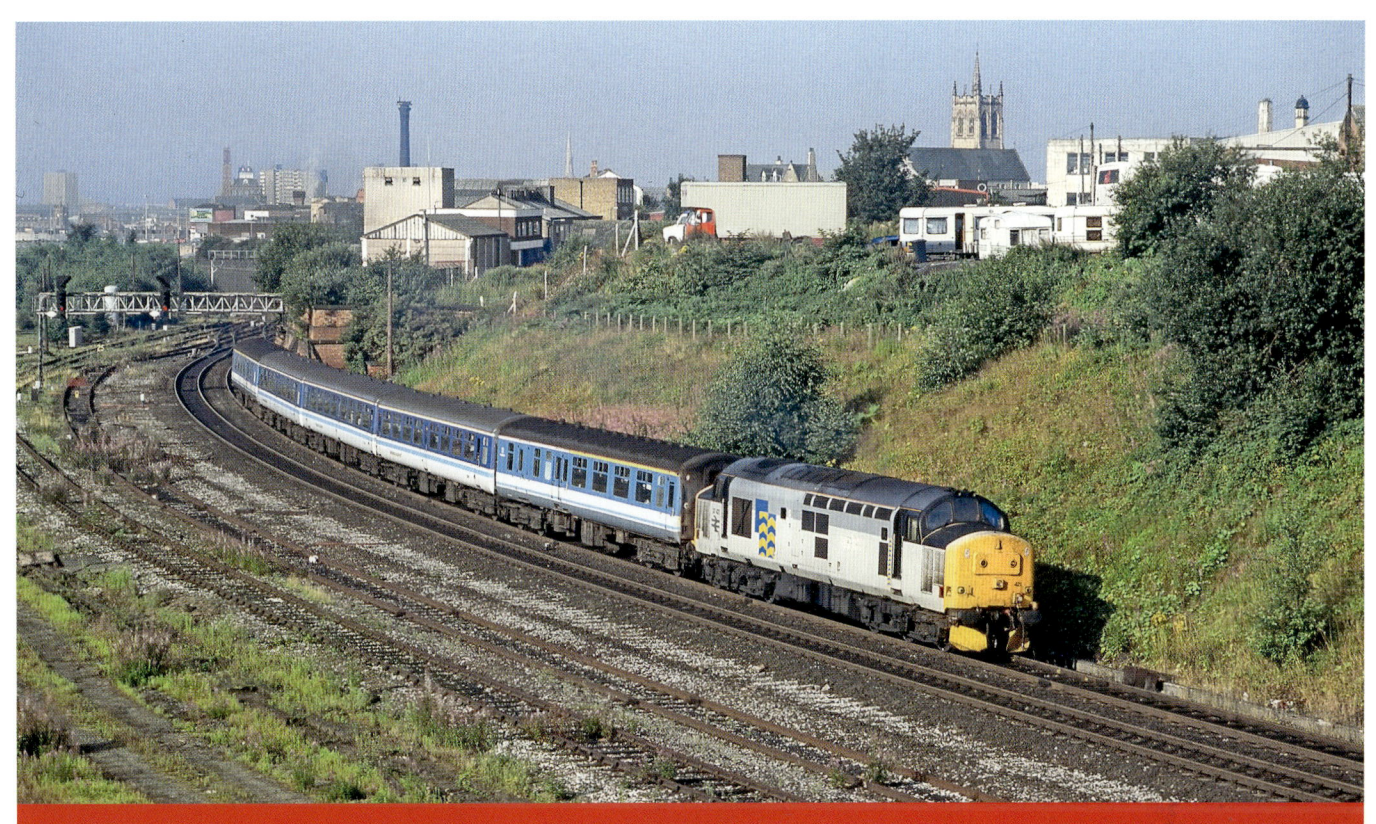

ABOVE: Even well into the second year of the revitalised loco-hauled trains, the colours of Regional Railways were not yet all prevailing. On August 17, 1993, 37421 was heading for Newton Heath as it passes the once-bustling but now closed carriage sidings at Red Bank with empty stock from Manchester Victoria. The five-coach set had run from Southport that morning and features three Mk.2a TSOs positioned between two brakes. The latter are Mk.2a BFKs transferred from NSE West of England services, with the leading example even still carrying the route badge at the left hand end, which have been downgraded to standard class BSKs. Neither has yet had the yellow first class stripe removed but the '1' symbols are gone from the doors while they are carrying the interim livery that saw the red NSE stripe overpainted with light blue, pending a full repaint. Meanwhile, the Railfreight Petroleum-liveried Type 3 was only three months away from its own date with tins of paint. *John Whiteley*

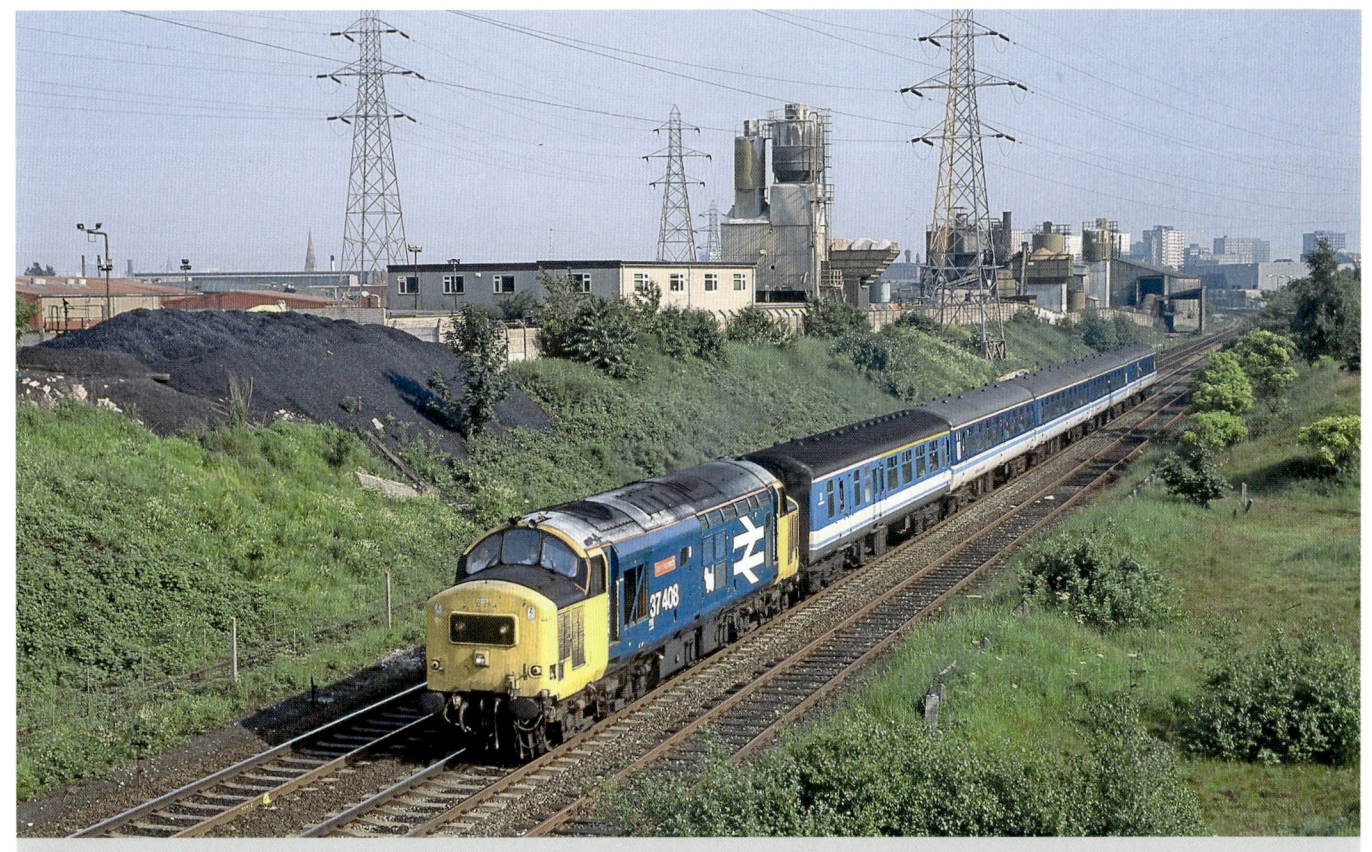

ABOVE: The enduringly popular and much-missed 37408 *Loch Rannoch* thrashes through the industrial surroundings of Agecroft and past the site of the demolished steam shed with the 17.14 Manchester Victoria to Blackpool North on June 8, 1993. The formation of its Mk.2a coaches is largely the same as that pictured with 37421 except that the rear brake is a BSO in Regional Railways colours. The leading ex NSE BFK is again downgraded and renumbered in the 355xx series. The Type 3 would lose its large logo blue colours five years later. *John Whiteley*

Modelling BR Locomotives of the 1990s 49

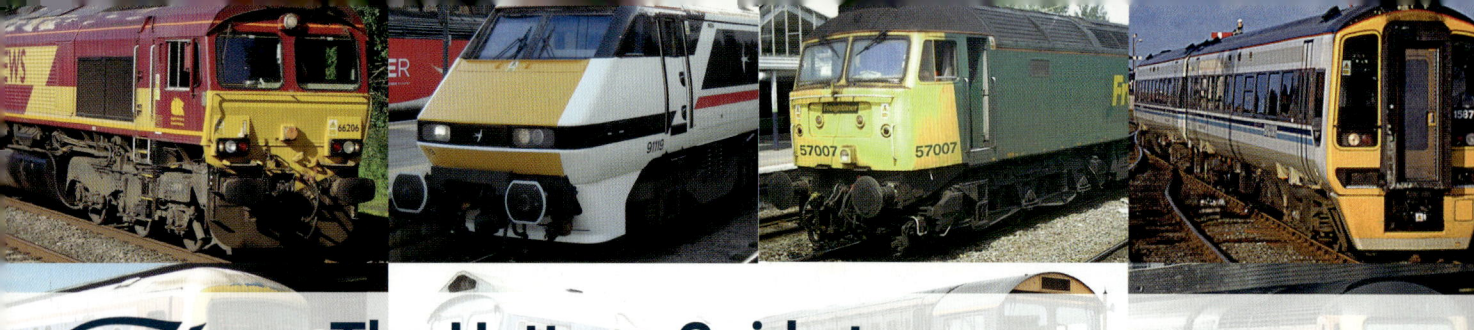

The Hattons Guide to... Britain's Railways in the 1990s

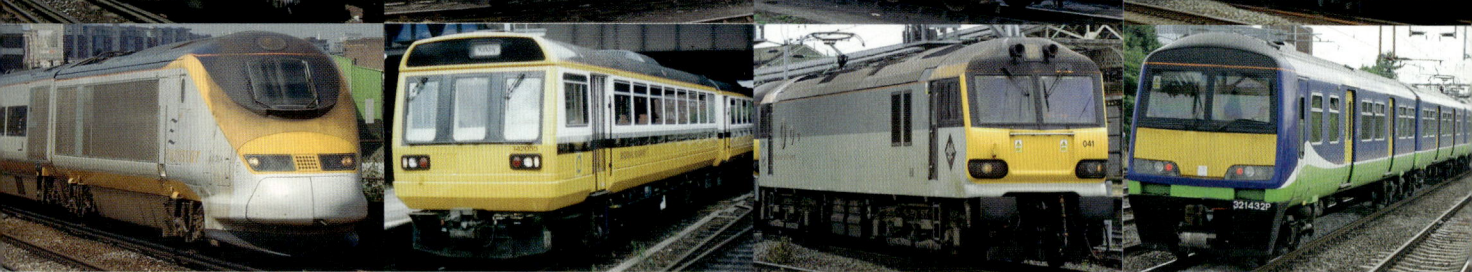

See more about the vehicles shown & models produced of them at **hattons.co.uk/directory**

Diesel Locos

New Locos for the 1990s

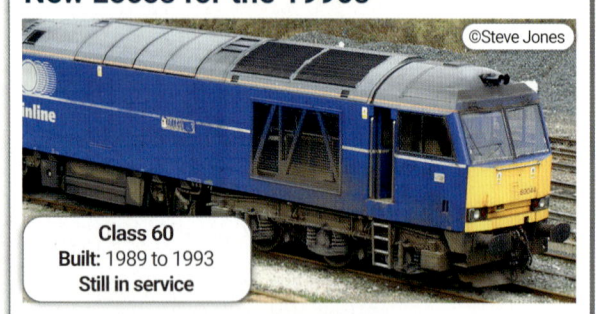

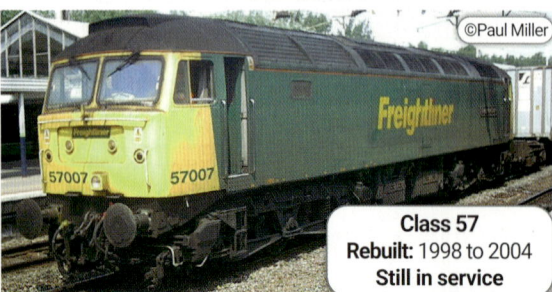

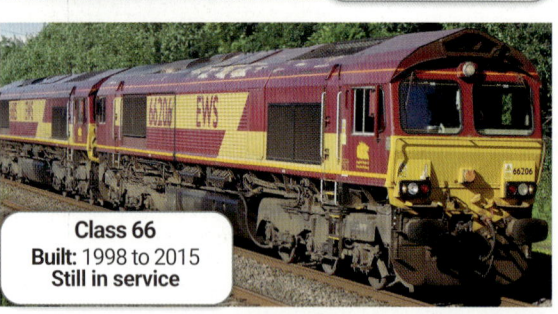

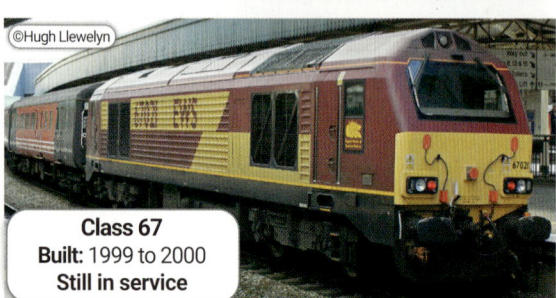

Class 60
Built: 1989 to 1993
Still in service

Class 57
Rebuilt: 1998 to 2004
Still in service

Class 66
Built: 1998 to 2015
Still in service

Class 67
Built: 1999 to 2000
Still in service

Other Operational Diesels

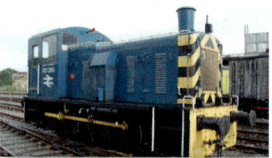

Class 03
Built: 1957 to 1962
Withdrawn: 1993/ 2008

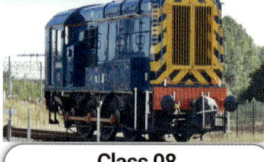

Class 08
Built: 1952 to 1962
Still in service

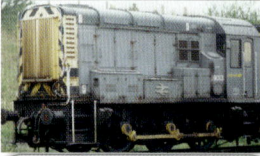

Class 09
Built: 1959 to 1993
Still in service

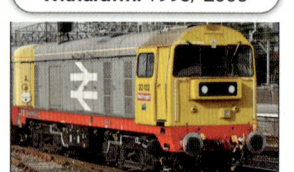

Class 20
Built: 1957 to 1968
Still in service

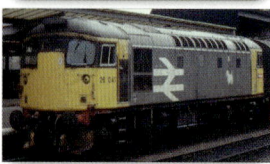

Class 26
Built: 1958 to 1959
Withdrawn: 1994

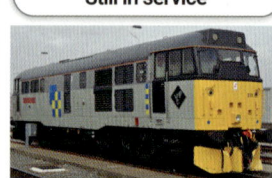

Class 31
Built: 1957 to 1962
Withdrawn: 2017

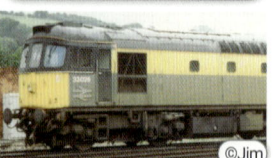

Class 33
Built: 1960 to 1962
Still in service

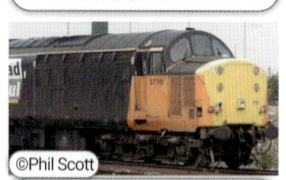

Class 37
Built: 1960 to 1965
Still in service

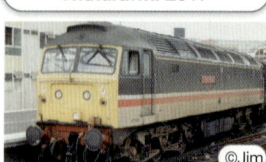

Class 47
Built: 1962 to 1968
Still in service

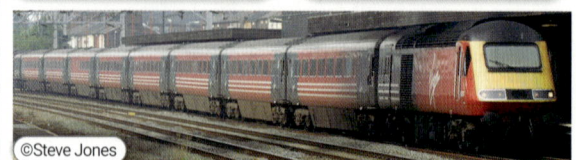

Class 43 (HST)
Built: 1975 to 1982
Still in service

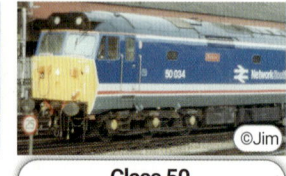

Class 50
Built: 1967 to 1968
Withdrawn: 1994

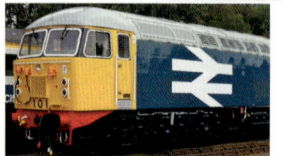

Class 56
Built: 1976 to 1984
Still in service

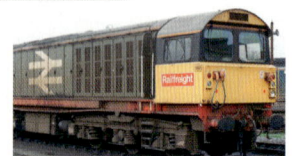

Class 58
Built: 1983 to 1987
Withdrawn: 2002

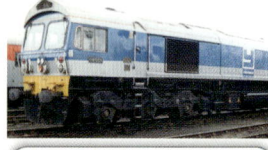

Class 59
Built: 1985 to 1995
Still in service

Photographs used under commercial use licences. Author information available at hattons.co.uk/directory. unless otherwise stated.

Learn more on the Hattons Directory...

BETA

The Hattons Directory is an ever-growing resource of information on real vehicles and the scale models that have been produced of them. Research vehicles and browse a huge range of products we have available or wishlist them & be notified about future stock updates.

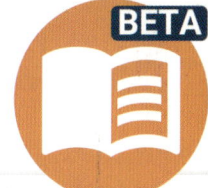

How it works:

1. **Full Prototype Information** — Facts & figures on real-life vehicles
2. **Scale Model Profiles** — Specifications & products produced
3. **Tooling Upgrades** — See changes to toolings over time
4. **Comparison Tool** — Compare models from different brands
5. **Liveries Produced** — See which liveries have been made
6. **Toolings in Each Scale** — Listings in OO, N, O, HO & more...

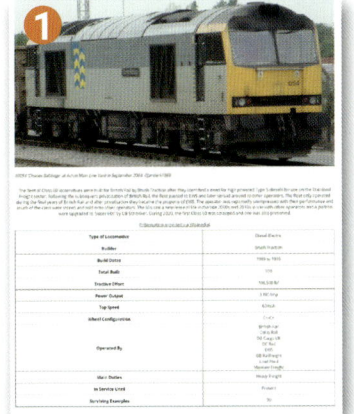

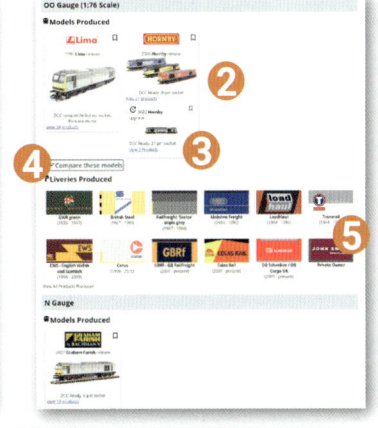

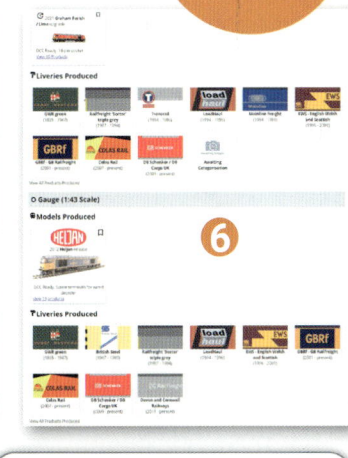

- Use our lightning-fast search to find vehicle & model profiles.
- Browse vehicles of all types from across the world.
- Over 175,000 scale products available to view
- Explore liveries & operators and see when they were in use

Explore full Vehicle, Tooling & Livery Guides at: hattons.co.uk/directory

---

Electric Locos

New Locos for the 1990s

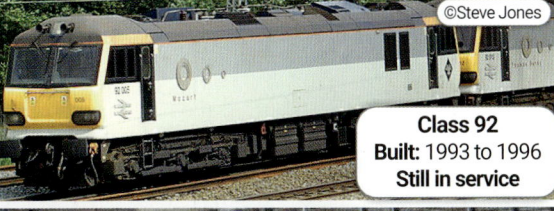

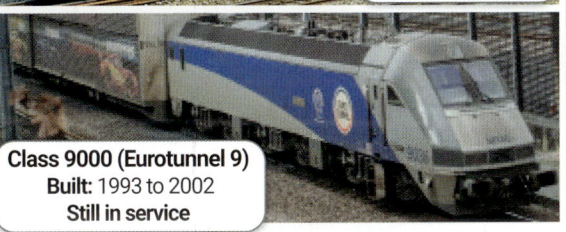

Class 92 ©Steve Jones
Built: 1993 to 1996
Still in service

Class 9000 (Eurotunnel 9)
Built: 1993 to 2002
Still in service

Other Operational Electrics

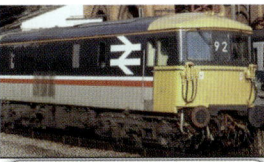

Class 73 Electrodiesel
Built: 1962 to 1967
Still in service

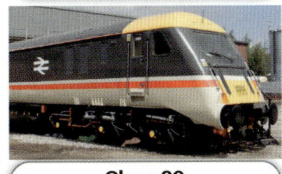

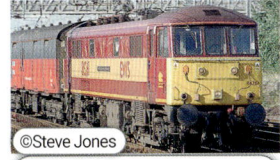

Class 86 ©Steve Jones
Built: 1965 to 1966
Still in service

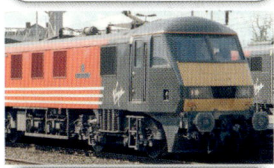

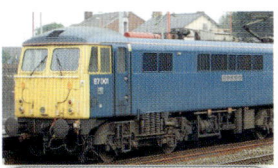

Class 87
Built: 1973 to 1975
Still in service

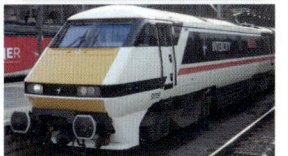

Class 89
Built: 1986
Withdrawn: 2000

Class 90
Built: 1987 to 1990
Still in service

Class 91
Built: 1988 to 1991
Still in service

Coaches

New Coaches for the 1990s

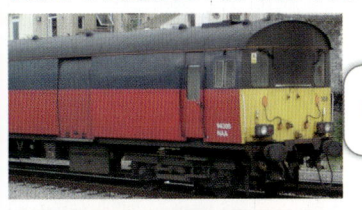

PCV
Rebuilt: 1994 to 1996
Withdrawn: 2004

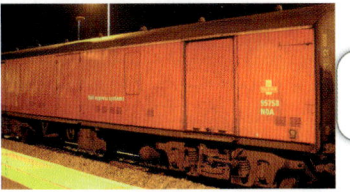

Super GUV
Rebuilt: 1993
Still in service

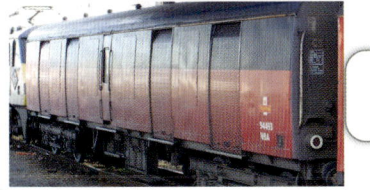

Super BG
Rebuilt: 1994
Withdrawn: 2004

Other Operational Coaches

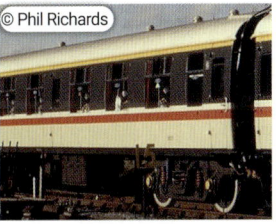

BR Mark 1 © Phil Richards
Built: 1951 to 1963
Withdrawn: 2004

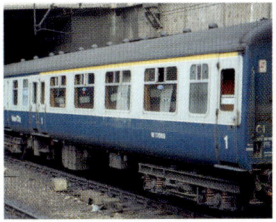

BR Mark 2 A - C
Built: 1963 to 1975
Withdrawn: 2003

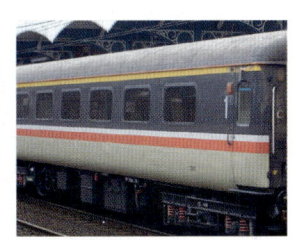

BR Mark 2 D - F
Built: 1963 to 1975
Withdrawn: Late 2010s

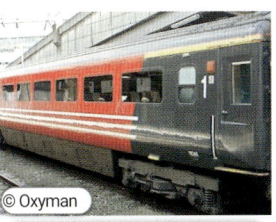

BR Mark 3 (HST) © Oxyman
Built: 1975 to 1988
Still in service

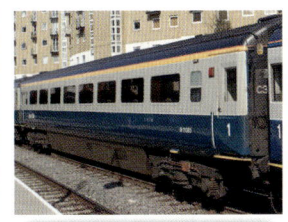

BR Mark 3 A
Built: 1975 to 1988
Still in service

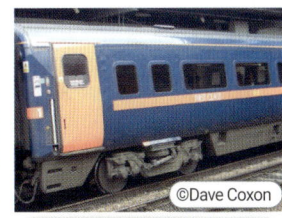

BR Mark 4 ©Dave Coxon
Built: 1989 to 1992
Still in service

Photographs used under commercial use licences. Author information available at hattons.co.uk/directory, unless otherwise stated.

Diesel Multiple Units

New Units for the 1990s

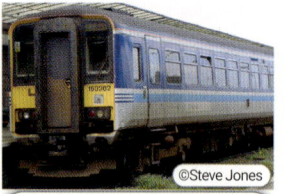

Class 153 Super Sprinter
Rebuilt: 1991 to 1992
Still in service

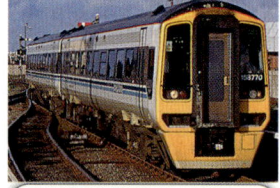

Class 158 Express Sprinter
Built: 1989 to 1992
Still in service

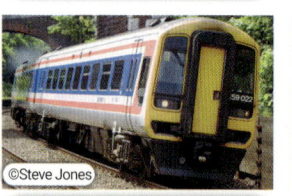

Class 159 South West Turbo
Built: 1989 to 1993
Still in service

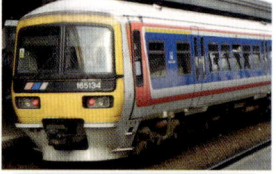

Class 165 Networker
Built: 1990 to 1992
Still in service

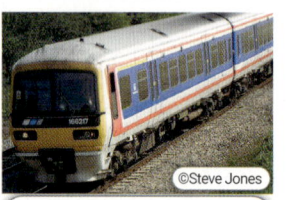

Class 166 Networker Turbo
Built: 1992 to 1993
Still in service

Class 168/0 Clubman
Built: 1998
Still in service

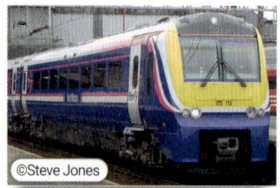

Class 170 Turbostar
Built: 1998 to 2005
Still in service

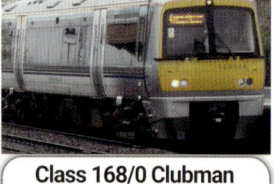

Class 175 Coradia
Built: 1999 to 2001
Still in service

Other Operational DMUs & DEMUs

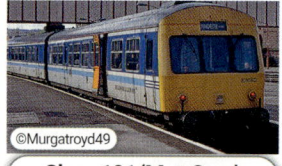

Class 101 'Met-Cam'
Built: 1956 to 1960
Withdrawn: 2003

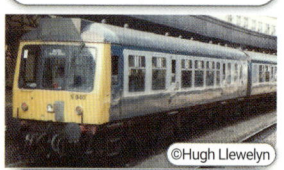

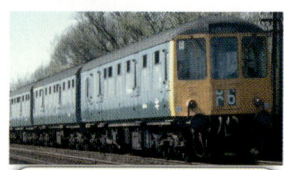

Class 104
Built: 1957 to 1959
Withdrawn: 1995

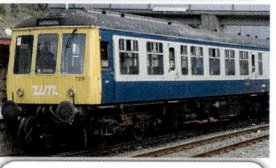

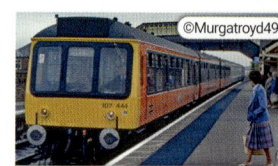

Class 107
Built: 1960
Withdrawn: 1992 (Sandite 95)

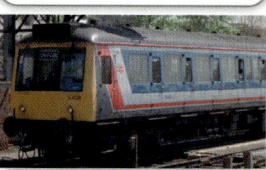

Class 108
Built: 1958 to 1961
Withdrawn: 1993

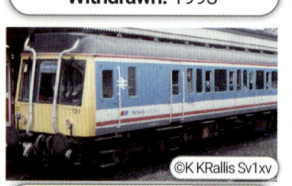

Class 114
Built: 1956 to 1957
Withdrawn: 1992

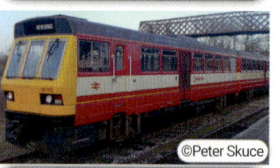

Class 117
Built: 1959 to 1961
Withdrawn: 2000

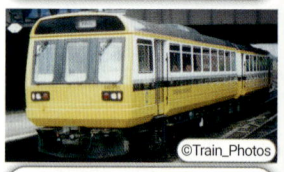

Class 121 Bubble Car
Built: 1960 to 1961
Withdrawn: 2017

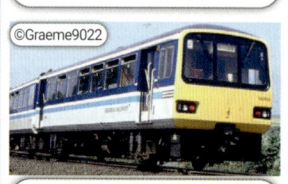

Class 141 Pacer
Built: 1984
Withdrawn: 1997

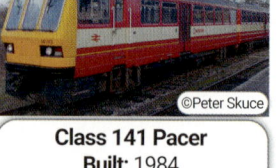

Class 142 Pacer
Built: 1985 to 1987
Withdrawn: 2021

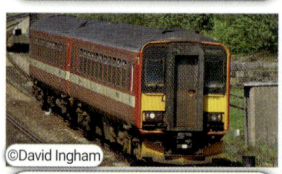

Class 143 & 144 Pacers
Built: 1985 to 1986
Withdrawn: 2020

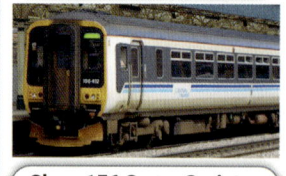

Class 150 Sprinter
Built: 1984 to 1987
Still in service

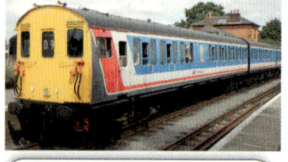

Class 155 Super Sprinter
Built: 1987 to 1988
Still in service

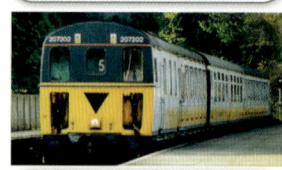

Class 156 Super Sprinter
Built: 1987 to 1989
Still in service

Class 205 Thumper
Built: 1957 to 1962
Withdrawn: 2004

Class 207 Thumper
Built: 1962
Withdrawn: 2004

🎨 Liveries of the 1990s 🎨

British Rail Liveries

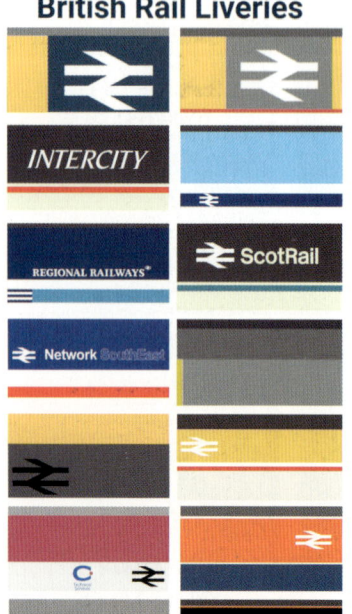

Privatised Passenger Liveries

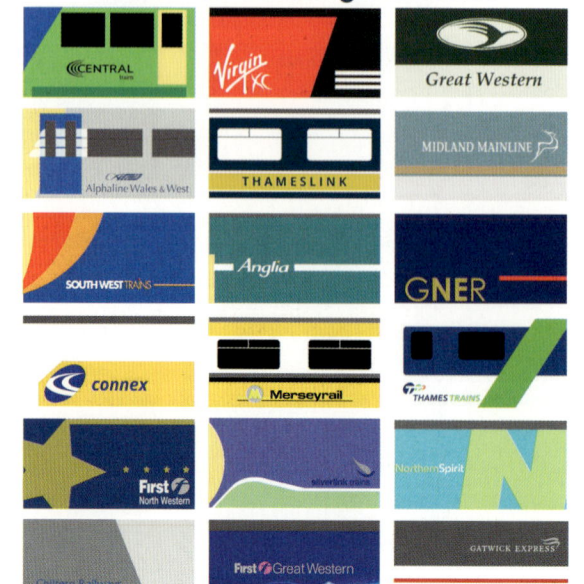

Privatised Freight & Hire Liveries

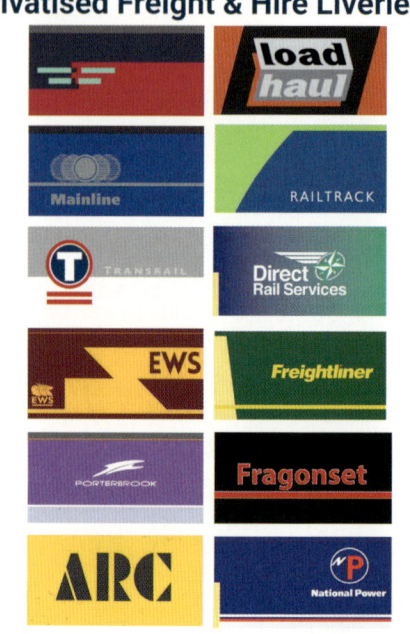

Explore more UK Railway Livery Profiles at hattons.co.uk/directory

Electric Multiple Units

New Units for the 1990s

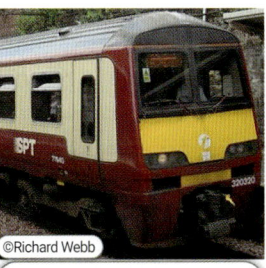

Class 320
Rebuilt: 1990
Still in service

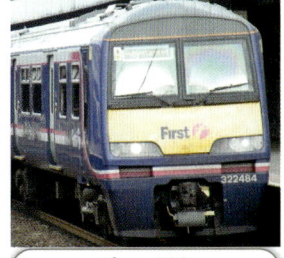

Class 322
Built: 1990
Still in service

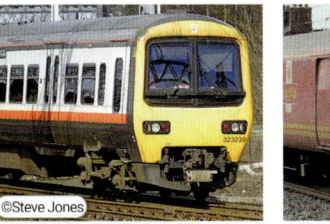

Class 323
Built: 1992 to 1995
Still in service

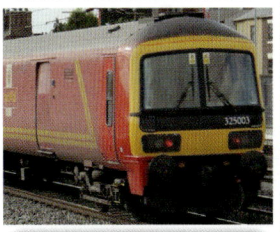

Class 325
Built: 1995 to 1996
Still in service

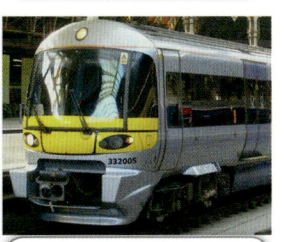

Class 332
Built: 1997 to 1998
Still in service

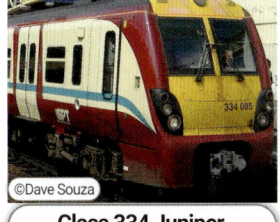

Class 334 Juniper
Built: 1999 to 2002
Still in service

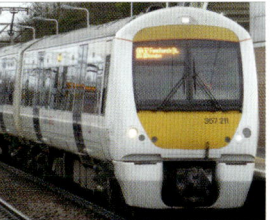

Class 357 Electrostar
Built: 1999 to 2002
Still in service

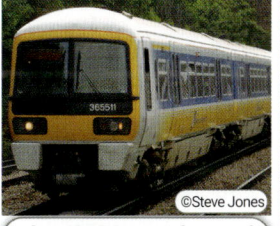

Class 365 Networker Exp'
Built: 1994 to 1995
Withdrawn: 2021

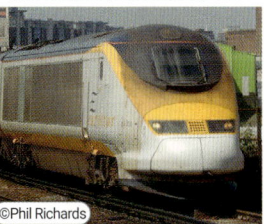

Class 373 Eurostar
Built: 1992 to 1996
Still in service

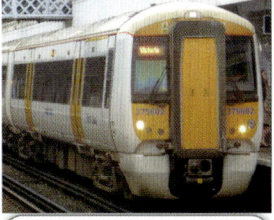

Class 375 Electrostar
Built: 1999 to 2005
Still in service

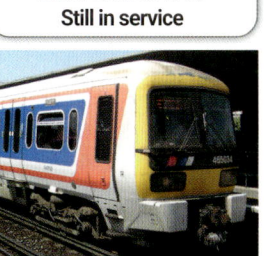

Class 465 Networker
Built: 1991 to 1994
Still in service

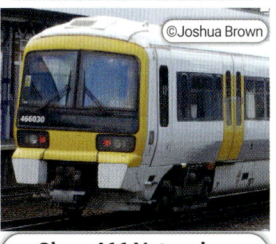

Class 466 Networker
Built: 1993 to 1994
Still in service

Other Operational EMUs

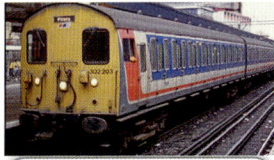

Class 302
Built: 1958 to 1959
Withdrawn: 1999

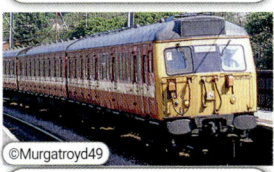

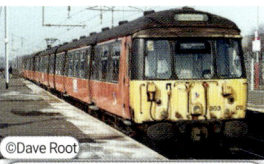

Class 303
Built: 1959 to 1961
Withdrawn: 2002

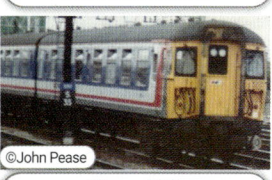

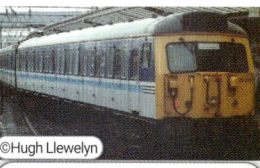

Class 305
Built: 1959 to 1960
Withdrawn: 2001

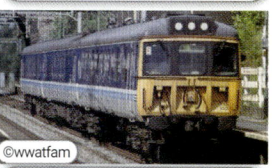

Class 308
Built: 1959 to 1961
Withdrawn: 2001

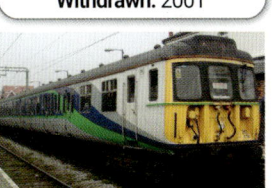

Class 309
Built: 1962 to 1987
Withdrawn: 2000

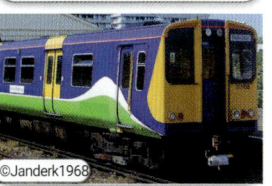

Class 310
Built: 1965 to 1967
Withdrawn: 2002

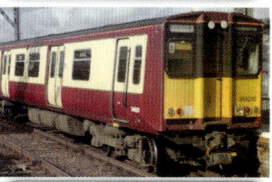

Class 312
Built: 1975 to 1978
Withdrawn: 2004

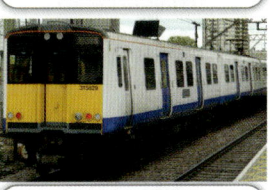

Class 313
Built: 1976 to 1977
Still in service

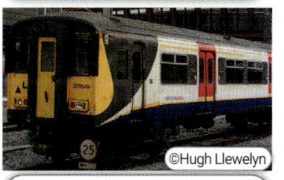

Class 314
Built: 1979
Withdrawn: 2019

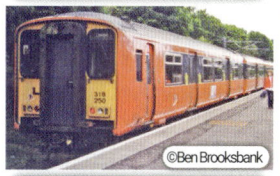

Class 315
Built: 1980 to 1981
Still in service

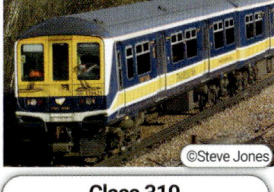

Class 317
Built: 1981 to 1987
Still in service

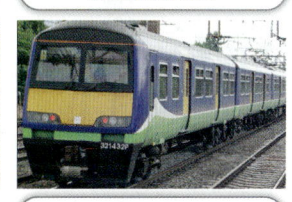

Class 318
Built: 1985 to 1986
Still in service

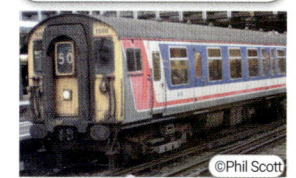

Class 319
Built: 1987 to 1990
Still in service

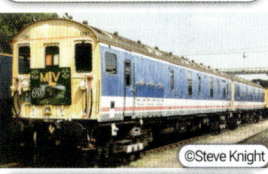

Class 321
Built: 1988 and 1991
Still in service

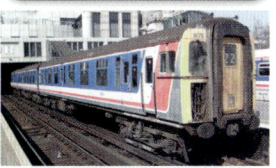

Class 410 to 412
Built: 1956 to 1963
Withdrawn: 2005

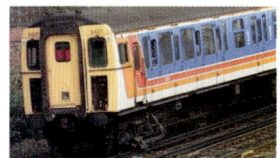

Class 419 MLV
Built: 1959 to 1961
Withdrawn: 2004

Class 420 to 422
Built: 1964 to 1972
Withdrawn: 2010

Class 423
Built: 1967 to 1974
Withdrawn: 2005

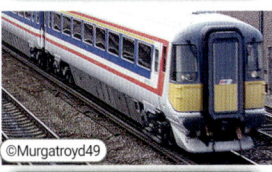

Class 442 Wessex Electric
Built: 1987 to 1989
Withdrawn: 2020

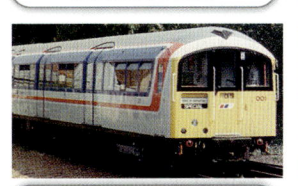

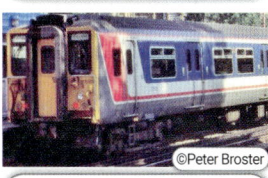

Class 455
Built: 1982 to 1985
Still in service

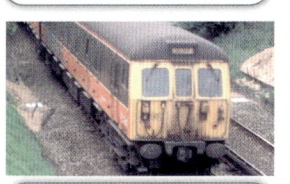

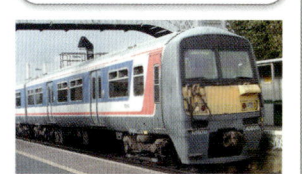

Class 456
Built: 1990 to 1991
Withdrawn: 2022

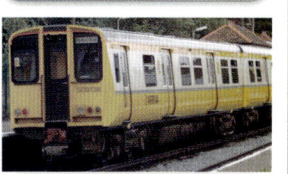

Class 483
Built: 1938
Withdrawn: 2021

Class 504
Built: 1959
Withdrawn: 1991

Class 507 & 508
Built: 1978 to 1980
Still in service

Photographs used under commercial use licences. Author information available at hattons.co.uk/directory.

Out of the shadows

The spring of 1994 saw much of the British Rail fleet recast as many freight locos were divided between three newly-created regional freight companies while the passenger locos passed to the ownership of a trio of leasing companies. **Simon Bendall** details the break-up and subsequent developments of the mid-1990s shadow privatisation period.

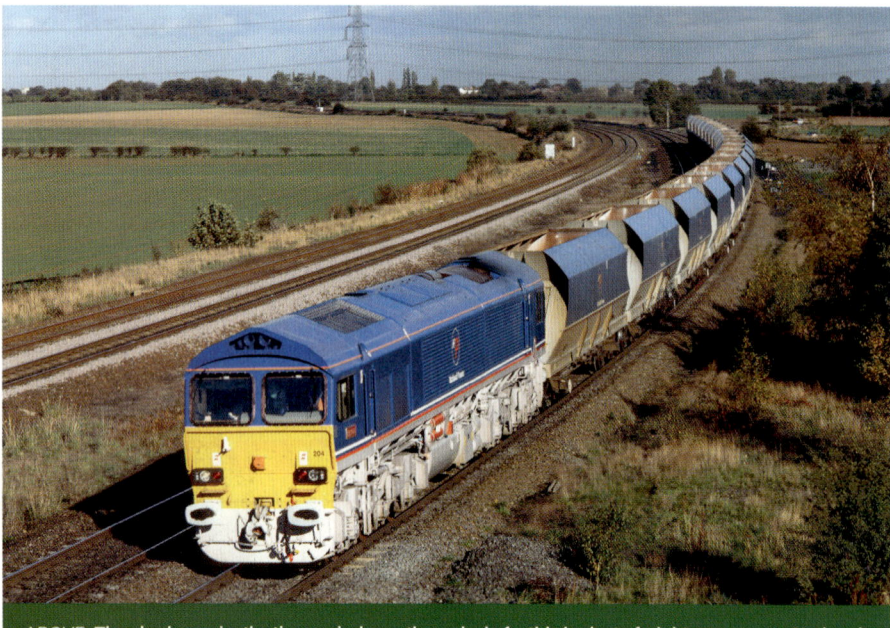

ABOVE: The shadow privatisation period saw the arrival of a third private freight operator as National Power introduced its own limestone and then coal workings to ensure certainly of supply during the turbulent reorganisation of the network. Finished in the company's superb livery, an almost brand new and yet to named 59204 powers through Burton Salmon on October 25, 1995, with the 6D92 11.30 Drax to Ferrybridge limestone empties. Martin Loader

March 1994 was a significant month for British Rail as it marked the abolition of the sectors and the transition to a structure of self-contained business units, these being deliberately independent so they could be packaged up and sold one by one by the government as part of the privatisation process. These units initially remained under the umbrella control of the British Rail Board but showed how the railway would look in just a few years, hence the term shadow privatisation.

The first change that arrived that month was the demise of the four Trainload sub-sectors of Coal, Construction, Petroleum and Metals. Their loco fleets were instead dispersed between three new freight companies that were created on a geographical basis. These were initially named Trainload Freight West, South East, and North East, each generally taking control of all the former Trainload locos that were based in their areas at the time.

There was some re-distribution of assets, for example the Class 60s were split as evenly as possible, but generally locos stayed where they were. After all, there was no point in taking the Class 58s away from Toton for example and sending them to new depots elsewhere in the country where maintenance staff and traincrew had no training on them. For this reason, the entire class remained as part of the Trainload Freight South East allocation but in turn, the company lost all of the Class 56s that had previously been based in the southeast and East Midlands.

Infrastructure recast

The three regional freight firms also took back all of the locos assigned to infrastructure work that had been under the control of InterCity, Regional Railway and Network SouthEast for the past two years, this somewhat uneasy fit having no place under the new structure. Trainload Freight West was also assigned the Class 31s and Class 47s that had previously been with Central Services for Civil Link duties and also took all of the Regional Railways Class 31/4s and Class 37/4s used on northwest and North Wales passenger trains. These were officially all infrastructure locos that just happened to spend much of their time hauling coaches!

Later in 1994, the three freight companies attained greater independence and were allowed to compete against each other for traffic. All three adopted new, more marketable identities, becoming Transrail, Loadhaul and Mainline Freight, this bringing new liveries as well.

Not all of the former non-passenger sectors engaged in the restructuring of 1994. For example, Railfreight Distribution initially remained untouched but would undergo its own difficult separation over the following two years as the Freightliner container division became an independent entity to be sold off separately, the division of assets between the two being somewhat acrimonious. Equally, Rail Express Systems saw no great change and was amongst the first to be sold off late in 1995.

Other operations that retained their independence included European Passenger Services, where the conversion of Class 37s for use on the ill-fated 'Nightstar' services was getting underway, and BR Telecommunications (BRT).

BELOW: Of the four Class 73/0s assigned to Merseyrail for infrastructure duties, two gained the company's yellow and brown departmental livery in January 1994. Seen at Hall Road depot in October 1996, 73001 had by now become 73901 to reflect modifications made for sandite use and exhaust alterations for diesel working in tunnels. The sandite duties involved powering two former Class 501 trailers in an unusual formation that saw the Class 73 sandwiched in the middle. The loco originally sported Regional Railways lettering in addition to the Merseyrail 'M' logos but this had been removed by this date. Simon Bendall Collection

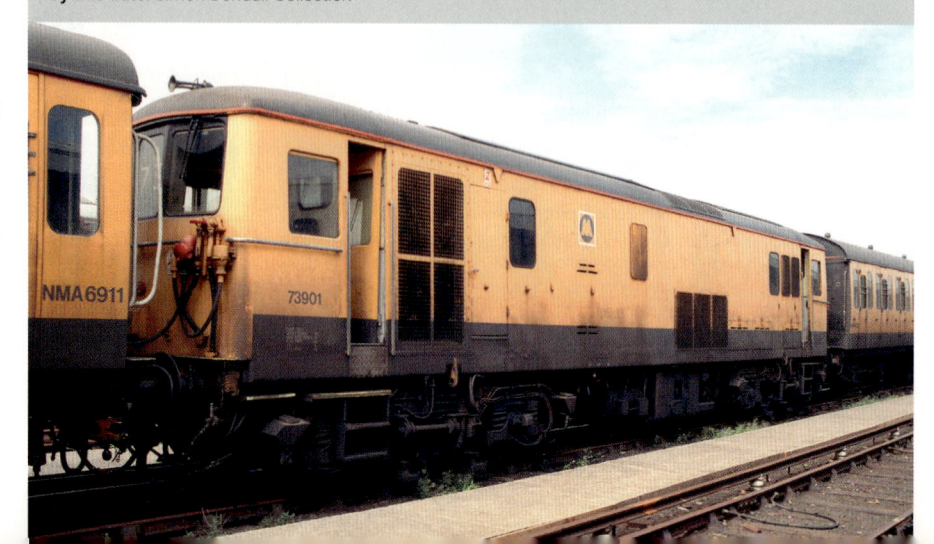

Out of the shadows

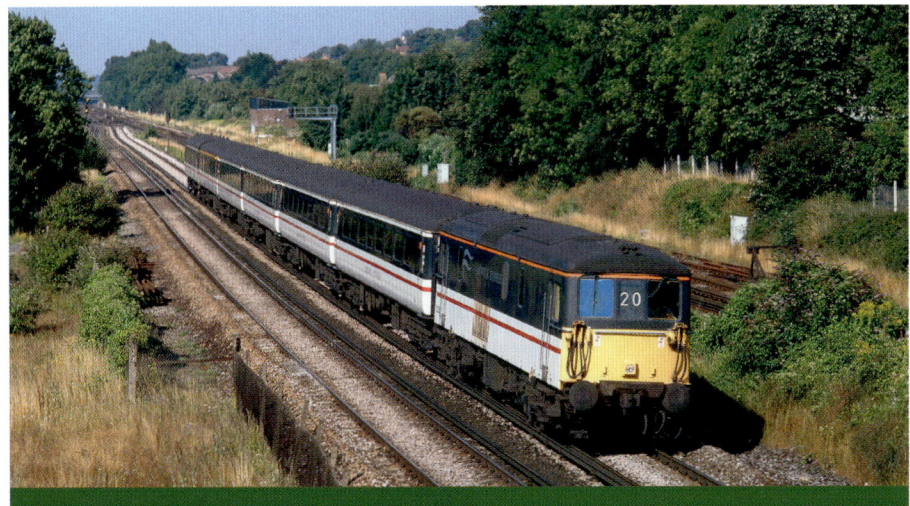

ABOVE: Of the various train operating units that took over the former InterCity routes, only Gatwick Express opted to amend the previous Swallow livery, changing the proportions of the red and white stripes, and adopting a new logo. On August 12, 1995, 73235 passes Coulsdon with the 16.15 Victoria-Gatwick formed of Class 488/3 and Class 488/2 trailer sets and a Class 489 GLV driving trailer. Dapol has produced its Class 73 in this livery in both N and OO while the passenger stock can be modified from Mk.2f coaches in both scales. The GLV is available ready-to-run from Britannia Pacific Models in OO gauge and as etched components from MJT while N gauge options include the discontinued CJM model and overlays for a Farish Mk.1 from Electra Rail Graphics. *Martin Loader*

Lease back

More controversial was the route taken for locos assigned to passenger operations, which now amounted to the former InterCity fleet of Class 47s, Class 73s, AC electrics and HSTs. These were divided up amongst the ownership of three newly-created leasing companies, named Eversholt, Porterbrook and Angel, and then leased back to the train operating units (TOUs), the same system being put in place for multiple units and passenger coaches.

The ownership division was done on a route basis rather than by class so, for instance, the HST power cars ended up divided between Porterbrook, which took the CrossCountry and Midland Main Line examples, while Angel was handed the East Coast and Great Western fleets. Eversholt did take all of the former InterCity Class 86/2s, these being split between CrossCountry, Anglia and the West Coast, along with the Class 91s. Meanwhile, Porterbrook was given the Class 47s used on CrossCountry duties with a few soon hived off to Great Western along with the West Coast electrics of 87001-35 and 90001-15, not to mention the Gatwick Express Class 73s.

This left a few stragglers, particularly Class 08/09 shunters and 03079 on the Isle of Wight, which were assigned directly to the passenger TOUs for depot duties. These were not leased but owned outright by each operating company and a few still have this status today. Five Class 73s were also given the same treatment, 73109 going to the South Western TOU while 73001/02/05/06 were allocated to Merseyrail for depot and infrastructure duties.

Private operators

Changes were also underway amongst the operators of the Class 59 fleets with October 1993 having seen Foster Yeoman and ARC reach agreement to pool their rail operations in order to create operational and economic efficiencies. This brought the creation of Mendip Rail, which took over responsibility for the Class 59/0s and Class 59/1s along with all shunters, wagons, and rail staff.

Under the agreement, the two fleets were merged into one with no operational distinction between them, bringing the sight of ARC locos and wagons working Yeoman flows and vice versa. With greater wagon utilisation achieved, Mendip was able to dispense with over 200 vehicles, bringing obvious savings. Operationally, maintenance of the Class 59s was concentrated at Merehead with Whatley taking over much of the wagon repair work. During 1994, Mainline Freight became responsible for providing drivers to Mendip Rail under a continuation of the manning agreement previously held with British Rail, this duly passing to EWS from 1996.

Early 1994 saw National Power enter the rail market with the delivery of 59201 and 21 high-capacity JHA hoppers, the electricity generator seeing this as a way of reducing its transport costs. The new rolling stock was destined for use on limestone traffic from the Peak District to Drax Power Station, where it was required for use in newly-installed de-sulphurisation equipment.

With National Power having concerns about privatisation and disruption to supplies, it took delivery of a further five Class 59/2s, 59202-06, in August 1995 along with 85 JMA bogie hoppers. The commodity being targeted this time was coal, with trains envisaged as principally operating from the vast Gascoigne Wood complex near Selby to various power stations belonging to the company. Operations commenced that November, mainly to Drax and Eggborough.

Special trains

One of the first sales in the embryonic privatisation process was the InterCity Charter Unit, this passing to the ownership of Waterman Railways from April 1995, although initial agreement for the sale had been reached the previous May. This gave the company ownership of some 200 coaches, including the white-roofed VIP charter fleet, but also six of the ex push-pull Class 47/7s, 47701/03/05/09/10/12 being surrendered by Rail Express Systems. Ambitious plans to run some 1,500 specials a year were duly announced, these ranging from steam-haulage and landcruises to simple day trips and wine and dine excursions. Further locos were envisaged to be used as well, beginning with Class 46 'Peak' D172 *Ixion*, which had returned to action on the national network in 1994.

A new image was also rolled out, based on Pete Waterman's liking for the London & North Western Railway. Locos would receive all-over LNWR 'blackberry black' with light grey and red lining while three liveries were devised for coaching stock, these ranging from all over plum with lining for everyday stock though to 'plum and spilt milk' for some Mk.2 air-conditioned vehicles and finally the fully-lined West Coast Joint Stock scheme for premier charter vehicles and *Ixion's* support coach.

In the event, only 47703/05/10/12 would be repainted in black along with reinstated 47488. As part of a maintenance agreement with Rail Express Systems, the Waterman Class 47s could be used as needed on mail trains when not required for charter traffic. Sadly, the early optimism soon evaporated as politics, red tape and ever increasing access charges took their toll with Waterman Railways broken up during 1996/97, the bulk of the coaches passing to Rail Charter Services and most of the Class 47s to Fragonset.

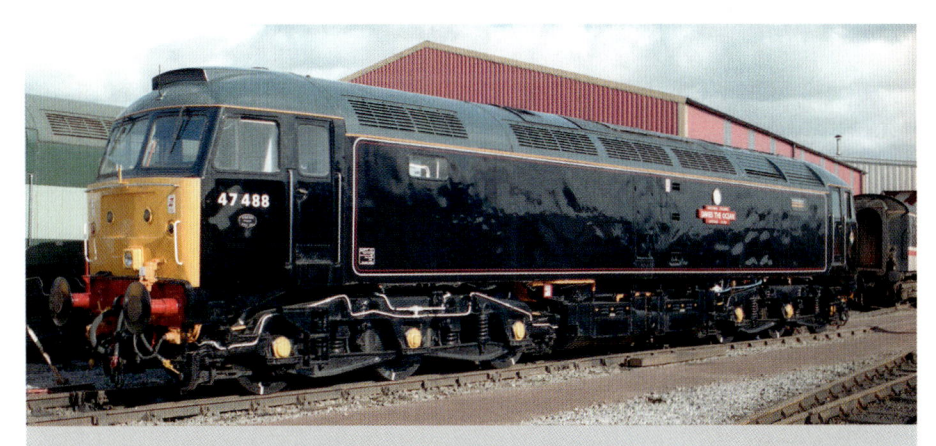

ABOVE: The Waterman Railways livery was a simple but stylish affair, as seen on newly-repainted 47488 *Davies The Ocean* at The Railway Age, Crewe, on March 18, 1995. The loco would spend part of the year and 1996 as well on hire to Cardiff Valleys as loco-hauled workings returned to the Rhymney line to increase capacity. The loco had been withdrawn from the RES fleet in October 1993 before passing to Waterman ownership, it being reinstated to work alongside the six tired Class 47/7s that came with the purchase of the InterCity Charter Unit. *Simon Bendall Collection*

Modelling BR Locomotives of the 1990s **55**

Out of the shadows

RIGHT: **It may be Christmas Eve 1996, but London's refuse still needs disposing of to landfill as 60044** *Ailsa Craig* **passes Kempston with the 6A61 08.25 Cricklewood to Forders Sidings 'binliner',** where the containers would be emptied into the pits of a former brickworks. Like the other London-based trains, this was formed of FUA/FYA container flats renumbered from FFA/FGA, as produced to a high standard in 4mm by Bachmann albeit with slightly different bogies. The leading container, complete with obsolete Trainload Construction logos, was used during propelling moves at the sidings, giving the shunter somewhere to ride and control the brakes. The distinctive refuse containers are available as resin castings in 4mm scale from Harburn Hobbies, albeit without the nameboards. Only three Class 60s received the attractive Mainline blue livery, the others being 60011 and 60078.
Martin Loader

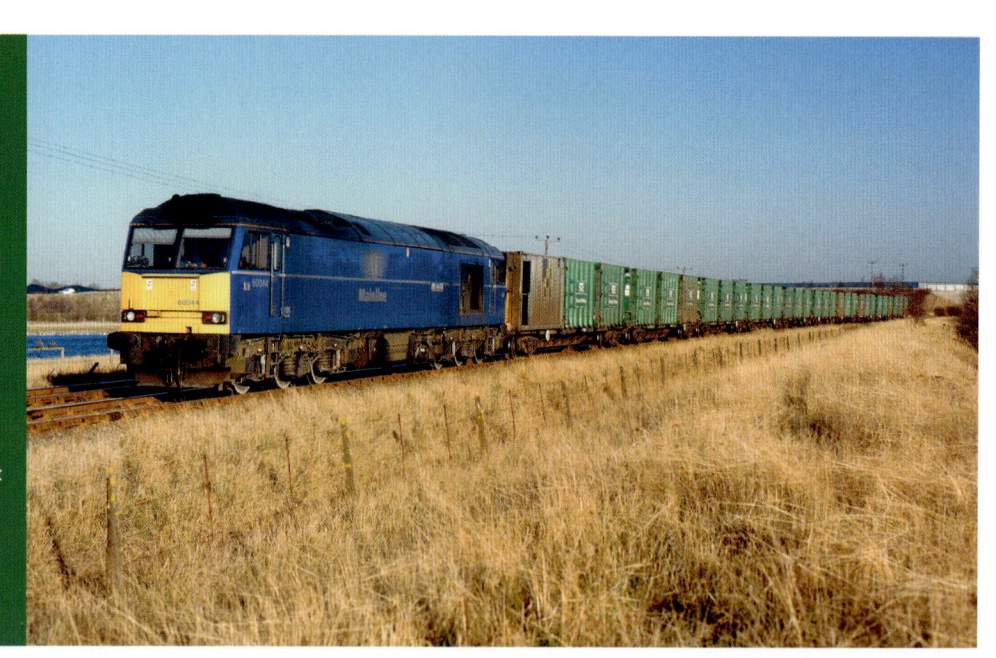

RIGHT: **With Toton Yard in the background and the TMD in the far distance, Loadhaul-liveried 37513 gets underway with the 6T18 08.00 departure to Chaddesden Yard, Derby, on July 13, 1999.** The train of two-axle ballast wagons is carrying spoil and features a mix of BR and privatisation era types. Making up the former are the engineers' grey/yellow-liveried ZBA Rudd, which are available in 4mm from Hornby and as a kit from Parkside but currently not in 2mm. The Railtrack green-liveried PNAs were built on a wide range of donor chassis with Bachmann offering a couple of variants in OO while in 2mm, the N Gauge Society offers a simple kit for another. Finally, the EWS wagons are MHA Coalfish built on HAA chassis, these being the earlier body variant as produced by Hornby in OO gauge rather than the later version with less ribs as newly released by Accurascale. Again, this is a gap that **remains in 2mm.** Paul Robertson

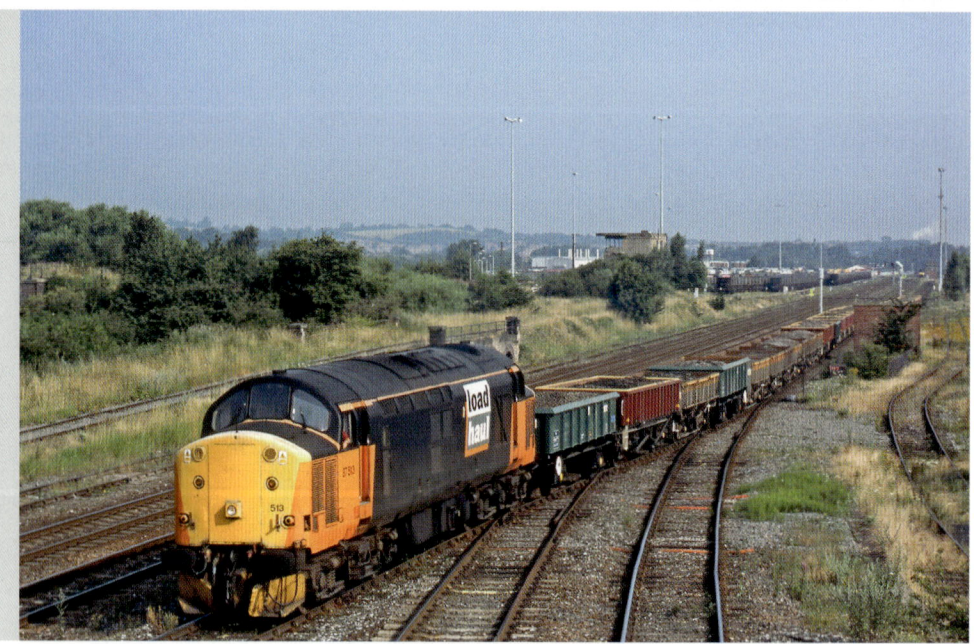

RIGHT: **Following the traction reallocation between the three regional freight companies, the heavy freight Type 5s could often find themselves deployed on workings that did not require their full capabilities, which was something that continued under EWS. One such occasion is illustrated on June 15, 1996, as Romanian-built 56025 heads the 6E41 13.24 Warrington Arpley to Dee Marsh 'Enterprise' trip,** the timber being destined for Shotton paper mill. Timber had been removed from Railfreight Distribution's portfolio in 1994 as had the OTA wagons as the core workings at the time fell squarely within Transrail territory. On this day, all nine of the wagons were converted OCAs, which are available from Hornby and as a kit from Cambrian in 4mm while Chivers Finelines does a 2mm kit. Bachmann also offers a 4mm model, this depicting the OTAs converted from VDA vans, the two types usually mixing together.
Martin Loader

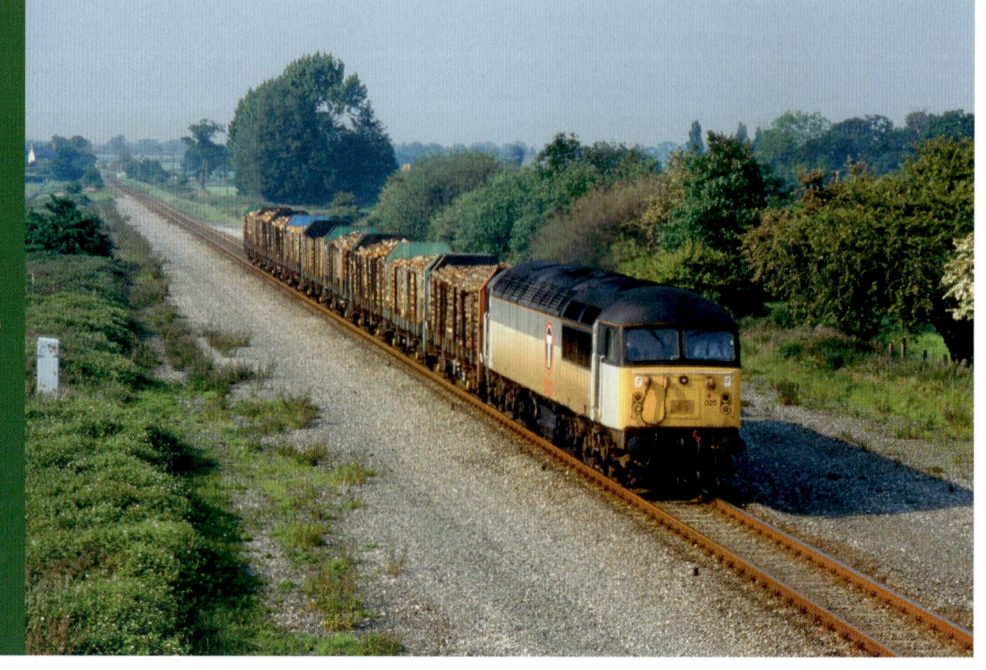

Out of the shadows

Freightliner reborn

As part of the set-up for privatisation, the decision was once again taken to separate Freightliner from Railfreight Distribution, creating an independent company. The division also saw the locomotive fleet split between the two, the newcomer taking both diesels and electrics as Simon Bendall details while Timara Easter re-liveries a Bachmann Class 90.

As part of the privatisation process of British Rail, June 1995 saw the Freightliner container division separated from Railfreight Distribution, reversing the merger of seven years earlier, as the intention was to sell the two freight units as separate companies. Predominately responsible for the movement of deep sea containers, Freightliner passed into private ownership in May 1996, the protracted process seeing the company secured by a management buyout with backing coming from private investment groups. Notably, Freightliner was the only one of the main BR freight businesses not to pass into the control of EWS.

As part of the divesting procedure, Freightliner was given a share of the Railfreight Distribution locomotive fleet. However, while this included ten of the then still relatively new Class 90s along with the bulk of the Class 86/6s, the company, despite strong protests, was lumbered with the dregs of the Class 47 fleet, with many of the Type 4s long overdue for works overhauls and in generally desperate external condition. Upon completion of the 1996 buyout, Freightliner sold all 70 of the locos in its fleet, along with 345 wagons, to Porterbrook in a lease-back agreement in order to raise finance for investment. Some of this was duly used to further expand the motive power roster in the form of additional Class 47s acquired from EWS and Railfreight Distribution along with the remainder of the Class 86/6s.

Following the split from Railfreight Distribution in 1995 and prior to the company's sale, a new image was adopted for Freightliner, although, in reality, it was actually the fusion of two existing schemes. In terms of paintwork, the Railfreight triple grey livery was retained, primarily because the vast majority of the loco fleet was already in the scheme. In theory, this would simply allow the removal of sub-sector emblems and their replacement with new Freightliner logos. However, such was the shabby condition of the fleet that largely without exception, locos received a full repaint into triple grey anyway. This provided the somewhat bizarre spectacle of Class 47s and Class 86/6s that had previously swapped triple grey for the Railfreight Distribution European scheme being returned to triple grey again.

Heritage re-called

For its new logo, Freightliner dipped into its past and adopted the red triangle emblem that had appeared on containers during the late 1970s along with the bold black lettering of the same period. The new livery made its public debut in August 1995 at the Crewe Basford Hall open weekend, 47376 being named *Freightliner 1995*. By the end of the year, it had been joined by 47157, 47270 and 47301.

Repaints of Freightliner's two AC electric classes commenced at the end of 1995 with 86637 the first to be outshopped. Notably the work was contracted out to Waterman Railways, the locos being re-liveried at its workshops at The Railway Age, Crewe. The first four months of 1996 saw half of the Class 90 fleet treated in the form of 90143/46-48/50 but well over a year passed before the other five machines, 90141/42/44/45/49, were similarly repainted, by which time their dirty and unbranded triple grey was a poor advert for the company.

Somewhat surprisingly, many of the repainted AC electrics initially retained their cast BR arrows and Crewe Electric depot plaques even after repainting while, in contrast, only 47301 and 47376 initially kept their Crewe Diesel plaques among the Class 47s. Another 40 or so of the Type 4s would be painted over the next three years with 15 more Class 86s completed. The use of the triple grey livery ceased in the second half of 1998 following the introduction of the new green and yellow scheme on re-engined 57001.

Modifications reversed

When acquired by Freightliner, the ten Class 90s were still in their freight-only specification with the electric train supply isolated and 75mph speed restriction in place. However, opportunities to hire the locos to passenger operators to bolster their own fleets would soon arise, beginning in 1999 when 90142 and 90146 were periodically loaned to Virgin Trains for use on West Coast services.

This saw the ETS equipment recommissioned, and speed restriction lifted, although the retractable buffers and central rubbing plate were not reinstated. The duo was also not initially renumbered back to their original numbers of 90042 and 90046 despite the reversal of the alterations, this finally taking place in 2001, the year before their hire ended.

The start of the 2000s brought further loan opportunities with both GNER and Anglia Railways to, respectively, cover for Class 91s undergoing overhaul and poor availability of the Class 86s. As a result, Freightliner took the decision to reinstate the ETS and 100 mph maximum speed on all of its remaining Class 90s, renumbering back to 90041/43-45/48-50 taking place in the summer of 2002. The odd loco out was 90147, which did not revert to 90047 until the end of 2004 as it returned from long-term repairs to fire damage.

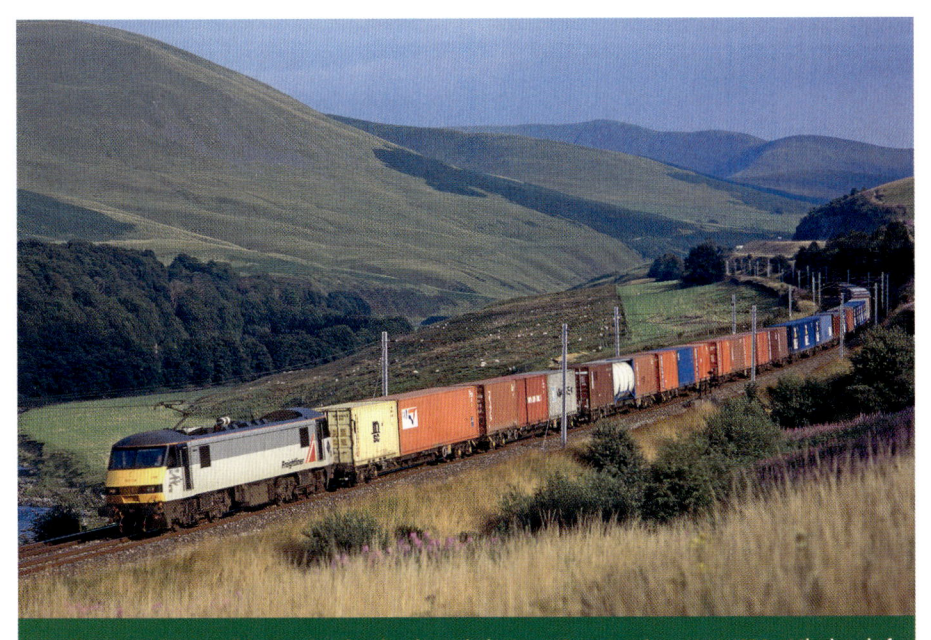

ABOVE: In perfect conditions, 90145 hurries through the Lune Gorge on August 14, 1996, at the head of the 4S87 Felixstowe to Coatbridge, the visible load mostly being 20ft boxes with the odd 40ft example also present along with a single tank-tainer. The leading ten wagons are all FSA flats formed as twin-sets, these dating from the start of the decade and still carrying their Railfreight Distribution logos. A RTR model of these is under development in both N and OO by Realtrack Models. *David Dockray*

Out of the shadows

Modelling the red triangle

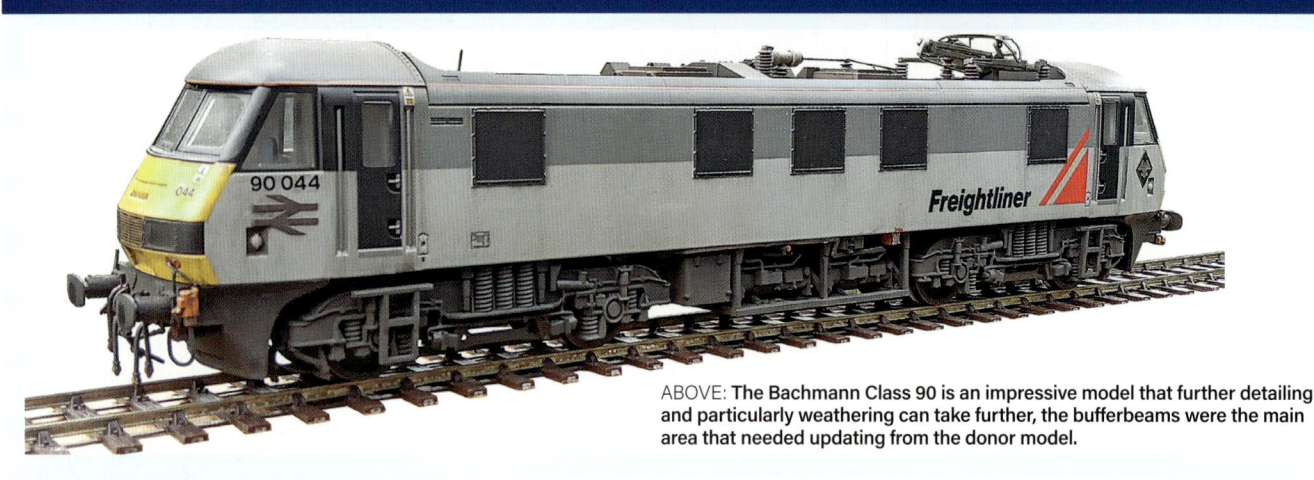

ABOVE: The Bachmann Class 90 is an impressive model that further detailing and particularly weathering can take further, the bufferbeams were the main area that needed updating from the donor model.

Like many modellers of AC electrics, I had been eagerly awaiting the arrival of Bachmann's OO gauge Class 90. Not long after the models appeared, a friend commissioned me to model a Freightliner grey example, this being depicted during the mid-2000s and following re-numbering back to '90/0' condition. Bringing the model forward in period was fairly straightforward with only a few detail changes required to reflect the period modelled.

On the body, the printed Railfreight Distribution markings came off without much in the way of fuss, being carefully scraped away with a home-made chisel-cum-scraper and the remainder was wiped off with Microsol. Replacement Freightliner transfers came from the Fox range as well as the cabside numbers, while the supplied etched double arrows were retained, and Shawplan Crewe Electric depot plaques fitted.

The only major livery difference was with the cab corner pillars, which needed to be repainted black instead of yellow. Post-1998 overhead warning flashes from the Modelmaster range were added where appropriate. At the No.1 end, the upper elements of the horn grille were carefully bent down to represent damage as these occasionally suffered from bird strikes. The TDM cable receptacles were also relocated to the revised position on the sides of the bufferbeams with replacement cables made from fine wire.

ABOVE: Several of the Freightliner Class 90s retained the triple grey livery until relatively recently, 90044 going straight to the current orange and black in January 2020.

Freight specification

Moving to the chassis, the gangway rubbing plates and associated mounting points were very carefully removed from the bufferbeams, so as to preserve the triangular baseplates, which remain clearly visible on the majority of the fleet. The excellent Hornby Class 60 buffers were chosen to represent the clipped oval style used after 1993 for freight-only locos.

Weathering was relatively straightforward with a coat or two of Johnson's Klear floor polish applied first to protect the transfers. The slab-sided nature of the bodysides means that there is nowhere apart from the grilles for dirt to collect. The main job was therefore to add lots of vertical streaking, especially under the corners of each grille. Several fine misted coats of dirt were airbrushed on and washed off with white spirit until the desired effect was attained.

The chassis was mostly weathered with the bodyshell removed before being reunited for a final quick waft to homogenise everything. Some paint was stippled on the faces of the buffers and a few areas dry-brushed, such as the bogie steps.

Model availability

In OO gauge, a Class 90 was first released by Hornby around 1989 and this continues to serve in the range today. Bachmann's version with all the expected modern refinements debuted in 2019 and has quickly appeared in many of the key liveries from the 1990s, including the initial trio of schemes: InterCity Swallow, Mainline, and Railfreight Distribution. This has been recently followed by Rail Express Systems and Freightliner triple grey, although the latter is with factory-applied weathering. Considerably older and much less-refined is the N gauge offering that resided in the Graham Farish range, this having appeared in most of the key sector colours over its lifetime. Now discontinued, it can still be found second-hand.

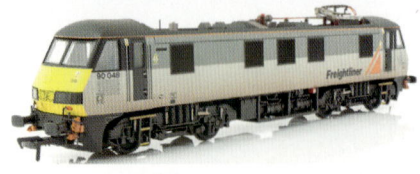

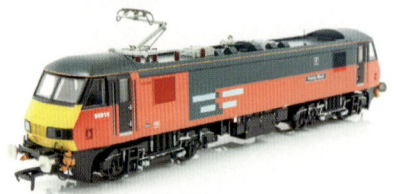

ABOVE: The class looked good in Rail Express Systems colours; 90016-20 all being painted in 1991/92 with some lasting into the mid-2000s. The Bachmann model is of 90019 *Penny Black*.

LEFT: Somewhat ironically, a Freightliner triple grey example has now appeared in Bachmann's range, although this portrays 90048 in more recent years with the BR arrows and Crewe depot plaques removed and the scars painted over. The company's 'zero injuries' safety slogan is also carried by the cab doors. The loco was only repainted in orange in June 2021.

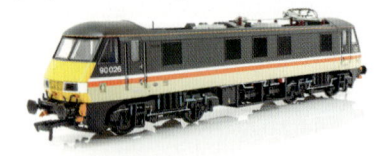

ABOVE: Often over-looked, it was pleasing to see the Bachmann model appear in Mainline colours so early in its production run, Applied to just 11 locos, 90026-36, when built, the model is of the first of the batch, which was repainted in RfD in January 1993. *All images courtesy Kernow Model Rail Centre*

Out of the shadows

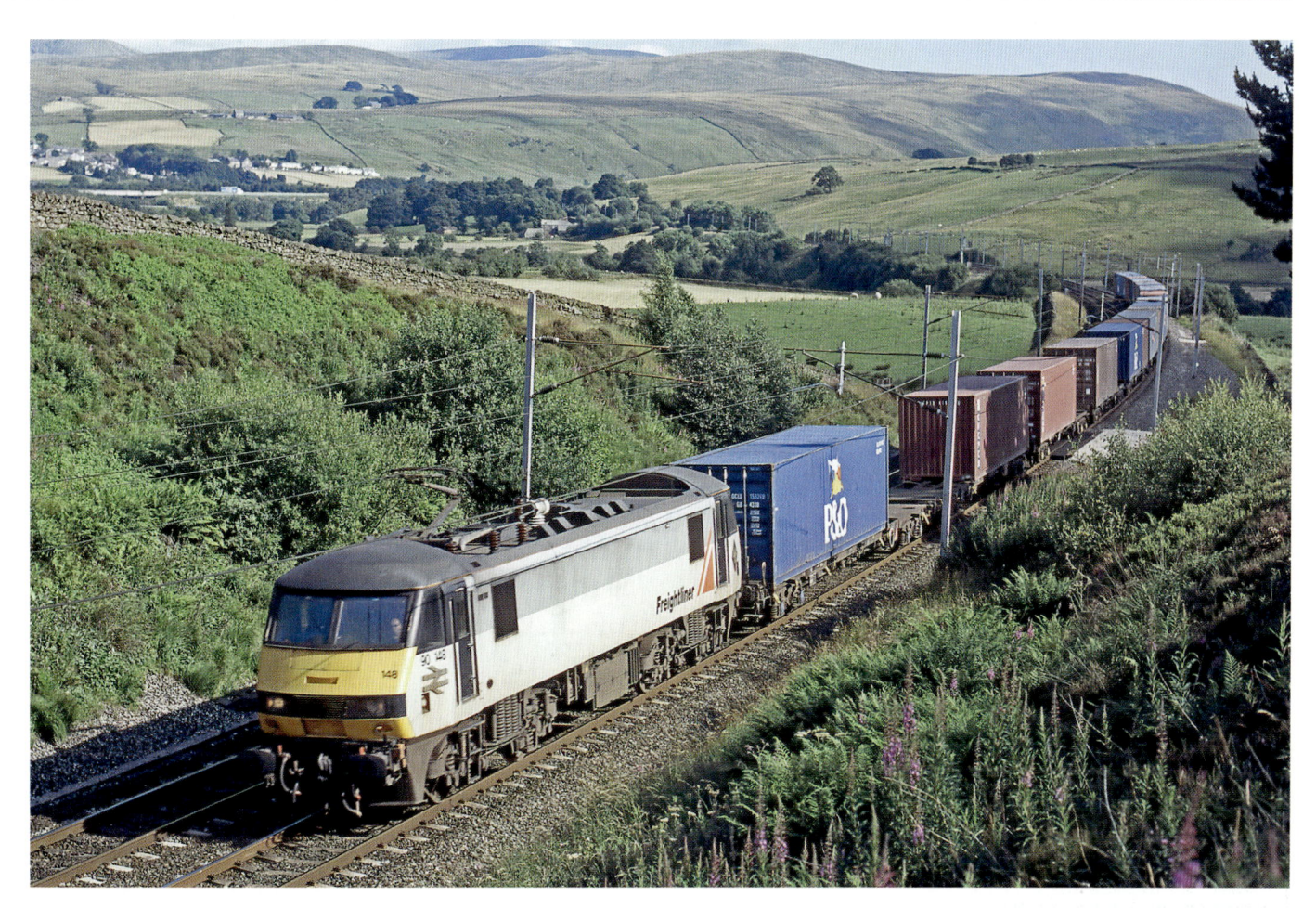

ABOVE: Another Freightliner working traverses the northern fells of the West Coast Main Line as 90148 passes Greenholme on the climb to Shap on July 20, 2000. It was in charge of the 16.18 Crewe Basford Hall-Coatbridge, the relatively short train again being formed of FSA outer and FTA inner 60ft flats but with Freightliner logo panels having replaced the original RfD ones. Repainted four years earlier, the loco would carry the same colours for a further 21 years. *John Chalcraft/Rail Photoprints*

RIGHT: With P&O containers prominent among the load, 90150 hums past Slindon on May 15, 1997, with the 4M54 12.35 Tilbury to Basford Hall. Again, a relatively short working, the visible portion is headed by an FSA twin-set then an FSA-FTA-FTA-FSA quad-set and another empty twin. Also notable amongst the boxes are the two open 40ft containers with high ends carrying substantial timber baulks. The loco would suffer serious fire damage in September 2004 and never work again. *Martin Loader*

RIGHT: Newly returned to Class 1 passenger action with Virgin Trains, 90142 propels the 15.45 Liverpool Lime Street to Euston through Castlethorpe on July 17, 1999, following the reinstatement of its ETS ability and maximum speed. Two years later, it would be doing much the same work for GNER partnered with Mk.4 sets. In OO gauge, Virgin-liveried Mk.3s have most recently been released by Oxford Rail with the DVT previously produced by Hornby. In N gauge, Dapol has released both the DVT and Mk.3s with Graham Farish just offering the passenger stock. *Antony Guppy*

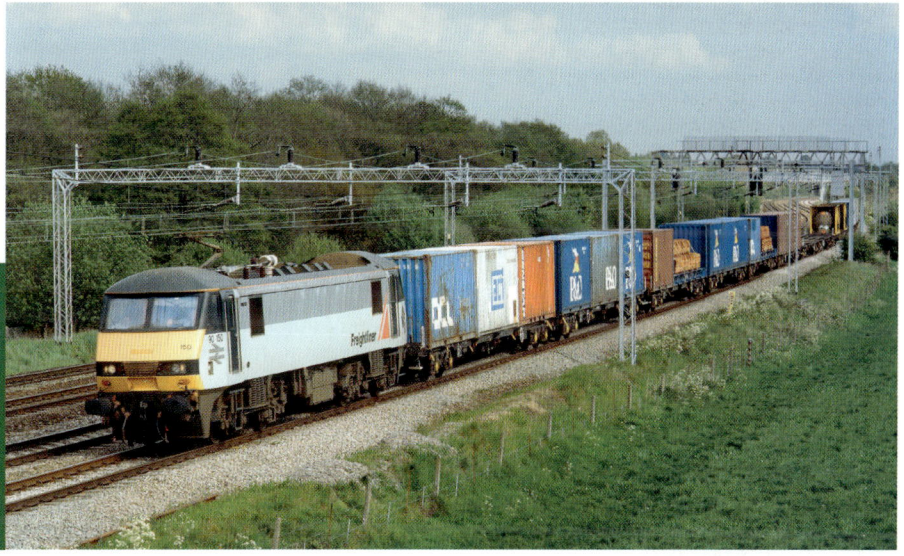

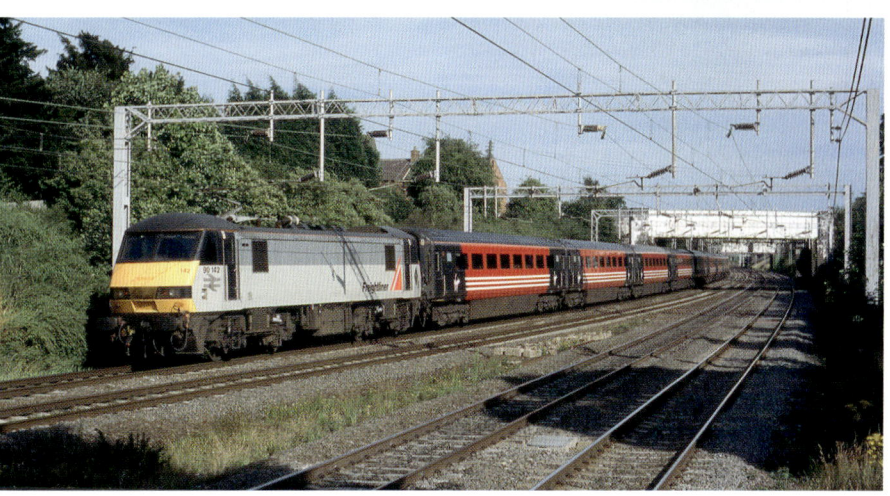

Modelling BR Locomotives of the 1990s 59

Out of the shadows

Channel carriers

With a bright future predicted for international freight services, the dual-voltage Class 92s were built to haul such traffic through the Channel Tunnel and onwards to UK destinations, as well as the 'Nightstar' sleeper services. Simon Bendall **details the type's early years while** James Makin **gets to work on the new OO gauge Accurascale model.**

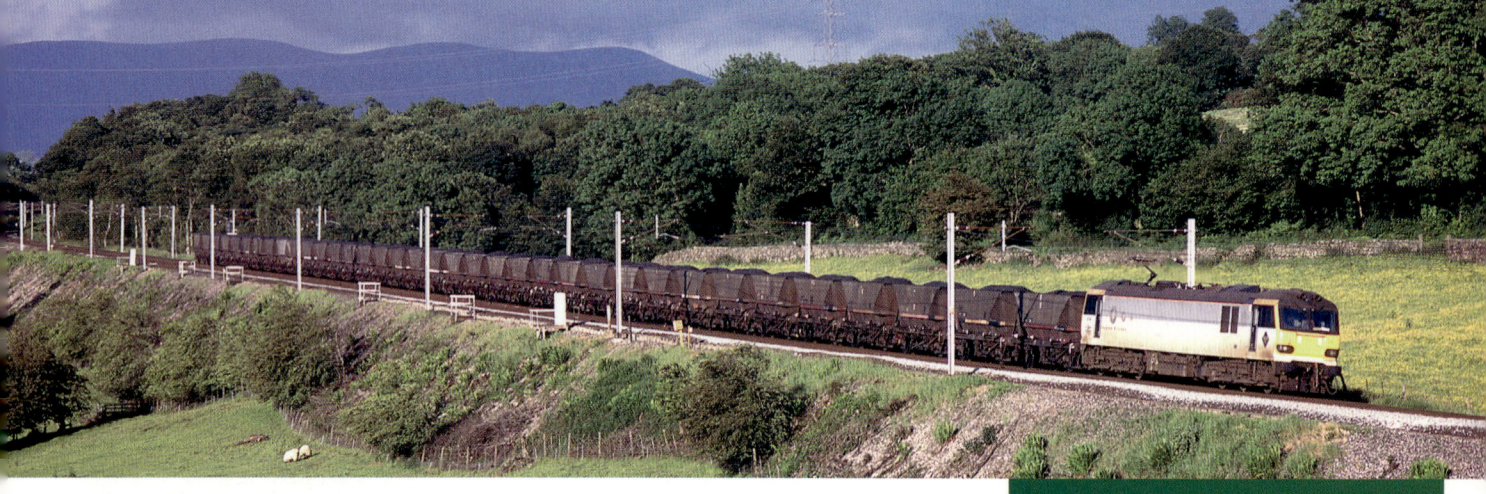

ABOVE: **The use of Class 92s on power station coal trains over the northern section of the West Coast Main Line was not uncommon under EWS ownership, their immense power aiding the climb over Shap, particularly on the loaded southbound workings. On June 14, 2000, 92041** Vaughan Williams **was in charge of just such a train as it passes Mealbank, near Kendal, which it would have worked between Carlisle and Warrington Arpley.** David Dockray

It was December 1993 when the first completed Class 92s were rolled out from the Loughborough workshops of Brush Traction, 92001 and 92002 heralding the arrival of the 46-strong fleet of electric locos designed for use through the Channel Tunnel. Ordered three and a half years earlier, they would become the last locos to be delivered to British Rail and also its most complex.

The Class 92s were the result of a development process that had begun some six years earlier to design and build a loco that would not only comply with the stringent safety and technical standards that would come to be applied to the Channel Tunnel but also be capable of operating on both the UK and French rail networks. The result was the largest electric loco yet seen in this country with the ability to work off both the 750V DC third rail system and 25kV AC overhead electrification.

Ownership was split between three operators with Railfreight Distribution (RfD) taking the bulk of the class in 92001-05/07-09/11-13/15-17/19/22/24-27/29-31/34-37/39/41/42 while French national operator SNCF took 92006/10/14/18/23/28/33/38/43. These were intended for use on freight trains while the remaining seven locos, 92020/21/32/40/44-46, were assigned to European Passenger Services (EPS) for use on the proposed overnight sleeper services from the UK regions to Europe, which were to be branded as 'Nightstar'.

Prolonged acceptance

The Class 92s were unfortunate to arrive at the same time as the rail industry was broken up for privatisation, this putting Railtrack in charge of the infrastructure and creating all manner of red tape for the acceptance of new vehicles when the expertise to manage the process efficiently was not necessarily there. As a result, the first run of a Class 92 under its own power on the UK network did not occur until November 1994 between Carnforth and Carlisle, while Channel Tunnel testing commenced early in 1995. The latter was satisfactorily completed by that March, allowing the class to commence freight operations between the yards at Dollands Moor and Frethun.

In contrast, it was a further 16 months before the Class 92s were approved to work on the third rail network, July 1996 bringing acceptance to run between Dollands Moor and Wembley Yard in North London. The same period had seen the last of the class, 92046, accepted for traffic following its release from Loughborough at the start of the year. Almost two more years would elapse before clearance was finally given in May 1998 for the electric locos to run under their own power on the West Coast Main Line, all transfers prior to this seeing the locos hauled dead in tow between depots.

However, while all of the class were in service, freight traffic levels were far below expectations while the 'Nightstar' operation had been abandoned in 1997 before a single passenger train had run due to concerns about viability in the face of competition from the budget airlines. The Railfreight Distribution fleet was also now under EWS ownership while the EPS operation was now restructured as Eurostar UK Ltd.

The seven Class 92s owned by Eurostar were stood down in April 2001 after EWS ceased to use them and four have not worked since. Similarly, SNCF stored its nine locos early in 2006, leaving EWS as the sole operator of Channel Tunnel freight traffic into the new century.

Livery alterations

All 46 Class 92s were delivered in the European Passenger Services livery of two-tone grey bodysides with a dark blue roof, this being a simple development from the existing Railfreight triple grey, just with a change of roof colour. All carried the Channel Tunnel 'polo mint' roundels on the bodysides and Crewe Electric depot plaques but only those owned by Railfreight Distribution featured cast BR arrows on the driver's cabsides, these being 92001-05/07-09/11-13/15-17/19/22/24-27/29-31/34-37/39/41/42. Eight of the French examples, 92006/10/14/18/23/28/33/43, instead carried cabside SNCF logos with 92038 the odd one out as it was never so branded.

The EPS examples were the least consistent in how they were branded, 92021 and 92040 both having silver logos on the cabsides while 92032/44-46 had nothing at all. More complex was 92020, which had EPS branding on the cabsides but also SNCF logos and Railfreight Distribution sub-sector emblems at opposite ends of the bodysides, it carried all three due to previous involvement in a handover ceremony in 1995. Its EPS logos would be removed within a couple of years but the other two remained until 2017. Again due to their involvement in ceremonies when still new, 92009, 92022 and 92030 gained Railfreight Distribution lettering and logos on their lower bodysides as well as red-backed cast nameplates, the latter also appearing on SNCF's 92023.

The first complete repaint occurred in the summer of 1998 with 92001 receiving EWS maroon and gold. The colours would only be applied to one more of the class, 92031 being repainted for its naming ceremony in June 2001.

60 www.keymodelworld.com

Out of the shadows

RIGHT: **The lightweight load bound for Mossend, will hardly trouble 92037** *Sullivan* **as it passes Shap Beck on August 22, 1998.** The three sets of FIA intermodal twins feature a single swapbody container and two transport flats loaded with pipes of different diameters, the smaller ones being coated while the larger size is unprotected and with surface rust as a result. These wagons are available in 2mm from Graham Farish and 4mm from Bachmann. Making up the rear of the train is a set of FHA 'Eurospine' wagons, these four-element vehicles being designed to carry specialised lorry trailers using the 'piggyback' concept. Owned by EWS, they only found use carrying Parcelforce trailers between London and Glasgow for a few years and it is this traffic in which they are pictured. No models of these are currently available in any scale. David Dockray

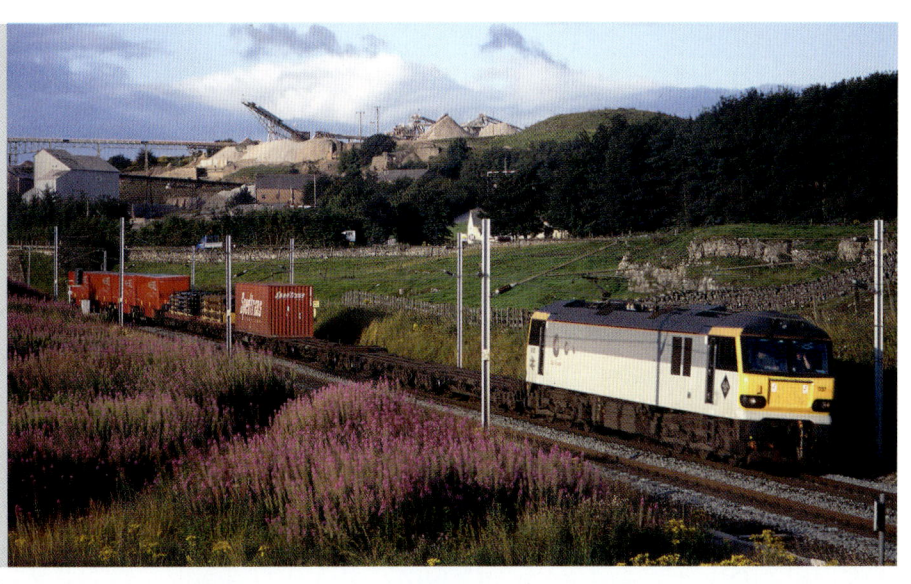

RIGHT: **It was not until May 1998 that the Class 92s received approval from Railtrack to run under their own power on the West Coast Main Line,** finally allowing the locos to move from their maintenance base at Crewe Electric to Dollands Moor and vice versa without being hauled by, typically, a Railfreight Distribution Class 47. Five months after this freedom was granted, 92009 *Elgar* leads 92038 *Voltaire*, 92029 *Dante*, 92046 *Sweelinck* and 92023 *Ravel* through Wandsworth Road on October 29. At this time, the class was effectively common user, allowing this mix of Railfreight Distribution, SNCF, and Eurostar (ex EPS) examples to run together. John Chalcraft/Rail Photoprints

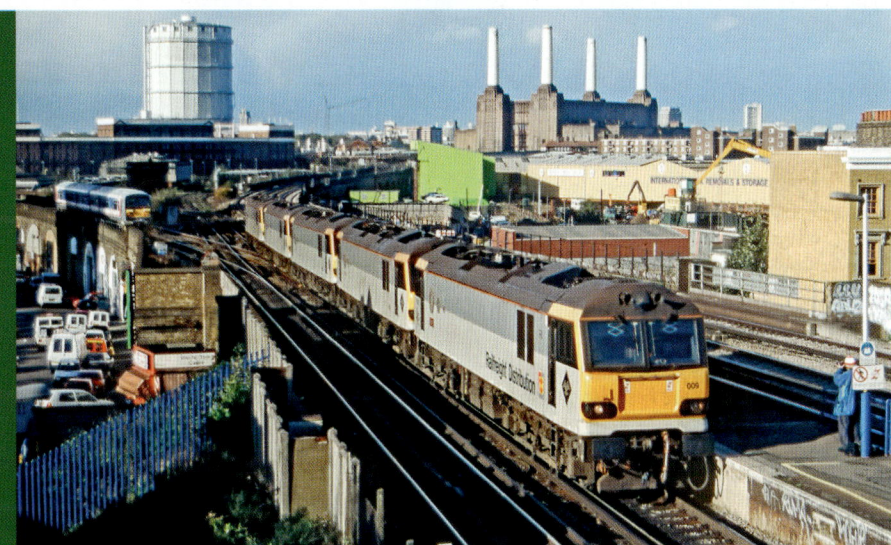

Model availability

In OO gauge, competing RTR models of the Class 92s arrived about the same time as the real thing, both Hornby and Lima going head to head to produce British Rail's final locomotive class. For many, the Italian offering was the best, both in terms of decoration and moulding quality. Today, it this model that resides in Hornby's range, its original tooling having long been retired.

The new Accurascale model is therefore the third rendering in the scale, sporting all the detail expected of a current generation loco, both inside and out. Of the initial 11 releases, three are relevant to the 1990s period, including 92003 *Beethoven* and RfD-branded 92022 *Charles Dickens*. Finally, there is class pioneer 92001 *Victor Hugo* in EWS maroon and gold, as applied in 1998.

In N gauge, a similarly modern and well-specified model has been produced by Revolution Trains, the first batch appearing at the start of 2021. This also included 92003 and 92001 in the same colour schemes along with an un-numbered and un-named two-tone grey example to allow it to be finished as any member of the class desired.

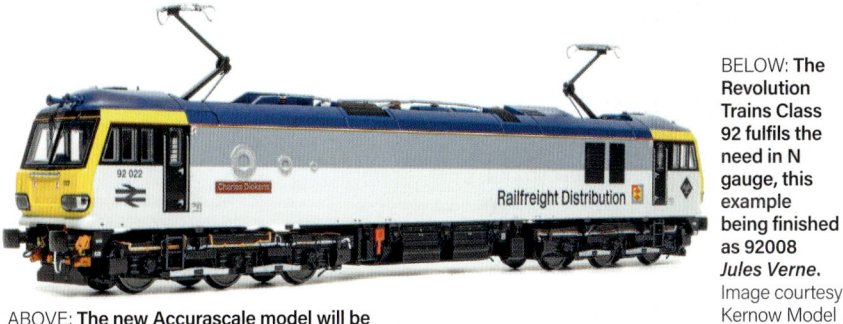

ABOVE: **The new Accurascale model will be available as 92022** *Charles Dickens*, **which was one of the few to be upgraded to cast nameplates and also receive bodyside RfD brandings.**

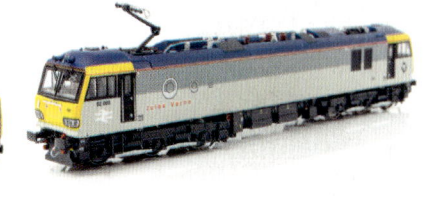

BELOW: **The Revolution Trains Class 92 fulfils the need in N gauge, this example being finished as 92008** *Jules Verne*. Image courtesy Kernow Model Rail Centre

LEFT: **Looking striking in EWS livery, 92001** *Victor Hugo* **was one of just two examples to receive the colours, their application causing some disquiet from the French at the time for what was a common-user fleet.**

Modelling BR Locomotives of the 1990s **61**

Out of the shadows

European enhancement

BELOW: **The weathering brings out the detail yet further on the Accurascale Class 92, this being finished as 92038 *Voltaire*. Although originally an SNCF-owned example, it was the only one not to carry the company's logos.**

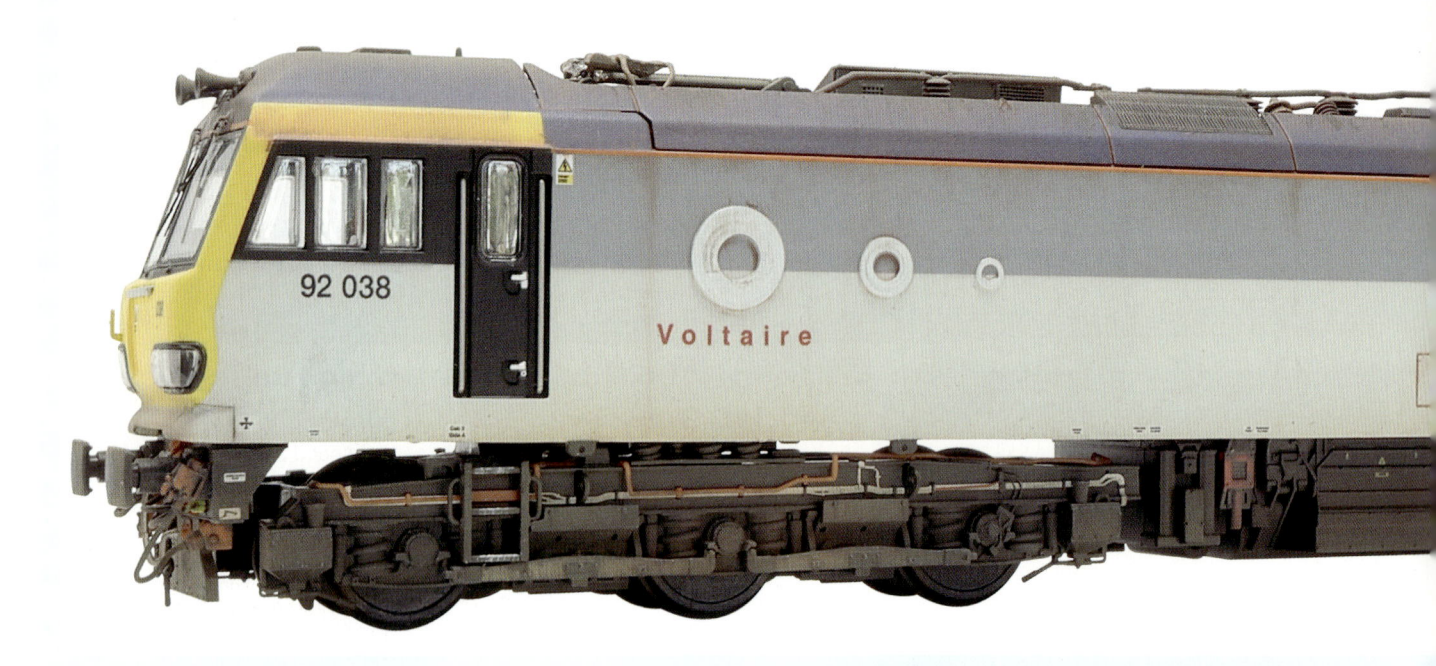

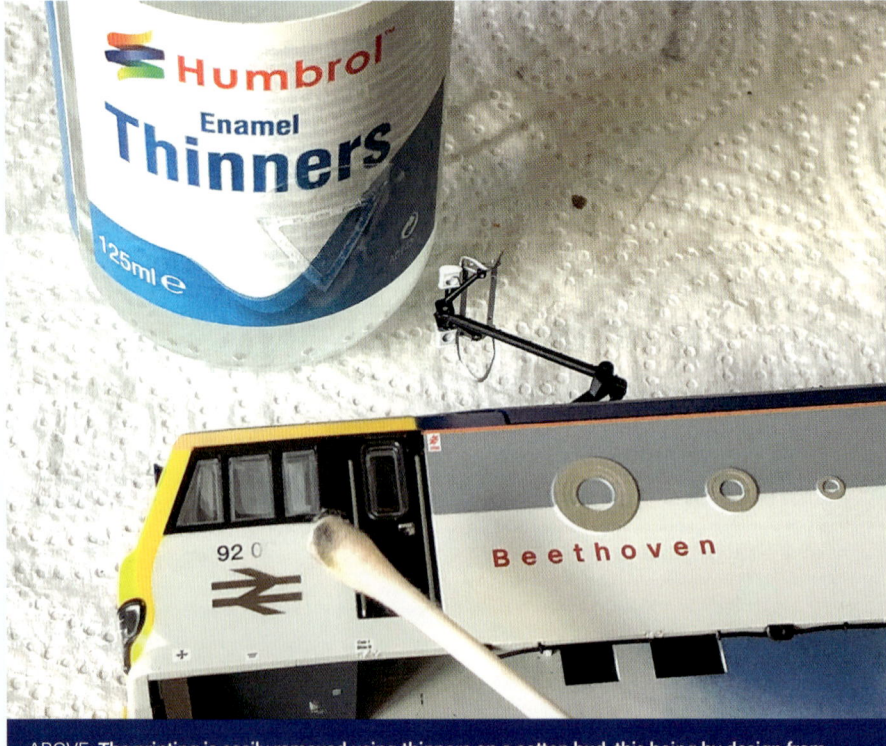

ABOVE: **The printing is easily removed using thinners on a cotton bud, this being by design from Accurascale to facilitate easy identity changes.**

With today's super-high specification models, it can be easy to think that some of the traditional fun of detailing locomotives has been lost, or that there is no scope for undertaking any further work. However, this article aims to demonstrate that a whole lot of joy can be had from personalising an already great model to make it a unique gem in a collection. The OO gauge Accurascale Class 92 worked on here is a pre-production painted sample so please be aware that some details may differ from the final batch of production locomotives.

Probably the hardest decision of the entire project was to actually select which member of the class to model. Accurascale will be releasing a range of names and numbers in its first batch, covering a wide range of liveries and timescales. My own modelling preferences date back to the late 1990s and early 2000s, when the class was in its infancy and just spreading its wings across the country, so an example in the original EPS two-tone grey livery was a must-have.

The names were a striking feature of the Class 92s, each receiving a cultural name that honoured composers, writers and so forth, so those with a real interest in this area can go to town on dedicating their models to their favourite cultural icons. Not quite being a man of culture myself, I just opted for 92038 *Voltaire*, simply as it was a loco that seemed to turn up at a variety of places during my trainspotting days!

Getting started

The Accurascale model was easy to take apart; a set of clips holds the bodyshell to the chassis and the cab interiors can be removed easily to allow the fitting of a driver later on. Care was taken to mask off each piece of glazing, including the light lenses, to protect these parts during the modelling process. Humbrol Maskol masking fluid was used for these elements along with Tamiya low-tack masking tape to protect the inside of the glazing.

As part of the identity change, the existing branding had to be removed. Given that this was a brand new product from a still relatively new firm, there was some trepidation in going about removing the existing name and number for fear of having to do a full repaint. Fortunately, I need not have worried as a cotton bud dipped in Humbrol enamel thinners made light work of the printing, which lifted in just seconds and left the underlying grey area in perfect condition.

62 www.keymodelworld.com

Out of the shadows

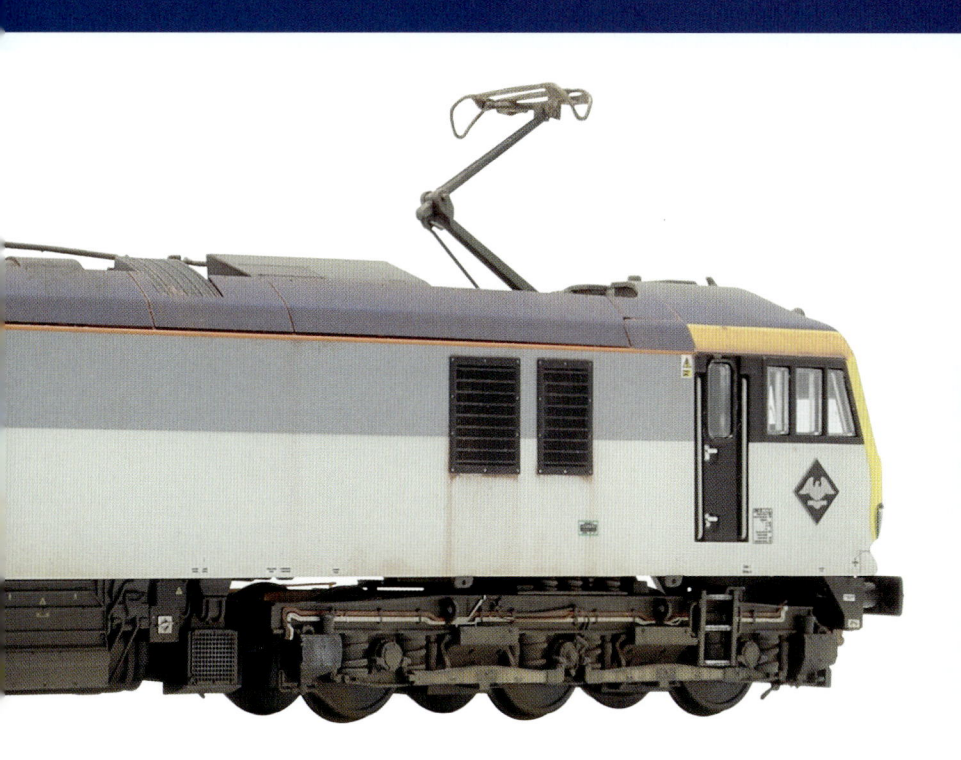

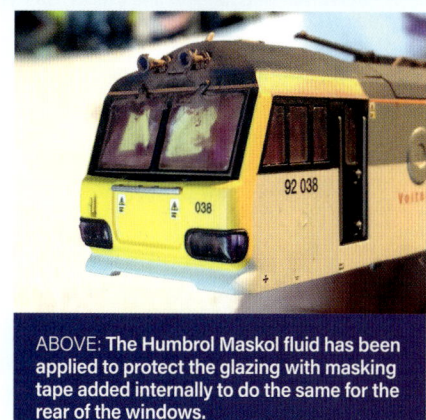

ABOVE: **The Humbrol Maskol fluid has been applied to protect the glazing with masking tape added internally to do the same for the rear of the windows.**

The donor model, 92003 *Beethoven*, was a version that already had etched BR arrows fitted but as my chosen prototype was an unbranded SNCF-owned example, these were gently removed with a curve-bladed scalpel. A small amount of paint came away with the glue, so this was gently touched in with Phoenix Precision's Great Western Trains silver-white and the whole bodyshell next given a coating of Railmatch gloss varnish.

Rebranding

Once the gloss varnish was dry, transfers could be added for the new name and number. These came from the Railtec range, the company offering a variety pack for certain class members as well as its new custom name and number sets that were recently announced. The waterslide decals sit nicely on the gloss finish of the bodysides while the overhead electrification flashes were also changed at this point, the model receiving the 1998-onwards revised yellow and white versions in place of the BR-era originals.

The bodyshell was then given a coat of matt varnish, again from the Railmatch range. My preference is for the aerosol version as it is a great way of quickly completing the task without resorting to airbrushing and the inevitable long clean-up stage afterwards! The varnished bodyshell was then left for a month to harden fully.

To start the weathering, an overall coating of Humbrol mid-brown (No.113) was applied, this being thinned to an approximately 70:30 ratio of paint to enamel thinners. This was liberally painted all across the roof and cantrail area of the model before being wiped away with a kitchen towel and cotton buds dipped in neat enamel thinners. Further paint was then removed by mottling on a paintbrush after it had been dipped in thinners, with the end result being a roof pantograph well

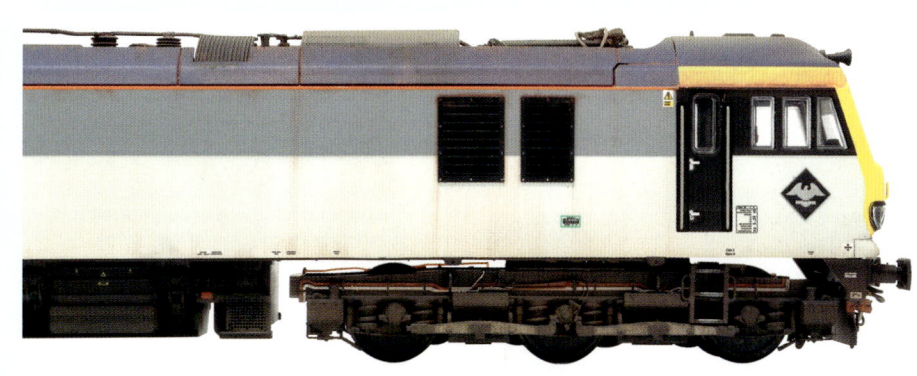

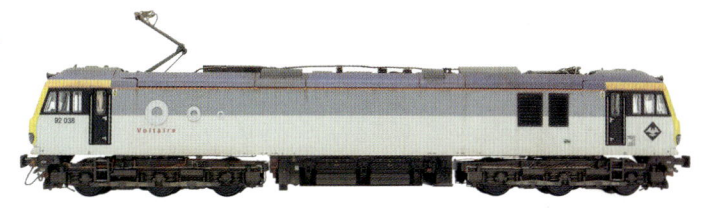

ABOVE: **The subtle streaking from the cantrail panel gaps and grilles is one of the main weathering effects that can be added, giving the model a look of a few years' service.**

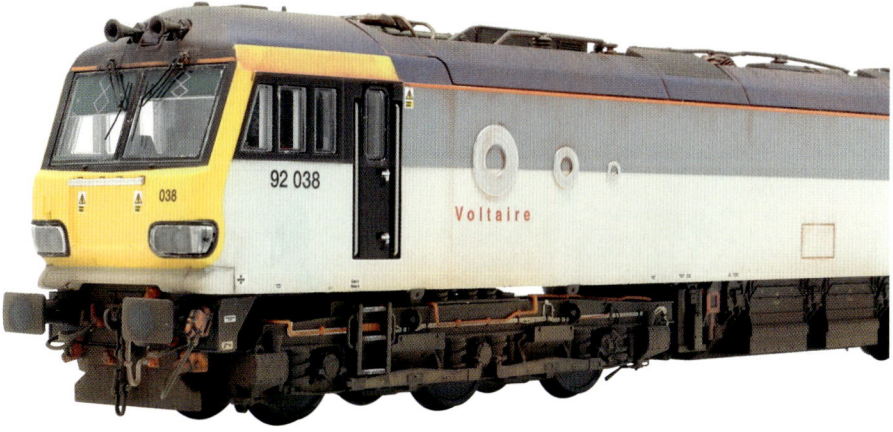

ABOVE: **The bufferbeam detailing fitted to 92038 is all supplied with the model, just requiring weathering to bring it to life. The windscreen blinds are homemade in two sizes and serve to bring further interest to the cab area.**

RIGHT: **The Class 92s were effectively designed to be two locos in one body to ensure reliability and the capacity to recover from failure while in the Channel Tunnel. This meant the body was largely a mirror image on the two sides.**

Modelling BR Locomotives of the 1990s 63

Out of the shadows

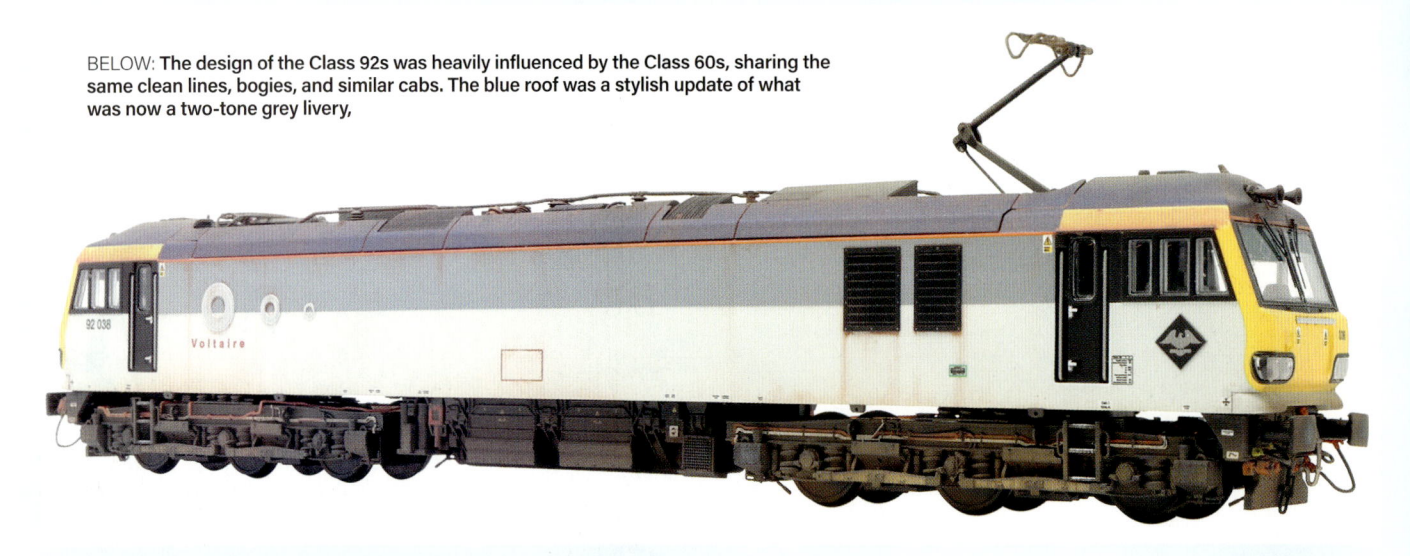

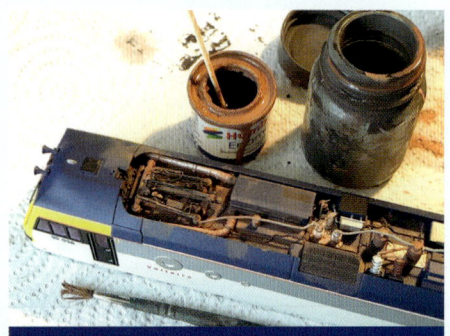

BELOW: The design of the Class 92s was heavily influenced by the Class 60s, sharing the same clean lines, bogies, and similar cabs. The blue roof was a stylish update of what was now a two-tone grey livery.

ABOVE: Both Fox and Railtec do the vinyl style of name used on the majority of the class, the replacement *Voltaire* transfers coming from the latter's range.

ABOVE: More detailed weathering of the roof components is in progress, this being a protracted process due to the need to treat all sides of the many parts.

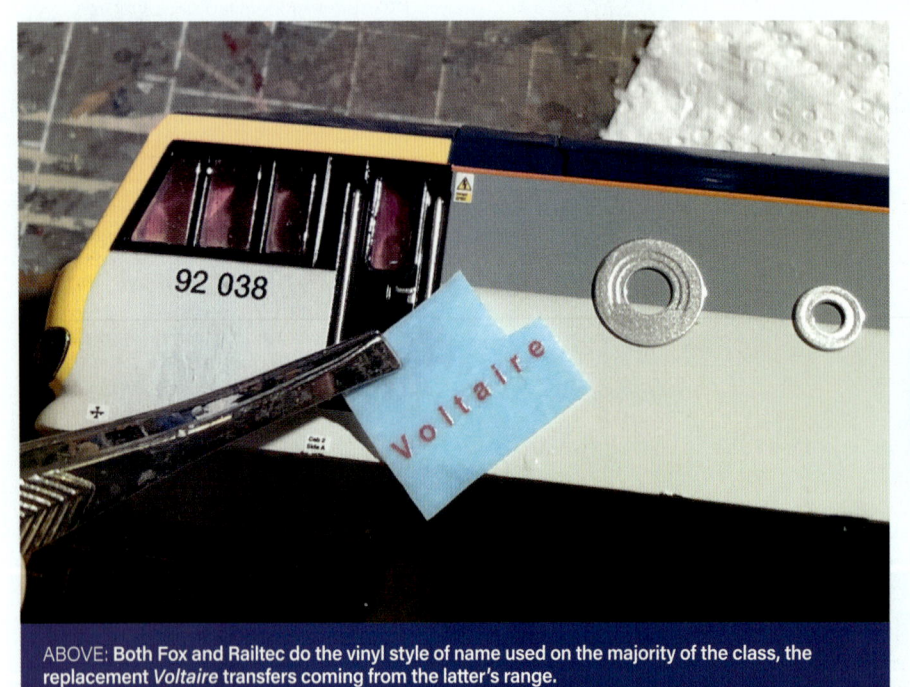

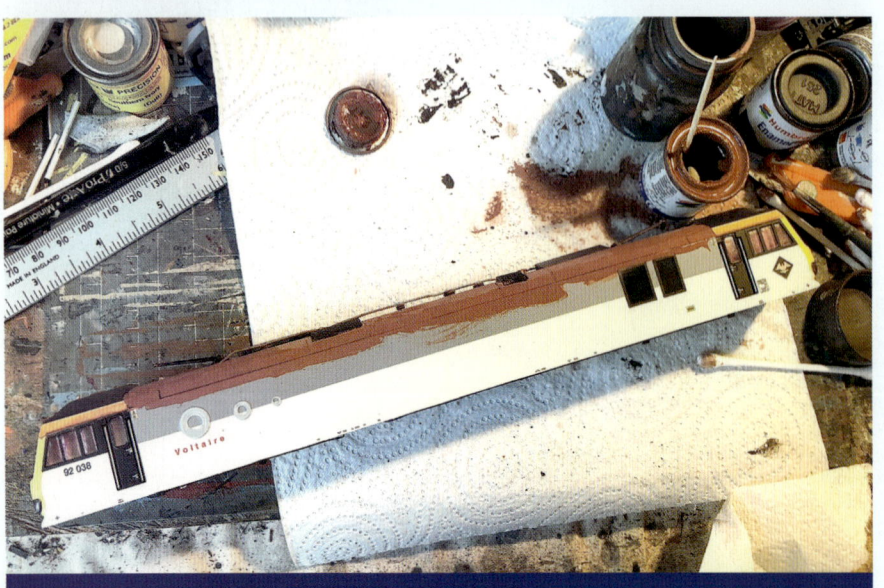

ABOVE: The thinned weathering wash has been applied to the cantrail sections. Although looking extreme, virtually all of this will be wiped away to just leave paint in the panel gaps and body crevasses.

that was generally clean in appearance but with grime gathered in sheltered areas.

Once left to dry thoroughly, this process was repeated with some other shades of sandy browns and darker browns, varying the amount removed so a layered effect was built-up on all the roof equipment. A lot of care was taken not to flood the fine etched grilles that can be found on Accurascale's model. The pantographs received an initial coating of dark brown paint followed by layers of darker browns and greys, which were then wiped away with cotton buds, leaving a multi-tone effect and darker colours in the recesses.

The whole roof and both pantographs were next dry-brushed with a range of light greys, earthy shades and Humbrol Metalcote gunmetal to gently highlight the edges on all the equipment, referring back to clear prototype photos of the roof at every stage to check if it matched and altering as needed.

More weathering

Turning to the bodysides, more paint was applied to help represent some of the light streaking that could be seen where dirt deposits from the roof were brought down by the capillary action of rainwater; these were frequently channelled down through the panel gaps in the roof and from the side grilles.

After having sifted through photos to find the desired appearance, neat dark brown paint was added to the bodysides and cantrail area, in this case Humbrol Nos.113 and 251, before being initially wiped back

Out of the shadows

BELOW: **An overview of the weathering applied to the roof, the many components and cabinets in the well being a trap for dirt along with cooper and carbon deposits.**

seat and then painted to represent the appropriate uniform of the period. With that, the model could be put back together, and all masking removed from the glazing.

An additional task was to draw up a representation of the sunblinds on the computer using CorelDraw, these being to two depths and with the scissor mechanism also represented. These can then be printed out on photo paper, cut out and secured to the inside of the windscreen glazing using PVA glue as desired.

Final tasks

Going by photos of 92038 *Voltaire* in late 1990s condition, the loco had a clean but well-used appearance, with traffic dirt gathered on the underframe and roof. Working with an airbrush, a dual-action Badger 175 Crescendo which is some 20 years old but still doing the job, a range of colours were sprayed on. Layers of Phoenix Precision's brake dust and track dirt shades were gently feathered onto the chassis, working slowly and carefully to build up the colours over the beautifully-highlighted pipework on the Accurascale bogies, only some of which needs to show through the grime. Small amounts of these shades were also sprayed on the roof area, merely dusting down to blend in with the hand weathering already undertaken.

Next, a tin of Phoenix Precision's roof dirt shade was opened and sprayed across the roof area, as was a gentle spray of Humbrol No.187, the slight green and sandy shades representing the distinctive copper and carbon deposits left across the roof where the pantograph is in contact with the overhead wiring.

The last jobs to be tackled were all by hand, including dry-brushing further Humbrol Metalcote gunmetal across the bogies to highlight the raised edges, adding oily grime shades onto the bufferheads, and a little touch of silver across the steps to replicate the wear and tear from use.

With the final weathering stages all completed, you are now rewarded with something truly personal that goes beyond even the high-specification of a modern-day ready-to-run release and ready for service on a layout. The model here will be running on third rail power on Worthing MRC's Loftus Road layout, heading up some of the lengthy Channel Tunnel traffic that could be seen through West London. Finally, thanks are due to Accurascale for supplying the sample featured here and for the company's dedication at pushing forward the standards of RTR models.

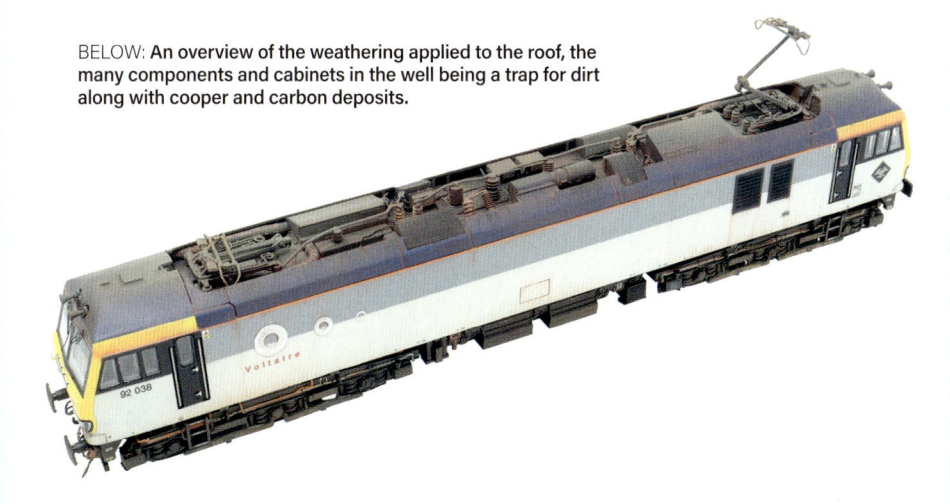

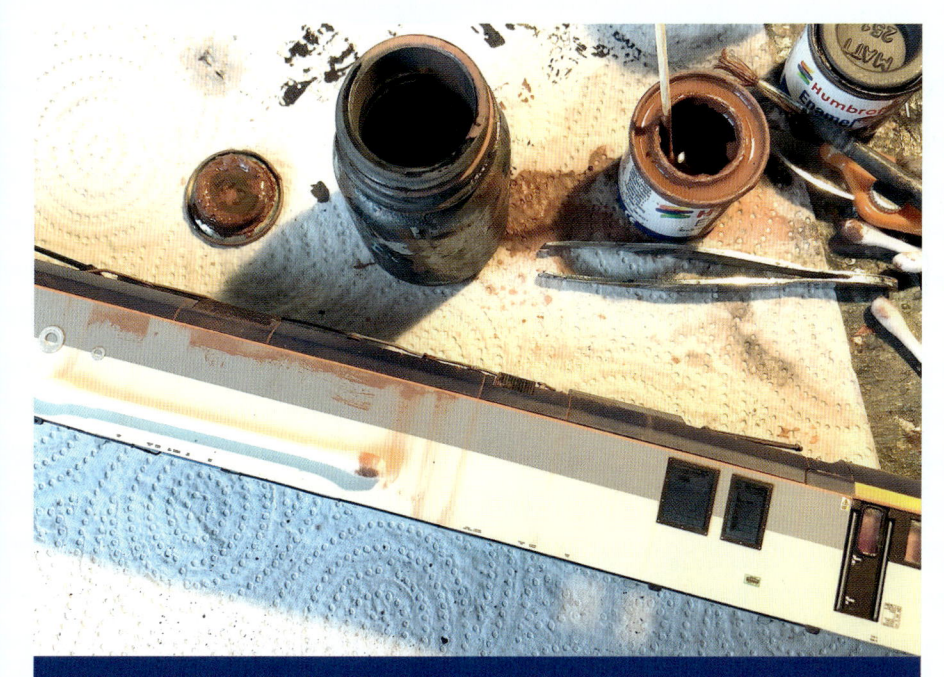

ABOVE: **The application of the bodyside streaks is in process, this again seeing the bulk of the thinned paint removed to leave behind subtle light streaks that do not overwhelm the model.**

with a kitchen towel to remove all but a darker patch on the paintwork. Working in a vertical up and down motion with a cotton bud dipped in enamel thinners, the area to the left and right of each streak was rubbed away, leaving a clean area around them. It is easy to over-egg the streaks, so the advice is to keep looking at photos and if they look too prominent, just give them a wipe with neat enamel thinners to either reduce the intensity or just start again with a more diluted paint wash until the required effect is achieved.

After the initial bodyshell weathering was completed, another coat of matt varnish was then sprayed over the body to protect the weathering and flatten down the finish. From experience, the paint-on and wipe-off stages described often leave a semi-satin finish and this can detract from the finished appearance if the varnish is not applied.

Little touches

Moving down to the chassis, comparatively little work needed doing with the Accurascale model already having a full complement of bufferbeam pipework. The silver third rail shoebeams were toned down in appearance by painting on a layer of dark grey (Humbrol No.32) and wiping it off in a vertical motion, this dulling the silver finish to a flatter grey.

At this point, the model was ready for reassembly prior to the last weathering stages. Before this occurred, a driver was added to one cab end, this being a cheap unpainted figure cut to fit into the driver's

RIGHT: **The home-produced windscreen blinds were drawn using grey-edged black diamonds on a black background, this representing the scissor mechanism. These were then printed out and trimmed to size.**

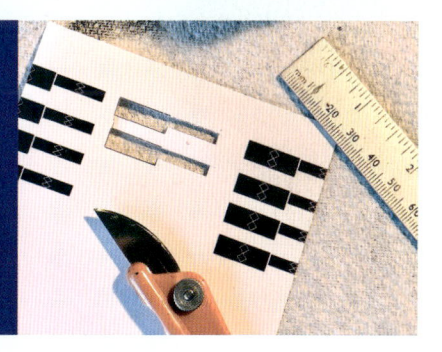

Modelling BR Locomotives of the 1990s **65**

Out of the shadows

Distribution updated

With the opening of the Channel Tunnel and the hoped for growth in international freight, Railfreight Distribution felt the need to update its image to be more 'European'. The company also continued as a separate entity beyond the 1994 creation of the regional freight companies as Simon Bendall recounts while James Makin models some suitably-liveried Class 47s in 4mm scale.

The origin of the Railfreight Distribution (RfD) European livery can be traced back to 1992. With the Channel Tunnel under construction, which would see RfD become responsible for operating freight services through to Europe, the freight company's management was looking at ways of 'Europeanising' its existing triple grey livery to create a new image. The end of the year saw the application of an experimental new livery to 90136 for evaluation by staff and managers alike. Based heavily on the SNCF 'Sybic' electric loco livery of two-tone grey and orange, which was already carried by 90130 following its part in the Freightconnection events of a month or two earlier, 90136 also sported the familiar RfD sub-sector emblems and red 'Railfreight Distribution' lettering.

While 90136 remained a one-off, behind the scenes RfD management continued to work on the new livery into 1993 with several ideas being considered before elements of the existing and experimental schemes were combined to create the new look. On the bodysides, the two-tone grey livery was retained but with altered proportions and tweaked shades of grey while the black cab window surrounds were abandoned in favour of full yellow ends. The dark blue roof colour was taken straight from the Class 92s while the 'Railfreight Distribution' lettering trialled on 90136 was kept, albeit enlarged, rearranged and with a change of colour to black.

The RfD 'red diamonds' were again retained along with cast depot plaques but, apart from a handful of locos, there was no place for the cast BR arrows. The positioning of the TOPS numbers created some problems as the very earliest repaints carried black numbers on the dark grey, directly beneath the cabside windows. However, as this affected their readability, the numbers were repositioned onto the light grey of the lower cabsides. A further addition, which was confined solely to some of the Class 47 fleet, were the small Channel Tunnel 'Polo mint' transfers on the upper cabsides.

Beyond dedication

The new RfD European livery debuted in the summer of 1993, 86608 being the first loco to be repainted during August followed a couple of weeks later by 47217. For the Brush Type 4s at least, the colours were initially intended to be confined to those locos dedicated to Channel Tunnel traffic but, in the event, it became a fleetwide scheme, soon spreading to the Class 47s used on automotive and other traffic flows. As a result, the class became by far the most numerous recipients of the livery as these now formed the backbone of the RfD diesel fleet following the decision to dispense with its remaining Class 37s.

In all, 49 of the Brush machines were repainted between 1993-96, which included a few non-standard applications. The most well-known of these was 47525, which had joined the Distribution fleet in the spring of 1995 along with 47555. With both in desperately scruffy InterCity Executive colours, a repaint was a necessity and 47555 was duly completed that August. However, with 47525 only part way through its repaint that same month, it was required for service so returned to traffic with fully painted RfD European cabs and rubbed-down InterCity bodysides! It remained in use in this condition until November when it was finally stopped at Tinsley to have the repaint completed.

Around the same time, 47150 and 47303 were both repainted into RfD European at the Yorkshire depot. In both cases, the repaint was something of a rushed job, far removed from Tinsley's normal standard, with neither loco receiving a blue roof or RfD lettering while 47150 was also denied sub-sector logos. In effect, this left 47150 in an unbranded version of the livery, an appearance that would later come to be shared by 47079, 47287 and 47370 as they were stripped of their RfD lettering and symbols following transfer to Freightliner in 1996.

A single fleet

During the course of 1996, the division of the Class 47s between Railfreight Distribution and Freightliner was finally satisfactorily completed. Thus, at end of that year, RfD just had a single pool of Class 47s for all of its duties, all but a handful of which were locos with the life extension modifications, including long range fuel tanks and cut back bufferbeams.

Those finished in RfD European colours, which were now reduced in number due to the losses to Freightliner, were 47033/49/51/53/85/95, 47125/46/86/88, 47200/01/17-19/28/36/37/41/45/58/85/86/93/97/99 and 47306/07/10/12/16/26/38/44/48/51/60/65/75. Completing matters were 47194, 47210/11/13/26/29/80/81/84/98 and 47304/13/14/28/35/55/62/78 which still retained the original RfD sub-sector scheme, 47276, 47363 and 47379 running in unbranded triple grey and finally Tinsley's depot 'pet' 47145 in is all-over European blue livery with RfD logos.

November 1997 saw EWS acquire Railfreight Distribution in the face of competition from Freightliner, this giving it access to the Channel Tunnel. The disliked Class 47s were targeted for early withdrawal as soon as deliveries of the Class 66s allowed with virtually all of the former RfD fleet out of traffic within two years.

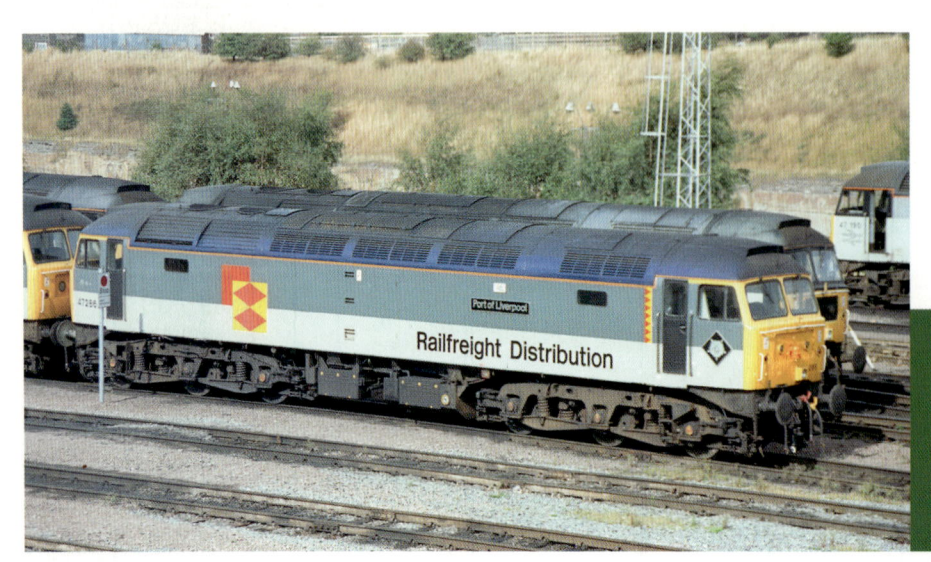

LEFT: Stabled at Tinsley in June 1995, 47286 *Port of Liverpool* shows off the full application of the RfD European livery, complete with the miniature Channel Tunnel 'polo mint' logo on the driver's cabside. This was one of the earlier recipients of the livery, being painted in December 1993, and also displays the life extension modifications of cut-back bufferbeams and extended range fuel tanks. Simon Bendall Collection

Out of the shadows

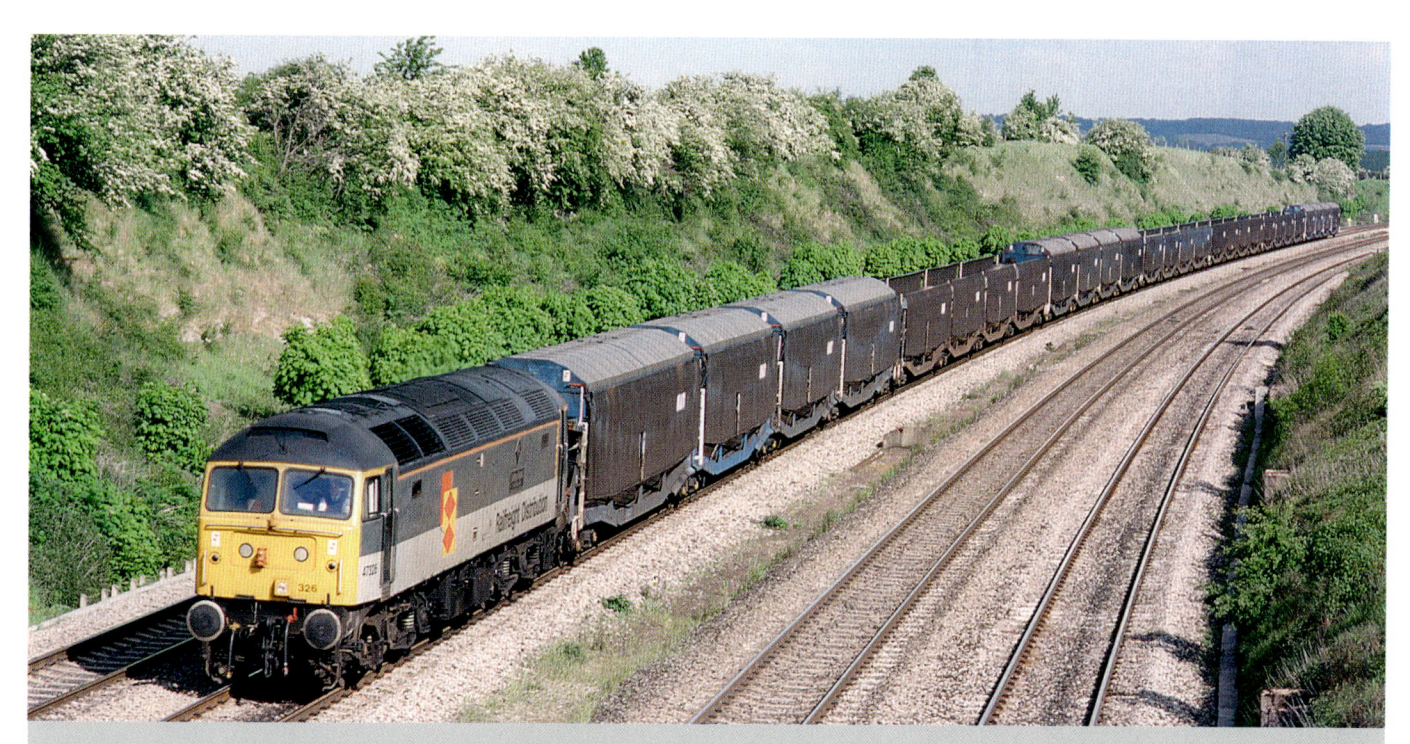

ABOVE: Automotive traffic made up a significant part of Railfreight Distribution's traffic portfolio in the 1990s. On May 7, 1995, 47326 *Saltley Depot Quality Approved* passes South Moreton with empty cartics returning from Southampton Western Docks to Cowley, Oxford, having previously taken new Rover cars for export. The train features seven sets of PJA Cartic-4 wagons owned by MAT, these all having the side protection screens while three have additionally received protective roofs in order to reduce instances of damage and vandalism to the vehicles. Revolution Trains is currently developing models of the Cartic-4s in both 2mm and 4mm, which will include a range of liveries and modifications. Simon Bendall Collection

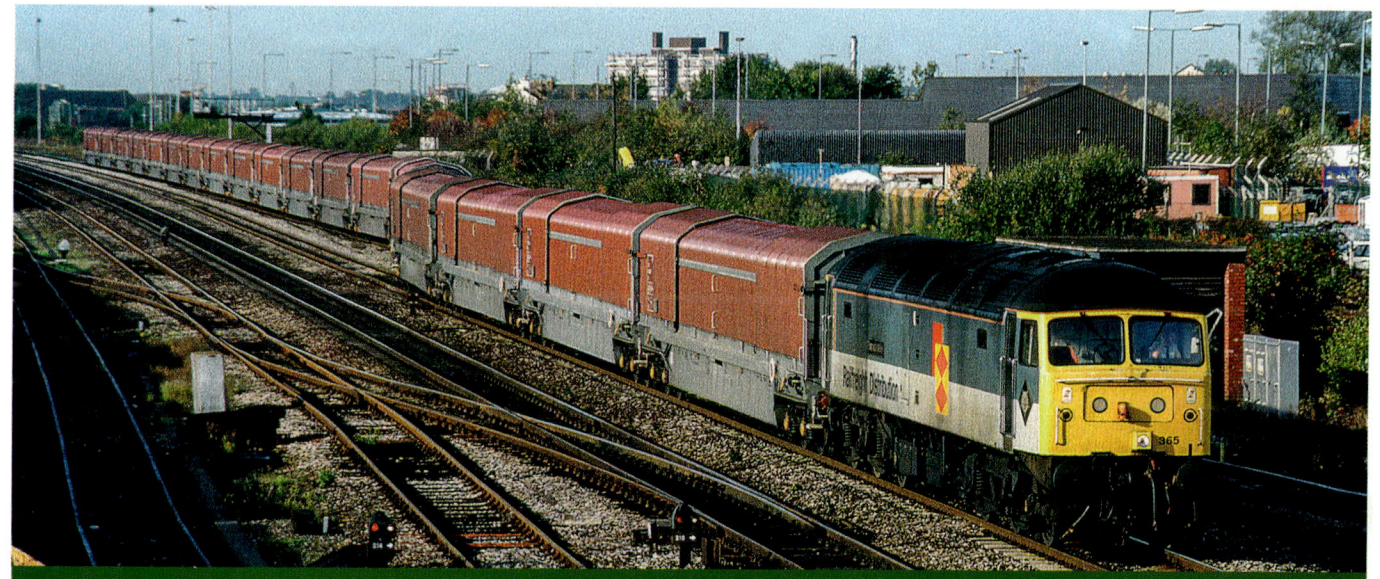

ABOVE: A further section of RfD's automotive portfolio was the transfer of Rover components between the manufacturing plants at Swindon and Longbridge, Birmingham. During October 1996. 47365 *Diamond Jubilee* gets underway as it joins the Great Western Main Line at Swindon with the 6M03 loaded working via Oxford. In tow is a uniform rake of KSA 'cube' wagons, these having been recently introduced to replace the previously used Cargowaggon vans and featured sliding canopies and hydraulic platforms so components could be loaded in the well between the bogies. A kit for these impressive wagons is available in 2mm from the N Gauge Society but they have yet to attract the attention of a manufacturer in 4mm. The Class 47's name referred to the diamond jubilee of ICI but with the original accompanying crest no longer carried, it was rendered rather meaningless. Simon Bendall Collection

RIGHT: During 1990, 47145 was adopted by Tinsley depot as its 'pet' loco, first receiving a fresh application of BR blue that was progressively embellished and the name *Merddin Emrys*. Four years later, the livery was updated using the European blue roof colour from the RfD scheme and with Distribution logos on the bodysides, it ran in this condition until stored by EWS. The loco is seen on the depot's fuel point on October 5, 1994, with plenty of useful detail on display. Simon Bendall Collection

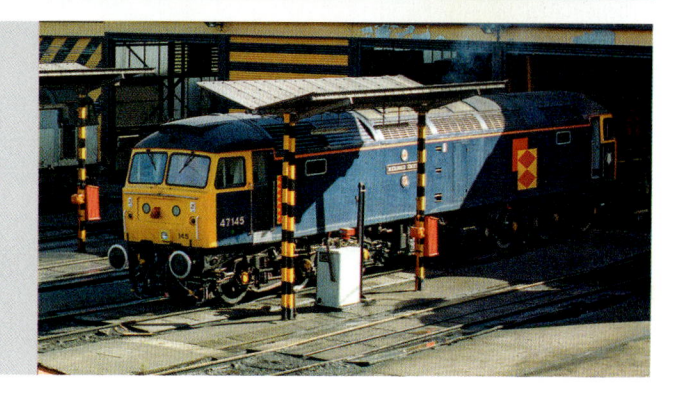

Modelling BR Locomotives of the 1990s 67

Out of the shadows

Distribution detailing

BELOW: Named *Dollands Moor International*, 47053 was entirely typical of a life-extended Class 47 in RfD European colours, gaining one of several names to mark the opening of facilities for Channel Tunnel freight traffic.

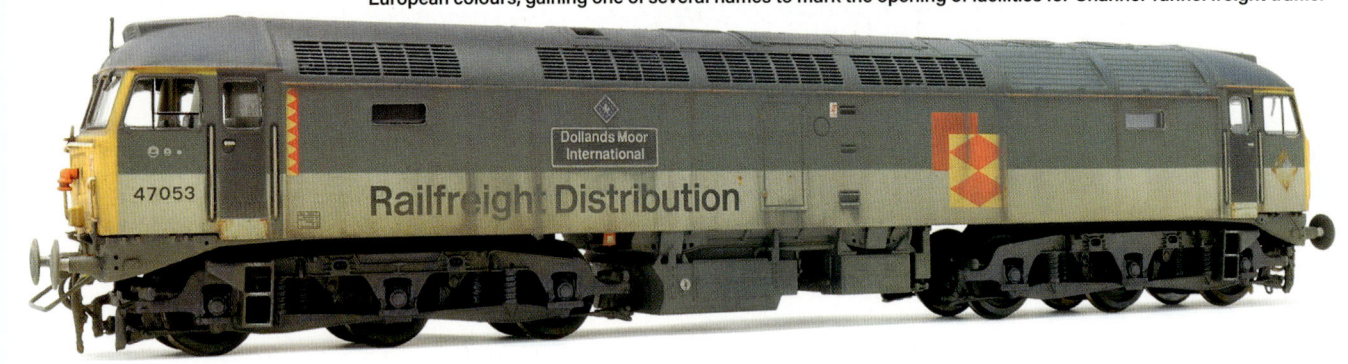

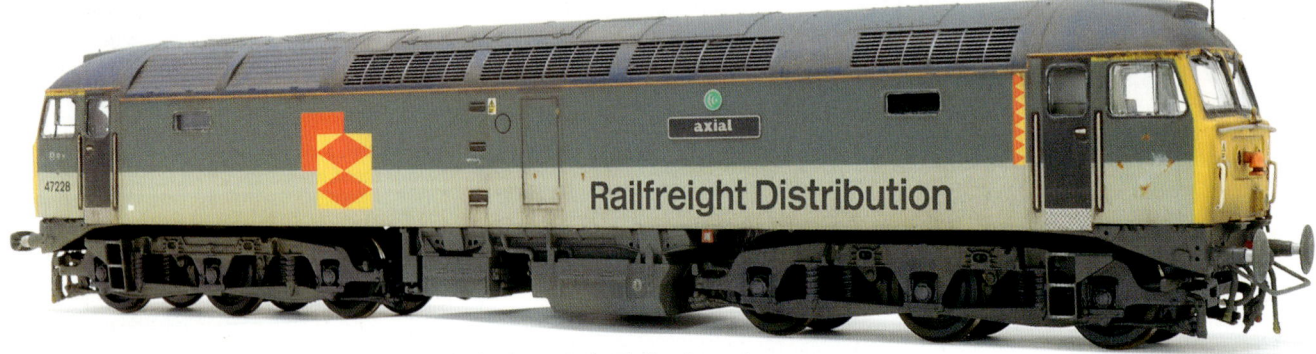

ABOVE: Following the takeover of Railfreight Distribution by EWS, the Tinsley depot plaques were generally removed, leaving a cabside scar. Otherwise, the loco's paintwork was in good condition at this time. The *axial* name was one of the more obscure, referring to a car transportation company.

The former Tinsley fleet of Railfreight Distribution (RfD) Class 47s has always been attractive from a modelling perspective. The bright, new 'European' colours contrasted with the earlier triple grey livery and the locos could be seen far and wide across the country on many different freight workings, often in double-headed formations on some of the heavier services. For my own modelling project, I sought to create an interesting cross-section of the fleet, these being accurate to the late 1990s period and just after the takeover of RfD by EWS,

RfD had a huge fleet of Class 47s, so it is sometimes tricky knowing where to even start to choose which ones to model. As a keen, young trainspotter in the late 1990s period, the natural place to start was to go through the old notes and model examples that I had encountered during some great days out at Didcot. I was attracted to the examples with large nameplates as the fleet started to receive a lot of corporate names during the decade, twinning the business with key customers and creating great public relations exercises.

While much-derided by enthusiasts of the time, as the years have passed, these names have become unique snapshots into the past as a lot of the businesses, locations or events featured have long since become defunct. Of course, there was one very special RfD locomotive that had to be modelled as well, 'celebrity' 47145 *Merddin Emrys*, the well-loved Tinsley machine that became the depot 'pet'.

Getting started

There is now a choice when it comes to Railfreight Distribution Class 47s with the 2021 release of Bachmann's all new model compared to the older version which can be found in plentiful supply at exhibitions and auction sites. The release of 47365 *Diamond Jubilee* in 2013 gave a great base model to start with, this featuring long range fuel tanks, cutaway bufferbeams and headcode panel recesses at both ends. The model did not appear to be a fast seller at the time so could be found heavily discounted in the major retailers at one stage, helping to create a sizeable RfD fleet for comparatively little outlay.

Having found a full selection of photos of the chosen prototypes via the internet, it was important to map out the planned work across the fleet. There would be a few instances of having to fill in headcode panels to create flush-fronted cabs, some changes to the fuel tank and battery boxes, as well as a couple of locos that required the original bufferbeam cowls or elements of these to be reinstated. All in all, some great fun lay ahead!

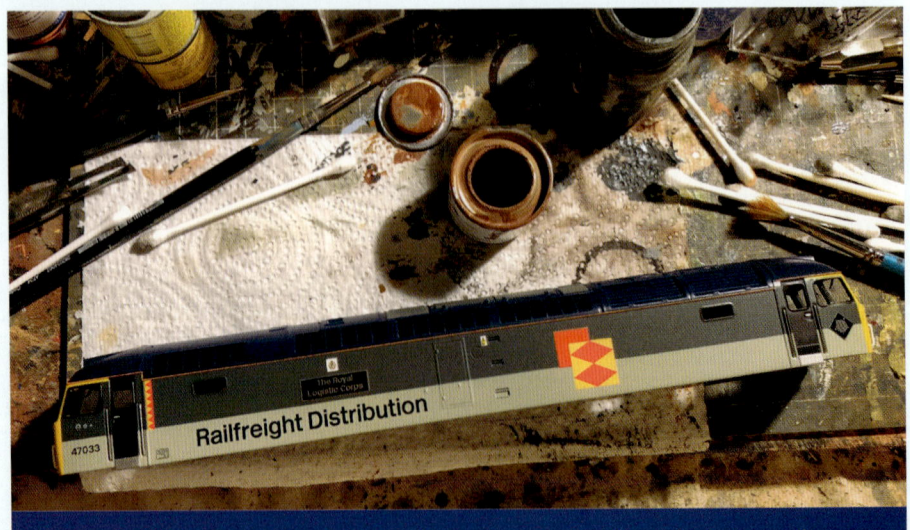

ABOVE: The body has been stripped down with an early stage of detailing being to remove the factory printing and then apply the new transfers and nameplates.

Out of the shadows

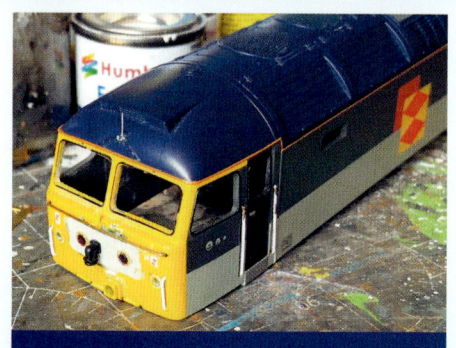

ABOVE: To create a flush-front, the headcode panel recess has been filled and smoothed and the marker lights reinstated using Shawplan etches. Also fitted is the 'green circle' multiple working connection.

The place to start was to take apart the locos and the glazing can then be removed or masked-up for the duration of the project. On my models, Humbrol Maskol was added to the glazing; this liquid sets to form a rubber mask and is ideal for avoiding the perils of having to remove glazing where it has been glued in hard by the manufacturer.

In each case, the printed numbers and nameplates were removed from the model. This was undertaken by dipping a cotton bud into Humbrol enamel thinners and gently rubbing across the printing, which will soon lift in one or two minutes. The black printing normally lifts first followed by the silver of the nameplates, but care must be taken not to rub too hard and go through the base paint layer. One alternative and successful method is to use a sharp, curved-bladed scalpel to gently scrape away at the printing, depending upon your preference. The Railfreight Distribution lettering and sub-sector logos were retained but it is worth observing prototype photos as there were some small variations in positioning across the fleet.

Body changes

Quite a few of the RfD machines had suffered from accident damage in their past lives and consequently had flush-fronted cabs, where they had been rebuilt without a headcode panel recess. With Bachmann's 47365 having headcode panels at both ends, this entailed filling in the recess with Humbrol model filler where this modification was required.

Firstly, the handrails were removed from the affected cab end along with the light lens glazing. With cocktail sticks temporarily added to mark out where the light lenses were, model filler was added into the recess and left to dry before being sanded-down smooth. Afterwards, Shawplan etched marker light surrounds were added to complete the look and the handrails re-attached.

Most of the RfD fleet received the life extension modifications in the early 1990s, this including the removal of the bufferbeam cowlings. Bachmann's model of 47365 already incorporated this alteration but a few locos avoided this alteration, included the selected pair of 47146 *Loughborough Grammar School* and 47348 *St Christopher's Railway Home*. For the latter, a Bachmann chassis was sourced with the original bufferbeam cowlings in place and then on the bodyshell, extra slivers of plasticard were added to the cut-back recess on all four cabsides to build the area back up to its

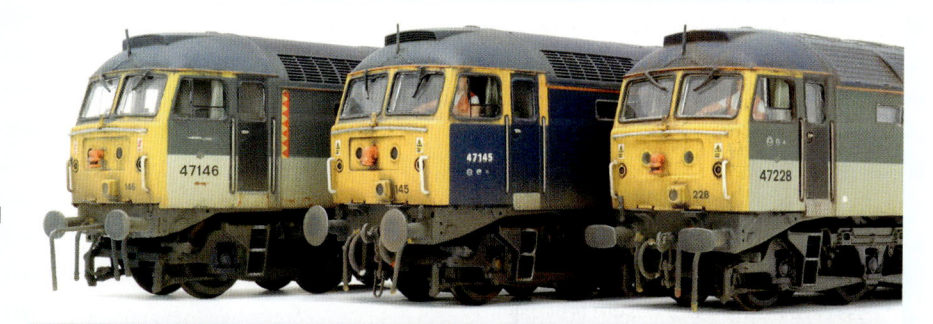

ABOVE: A line-up of 47228, 47145 and 47146 shows several differences, including the Class 60-style buffers on the former and the removed bufferbeam cowlings on all three but with 47146 still retaining its full depth cabsides.

BELOW: The model of 47145 *Merddin Emrys* employs the Bachmann limited edition and has received the same level of detailing and weathering as its sisters.

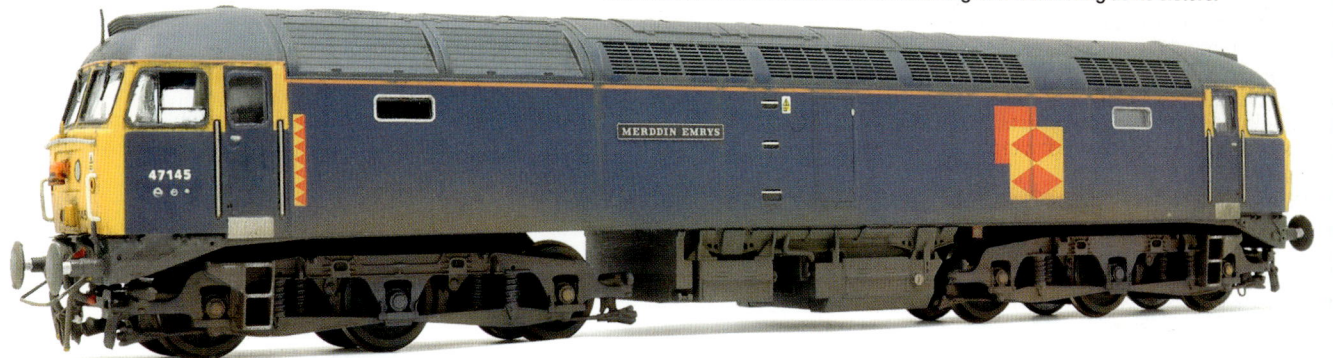

BELOW: One of the RfD Class 47s not to receive life-extension modifications was 47146 *Loughborough Grammar School*, this still having is obsolete water tanks rather than extended range fuel tanks.

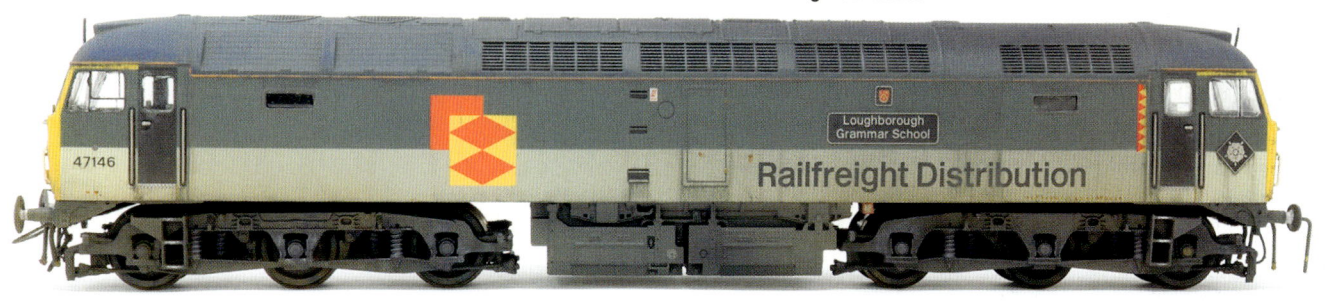

Modelling BR Locomotives of the 1990s **69**

Out of the shadows

BELOW: In contrast to 47228, classmate 47241 *Halewood Silver Jubilee 1988* is in particularly poor condition with extensive rusting on the bodyside and peeling lettering. The loco also has different buffer types on each end.

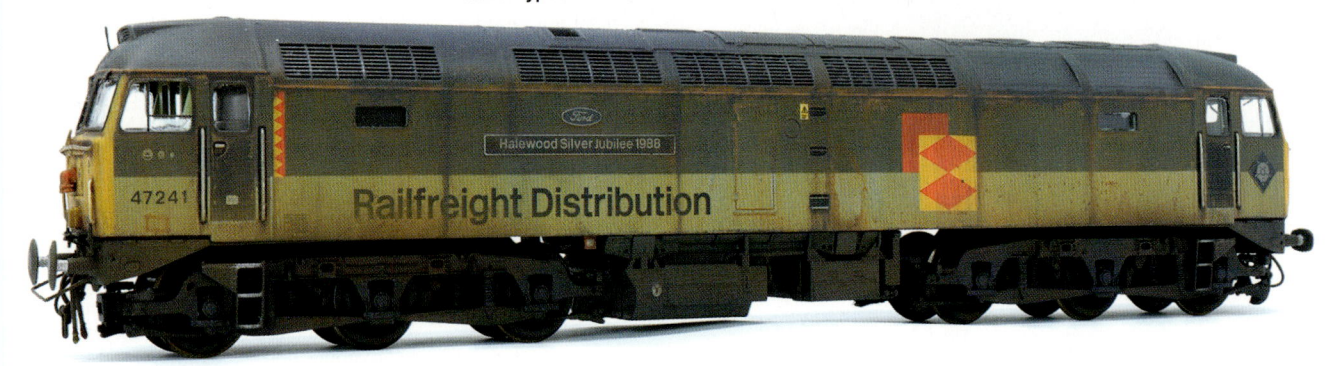

BELOW: In addition to international and automotive traffic, RfD also handled Ministry pf Defence workings during the 1990s. As a result, several Class 47s had military-themed names, including 47033 *The Royal Logistics Corps*, this being another life-extended machine.

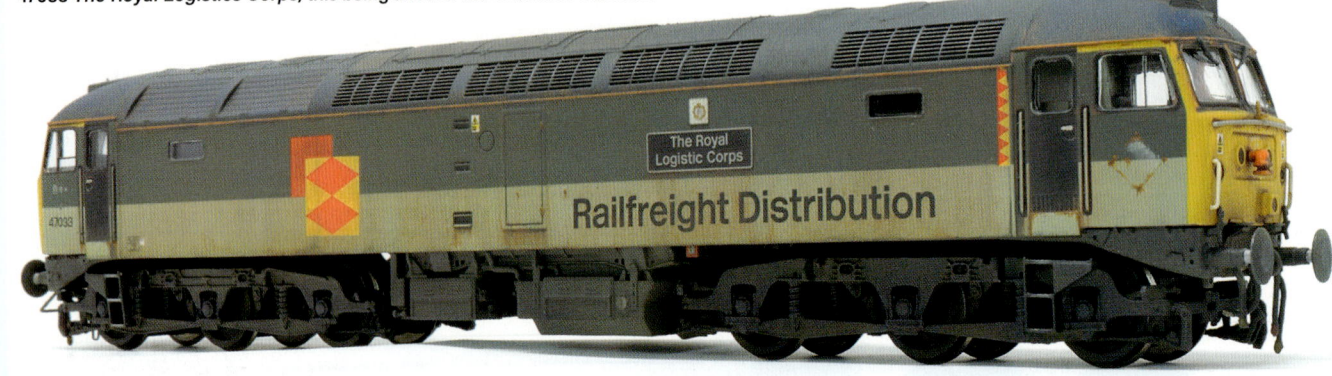

original depth. The additional plastic was painted Rail grey to match the Bachmann paint job using the Phoenix Precision shade.

However, 47146 was a unique half-way house, the loco having lost the cowls but retained the full-depth cabsides. Similar to 47348, slivers of plasticard were added to the sides and front of the loco and gently filed to shape with a needle file. While most RfD Class 47s had standard round Oleo buffers until the end, there were some that received the rectangular style as used on Class 60s. Shawplan whitemetal replacements were used in these instances while 47146 even had Class 37-style oval buffers at one end. Bufferbeam pipework was added from the supplied Bachmann detailing packs along with Replica Railways parts and some 0.45mm handrail wire for additional piping where needed.

Underframe boxes

The majority of the RfD fleet had the extended range fuel tanks fitted by the mid-1990s and this is the version that the Bachmann model of 47365 is supplied with. However, a few locos still retained the battery-box only underframe style while even less had the obsolete boiler water tanks in place. In both cases, spares were obtained directly from Bachmann.

This is also an area where extra detail can be added depending upon the time available and inclination. The areas between the battery boxes can be opened out, firstly by removing the centre piece of Bachmann's moulding. There is scope for recreating some of the pipe runs underneath, although it is worth checking that the added detail does not interfere with the swing of the bogies when navigating pointwork.

Smaller details can also be added; most noticeable on the sides are the underframe-mounted emergency fire extinguisher pulls, which are located just above the bogie towards the No.2 (non-radiator) end of the loco. To represent these, pieces of 1.5mm square plasticard can be added underneath the loco and the red frame painted on with a fine 5/0 paintbrush.

The Bachmann model has a few unwanted mould lines across the roof that can be gently filed down, notably over the top of each cab roof next to the horn vents and the horizontal lines at the No.2 end on the cantrail in the blank space between the grilles. The blanked-off boiler ports can be matched to photos of your chosen prototype, the Bachmann model having the rectangular plated version, but Shawplan produces etched brass parts for the other versions or, alternatively, these can be crafted from card or styrene.

Another option available is to replace the roof fan grilles with the etched versions from Shawplan, the only downside being that they are fragile and ideally should only be fitted right at the end of the detailing process. If fitted earlier, a tip is to apply masking tape to the inside of the grilles during the modelling stages to avoid accidentally sticking one's fingers right through the beautifully delicate mesh!

Finishing

With the major work completed, a layer of Railmatch gloss varnish was added to give a good surface onto which the transfers could be applied, using Railtec decals for the numbers and with etched nameplates supplied by Shawplan and Fox Transfers. The etched nameplates were secured using matt varnish, which is ideal to give a long drying time to allow straight positioning on the bodysides. The transfers were sealed with an overall coat of Railmatch matt varnish to protect the surface and the models were left for a month to allow the varnish to harden before starting the weathering process.

Each loco was studied in depth before starting the weathering with washes of thinned Humbrol paints applied to each bodyshell, these being painted on and then wiped away in a downward vertical motion using kitchen towel. The shades used were typically dark browns and greys from the Humbrol enamel paint range. Each layer of paint wash would leave a residue behind after being wiped down, and by using a clean cotton bud dipped in enamel thinners, it is then possible to remove the rest of the residue to just leave a streaky appearance in the areas where desired, this replicating where rainwater brings dirt down from the roof.

Rust patches and damage were added with fine 5/0 paint brushes, including where the Tinsley depot plaques were removed, leaving behind surface rust patches and bolt holes. By using the fine brushes to mottle on shades of brown, a rust effect was built up from light brown to dark brown at the epicentre of the patch, all the time following photos closely to get a realistic finish. Finally, the bodyshells received a top layer of matt varnish to protect the weathering. Cab detailing included painting the false floor of the moulding in black to disguise the lack

Out of the shadows

BELOW: Another Type 4 not to be modernised was 47348 *St Christopher's Railway Home*, this retaining full bufferbeam cowlings and only having the battery boxes underneath.

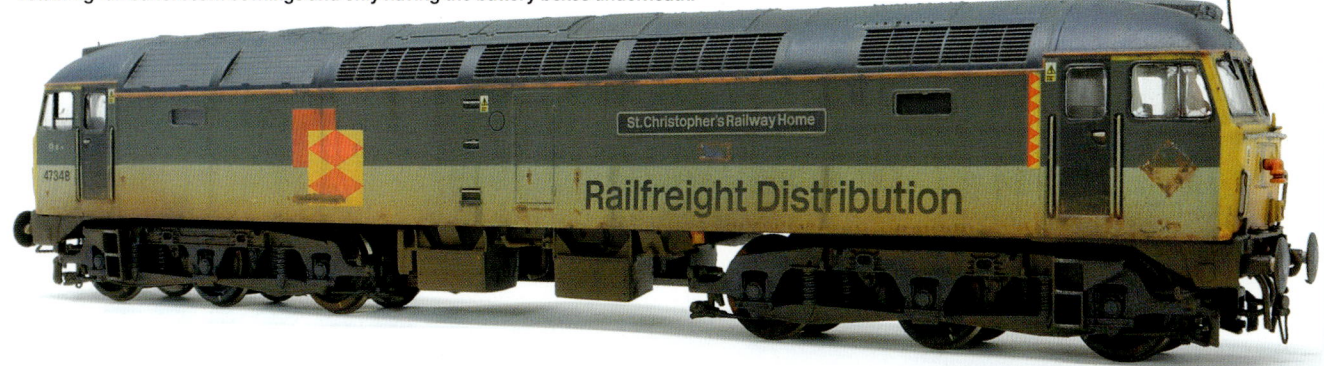

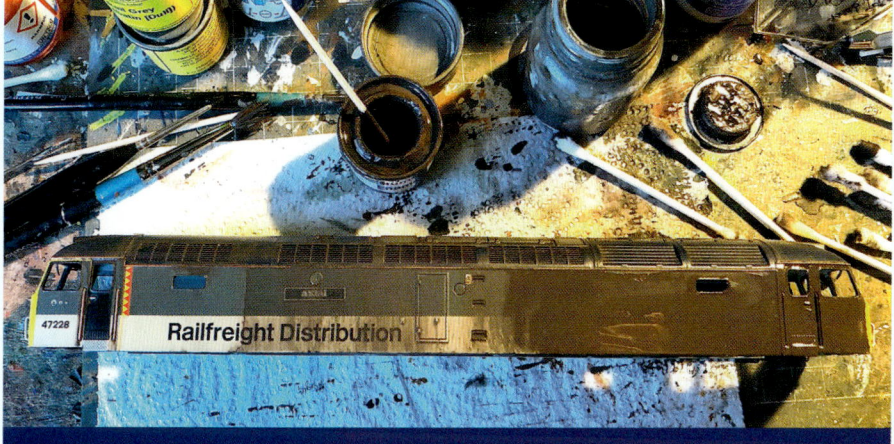

ABOVE: The various stages of bodyside washes are shown with the right hand side having the full wash applied, the central section being partly cleaned and the left hand with residual dirt left behind after further cleaning with thinners on cotton buds.

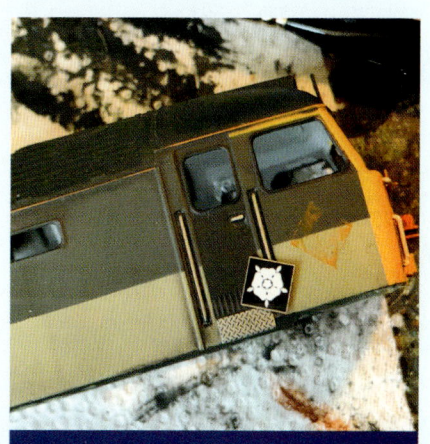

ABOVE: Using an etched depot plaque as a guide, this gives the dimensions for applying the rust patch left behind by a removed example.

of depth while the driver figure was also modernised to have EWS attire.

Following re-assembly, the locos received a final dusting of colours with an airbrush to represent the traffic grime and dirt from daily use, this being layers of Phoenix Precision brake dust, track dirt, roof dirt, dirty black and a custom mix of black and dark blue to represent the oily diesel exhaust deposits on the roof. With that, the locos were ready to be released into traffic and assume their work on my new Didcot project. In the meantime, they can be seen in action on Worthing MRC's Loftus Road layout, more of which can be found at www.facebook.com/LoftusRoadModelRailway.

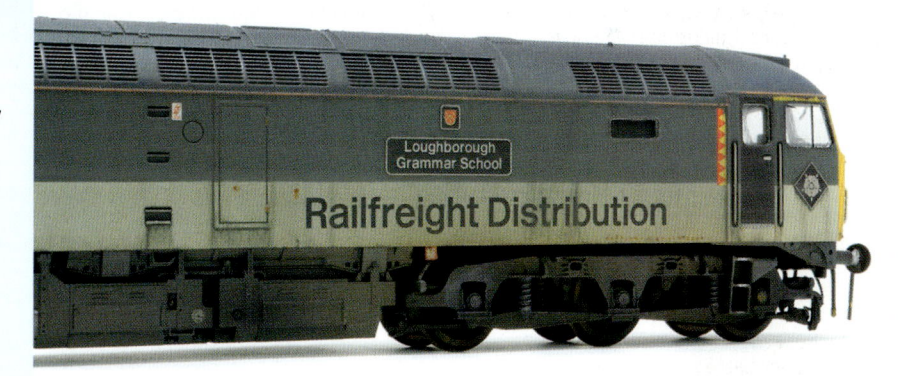

ABOVE: Most RfD European Class 47s retained paintwork in reasonable condition thanks to their relatively recent paint jobs. Thus, the application of traffic dirt is a main element of the work.

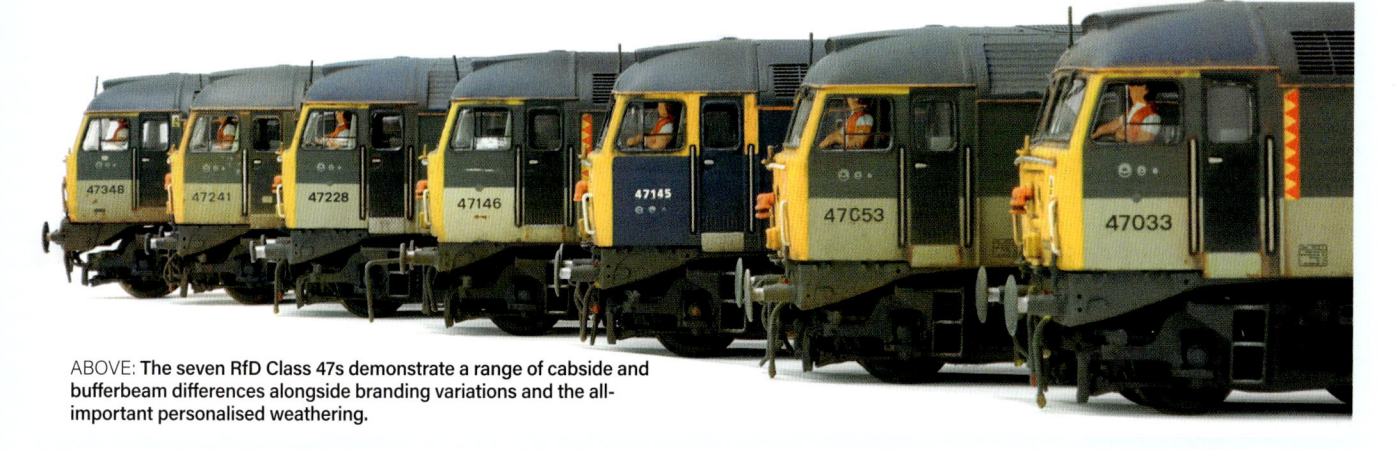

BELOW: The seven RfD Class 47s demonstrate a range of cabside and bufferbeam differences alongside branding variations and the all-important personalised weathering.

Modelling BR Locomotives of the 1990s 71

Out of the shadows

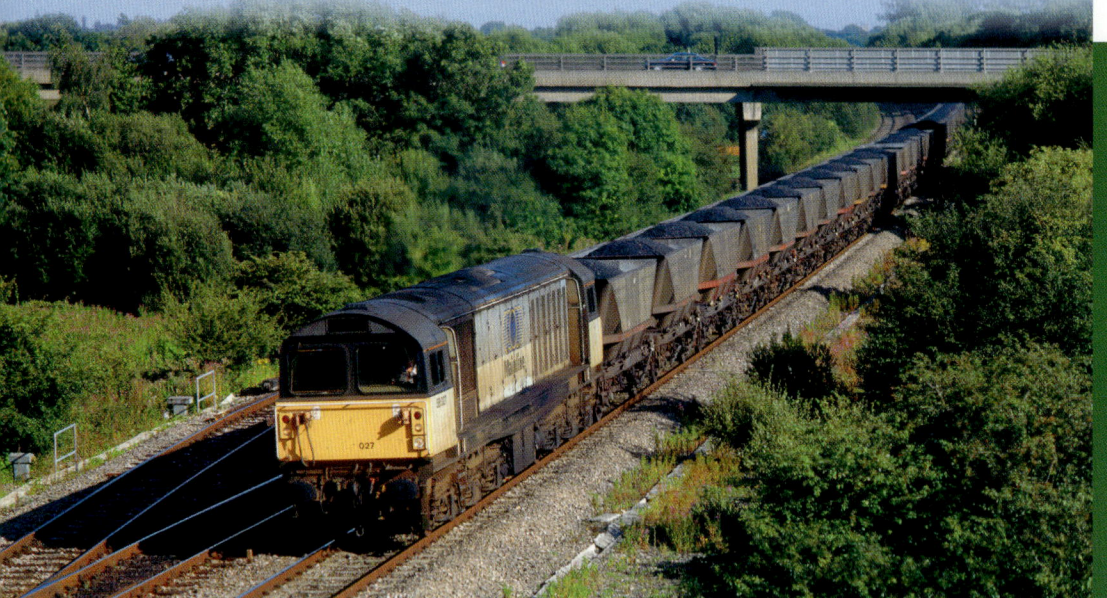

LEFT: The triple grey version of the Mainline Freight livery was arguably rather bland when compared to the full blue and silver application, but it was the more common of the two by quite some margin. On August 7, 1998, 58027 was still doing the job for which it was built, shifting vast quantities of coal efficiently. However, the nature of the flows had now changed with a greater reliance on imports. Where once it would have been heading loaded hoppers south at Wolvercote Junction to Didcot Power Station, it was now going north instead with the 14.30 departure from Avonmouth to Ironbridge Power Station.
Martin Loader

A 'Bone' expansion

Under British Rail ownership, the Class 58s were largely confined to working merry-go-round coal trains in the Midlands. With the coming of privatisation, the Type 5s saw a much expanded sphere of operation under Mainline Freight and use on a wider range of commodities. **Simon Bendall** details what was a welcome development while **James Makin** upgrades the OO gauge Heljan model.

The first of the new Railfreight operators created in the spring of 1994 was Trainload Freight South East, this name being something of a misnomer as its operating sphere extended far beyond what would typically be termed the southeast of the country. To the north, the company reached the Leicestershire quarries while its main depot was Toton in Nottinghamshire while in the west, the likes of Westbury and Swindon were both in its remit. Naturally, East Anglia, the Home Counties and everything south of the Thames were also on the company's patch.

Trainload Freight South East opted to rebrand itself as Mainline Freight from October 1994, design consultants Halpin Grey Vermeir creating its new 'rolling wheel' logo. Unlike Loadhaul, which plumped for a completely new livery from the outset, Mainline initially chose to retain Railfreight triple grey, just replacing the now defunct sub-sector decals with the new yellow and blue logo.

The new Mainline emblems had first appeared three months earlier when 37203 and 60079 were used for branding trials at Toton, the aim being to assess the visual impact as well as check sizes and durability through the washing plant. Once this was completed, the logos were removed again. For the next few months, no progress was made on the rebranding although, in the meantime, virtually all Mainline Freight-owned locos in triple grey were stripped of their sub-sector emblems in anticipation of receiving the new logos.

It was not until the Freightconnection 1994 event in London's Docklands on October 4 that Mainline Freight finally broke cover with the unveiling of 58050 *Toton Traction Depot* in a completely new livery. The loco cut a striking sight finished in a mid-blue colour with silver logos and bodyside stripe and an Executive dark grey roof. Painted amid much secrecy at Toton the previous week, the livery was intended for a short evaluation period prior to fleet-wide application.

Mass application

Just five weeks later on November 14, Mainline Freight was officially launched with a series of special events at a number of locations. To mark the occasion, a number of locos were repainted into the new blue livery at Mainline's principal maintenance depots. Stratford turned out mascot 37023, the loco taking part in events at Acton, Didcot and Hither Green as well as its home depot during the day. Not to be outdone, Stewarts Lane contributed both 37798 and 73114, the electro-diesel being named after its home depot while the Type 3 was despatched on tour to Eastleigh. In the Midlands, Worksop was host to namesake 58011 *Worksop Depot*, this being the first loco to receive the production yellow and blue Mainline logos on its existing triple grey livery.

Focussing on the Class 58s, the pace of blue repaints was not particularly quick, the second example, 58023, not appearing until May 1995 as part of its preparations for naming as *Peterborough Depot*. Five months later, 58021 also emerged from Toton for its christening as *Hither Green Depot*. The remaining 10 Class 58s to receive a coat of blue were all painted during the course of overhauls at Doncaster Works, the second half of 1995 seeing 58002/14/32/38/46 completed while

BELOW: Of the three regional freight companies, Mainline Freight was undoubtedly the most proactive in stripping off the Railfreight sub-sector logos. In contrast, Loadhaul really did not bother with such trivialities! Most of the Class 58s would run unbranded for a time as demonstrated by 58015 on October 8, 1994, as it surveys the previously unfamiliar surroundings of Hither Green depot in southeast London.
Simon Bendall Collection

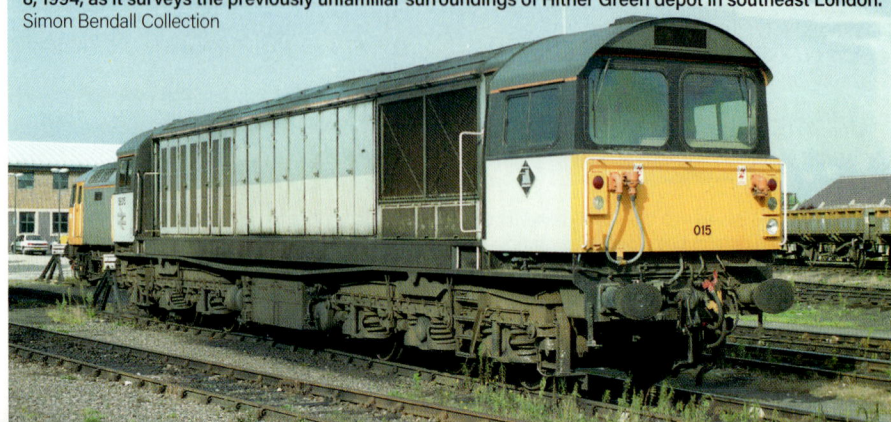

72 www.keymodelworld.com

Out of the shadows

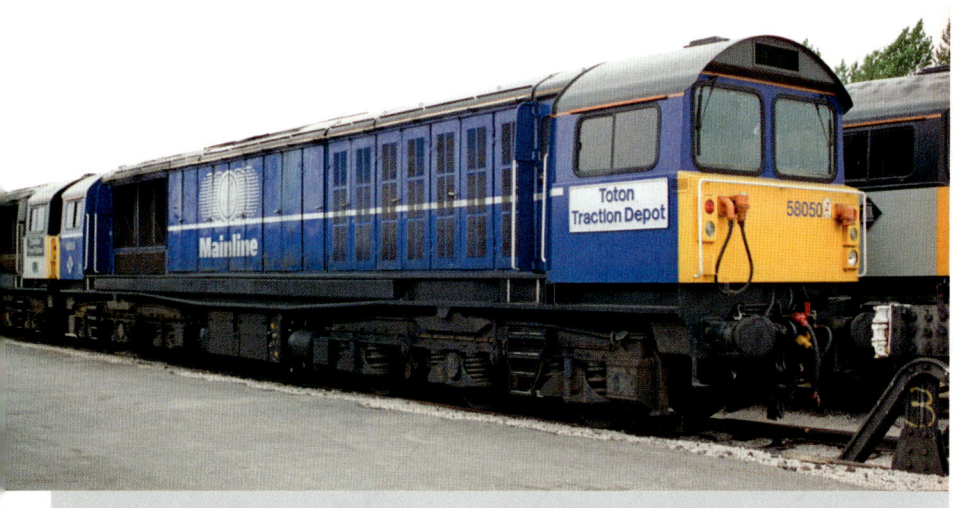

ABOVE: **The last of the class, 58050** *Toton Traction Depot* **is seen stabled at Worksop on July 31, 1996, awaiting its next duty. This loco was not only the first to carry Mainline Freight blue in October 1994 but also the first into Railfreight Coal exactly seven years earlier. The nameplate colour was initially blue lettering on a pale grey background for repainted locos but red plates with polished lettering would also be carried by a few locos.** John Turner/53A Models of Hull Collection

New duties

Under Mainline Freight ownership, all of the Class 58s remained based at Toton with power station coal traffic still their principal duty. However, the locos were no longer dedicated to these workings and began to appear on other flows originating from the East Midlands area. For example, this included the aggregates traffic emanating from the likes of Mountsorrel and Bardon Hill as well as cement traffic from Ketton.

They also began to appear regularly in previous uncommon territory, such as East Anglia and the southeast. This expansion became even more pronounced with the arrival of EWS, many of the class still carrying one of the two Mainline liveries. This even included use on the 'Enterprise' wagonload services that originated from Eastleigh and ran via Didcot, bringing appearances on such previously usual commodities as timber, china clay slurry, Ministry of Defence stores and even infrastructure wagons.

58005/08/36/42 were all squeezed in within the first three months of 1996. Last of all was 58013 in April 1996, two months after EWS had officially taken over but before a new livery had been decided on, this emerging in plain blue with no silver stripe or logos.

Turning to the application of the coloured Mainline Freight logos to triple grey locos, this began in earnest from April 1995, 58017 being one of the first done for its naming as *Eastleigh Depot*. Applied during normal maintenance cycles, the logos spread quite rapidly. Of the Class 58s, 58001-13/15-20/22/24-31/33-45/47-49 are all known to have received the coloured logos while 58014/50 did not. It is unclear whether 58021/23/32/46 did get the logos or not due to the short time between its introduction and the quartet going blue.

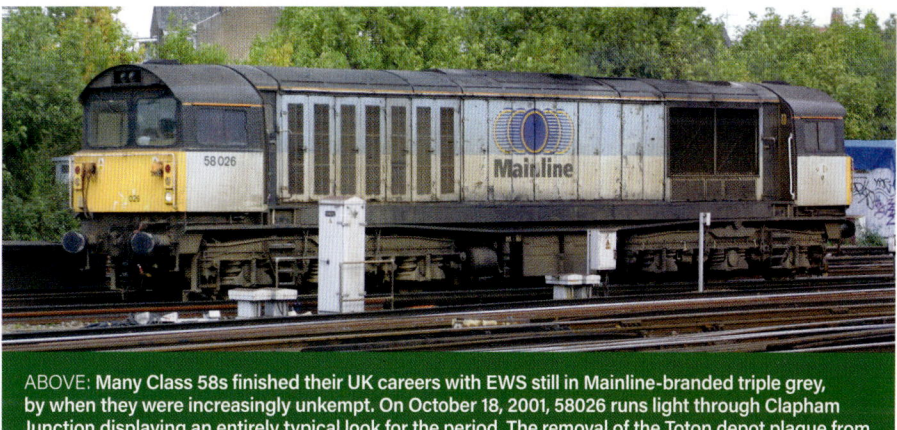

ABOVE: **Many Class 58s finished their UK careers with EWS still in Mainline-branded triple grey, by when they were increasingly unkempt. On October 18, 2001, 58026 runs light through Clapham Junction displaying an entirely typical look for the period. The removal of the Toton depot plaque from the secondman's cabside has left the inevitable scar.** John Turner/53A Models of Hull Collection

Model availability

It was not until 2007 that OO gauge modellers could enjoy a Class 58 to a modern specification, this usurping the Hornby model that was released some two decades earlier. Several batches of the Danish model have followed since, not always with the most accurate livery application unfortunately, with one of the more recent appearing in conjunction with Bachmann and packaged in EFE Rail boxes. All of the liveries have been produced at one time or another with the model reflecting some of the differences found between the 50 locos, such as the bogie sideframes with or without sandboxes and the fitting of handrail guards to later examples. It is much the same story in N gauge where Dapol has offered the Class 58 for a number of years, new batches periodically appearing in all the key colours.

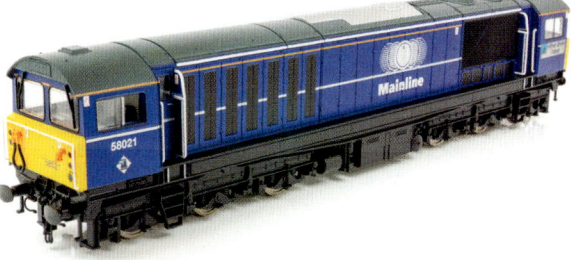

LEFT: **Mainline blue 58021** *Hither Green Depot* **was one of the OO gauge models released under the EFE Rail banner in 2020, these being to the same specification as the Heljan version but perhaps with a bit more attention to the livery application.** Image courtesy Kernow Model Rail Centre

BELOW: **Heljan has also produced the triple grey Mainline scheme as illustrated by 58009. If searching the secondhand market, it is worth noting that some triple grey releases have appeared without the cab doors being painted black or the bodyside grilles picked out in grey. This is one of the accurate ones.**

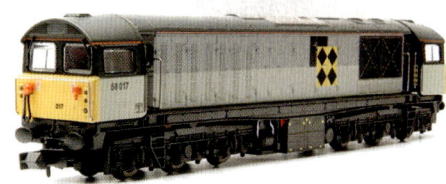

ABOVE: **All of the Class 58s carried Trainload Coal, 58049 being the last to be admitted for overhaul at the end of 1991 and losing its Railfreight Red Stripe livery in the process. This is the Dapol N gauge recreation of 58017.**

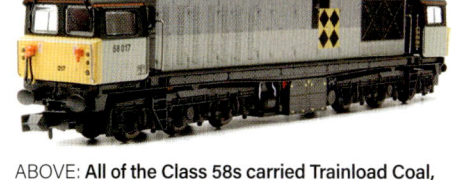

Modelling BR Locomotives of the 1990s 73

Out of the shadows

Class 58s for Didcot

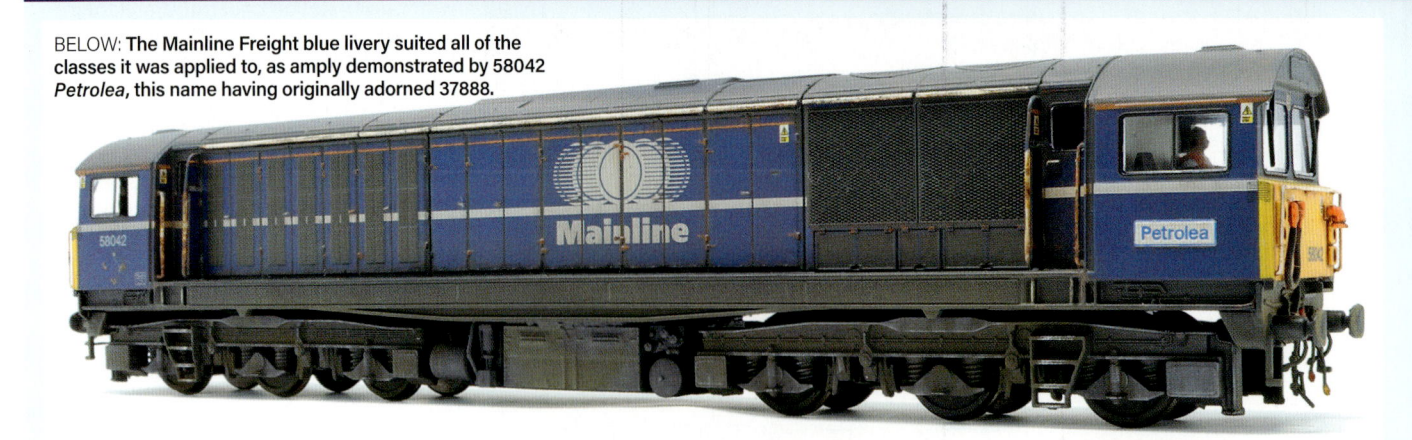

BELOW: **The Mainline Freight blue livery suited all of the classes it was applied to, as amply demonstrated by 58042** *Petrolea*, **this name having originally adorned 37888.**

Once solely the preserve of merry-go-round trains, the Class 58s managed to spread their wings later in their careers to a wide variety of workings under EWS ownership, including 'Enterprise' wagonload traffic and Ministry of Defence workings, alongside the odd appearance on Virgin CrossCountry services. This made them essential motive power for my layout based on Didcot using Heljan's OO gauge model as the basis.

The first step was to take the models apart, which initially involved unclipping the bodyshell from the chassis. By inserting a small flat-bladed screwdriver just above the bogies, you can start to ease away the bodyshell, repeating on each side until it is fully separated from the chassis. Next, the plastic light lenses need to be removed and then the tightly-fitted cab interior mouldings, which again can be levered out with a screwdriver. The glazing can either be taken out as well or, alternatively, Humbrol Maskol masking fluid can be applied over the windows to protect them.

The bodyshell requires minimal modifications but a worthwhile upgrade is to replace the roof fan grilles with the etched versions from Shawplan's Extreme Etchings range. One omission from the Heljan model are the door handles for the bodyside access doors, which are a small but noticeable detail on the otherwise flat sides. Tiny sections of styrene strip were cut, no more than 1mm in length, and individually glued to each door where the handle would be, these being affixed with Microscale 'Krystal Klear' glue. The reason for recommending this glue is that it is non-solvent based, so any excess can easily be removed without harming the paintwork. After fixing, the door handles were painted silver, touched in with a fine 5/0 brush.

Livery corrections

The Heljan number and name printing was removed very carefully using Humbrol enamel thinners, brushed onto the areas required and gentled rubbed further with a cotton bud dipped in thinners. Working very slowly and carefully, the printing should begin to lift within a couple of minutes. Heljan's base livery paintwork is very thin however, so it is important not to apply too much pressure or the plastic can easily be exposed underneath. One alternative method is to gently scratch away at the printing with a curve-bladed scalpel. However, extreme caution again needs to be taken to avoid going through the paintwork.

Eventually, with the printing removed, it was time to move on to giving the bodyshell a coat of Railmatch gloss varnish. A couple of passes of the aerosol will give a good glossy finish, which will come in handy to help with the paint corrections required as well as giving a good foundation for laying the waterslide decals on top later in the process.

Heljan has been known to make a series of livery errors and omissions with the Class 58s, all requiring fixing with a little patience and some fine paint brushes. For the Mainline grey examples, possibly the most infamous area that needs attention is the incorrect spelling

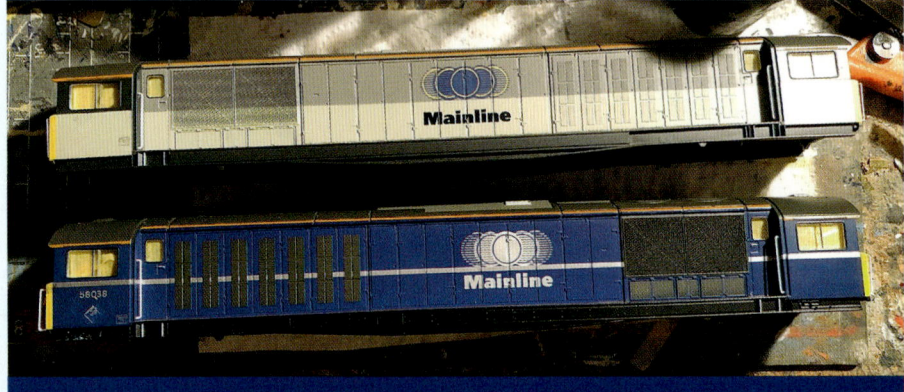

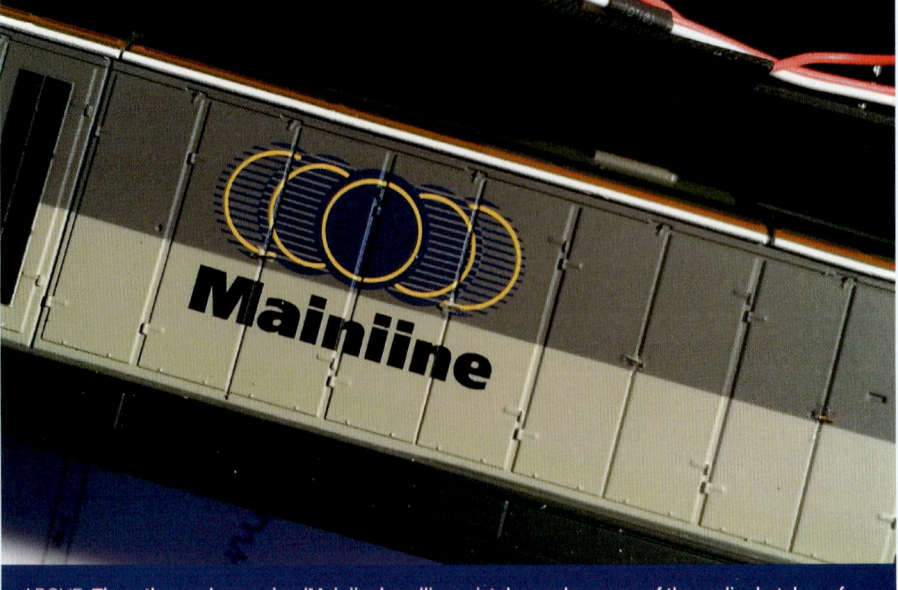

ABOVE: **Two of the Class 58 bodies are pictured following dis-assembly, masking of the glazing and removal of the printed numbers and other details.**

ABOVE: **The rather embarrassing 'Mainiine' spelling mistake made on one of the earlier batches of models. Fortunately turning the 'i' into a 'l' is straightforward with a bit of paint.**

74 www.keymodelworld.com

Out of the shadows

BELOW: 58034 carried one of the older Class 58 names in *Bassetlaw*, this being somewhat immortalised as it was the subject of one of Hornby's releases in the 1980s.

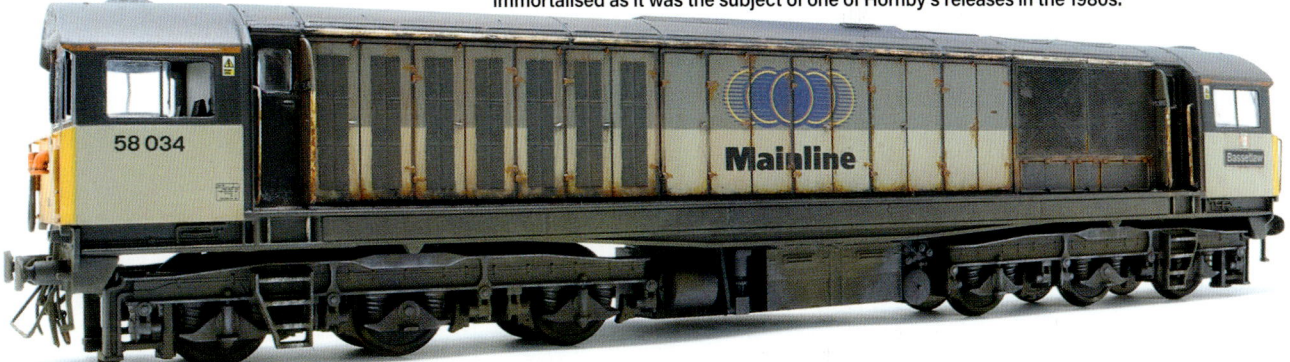

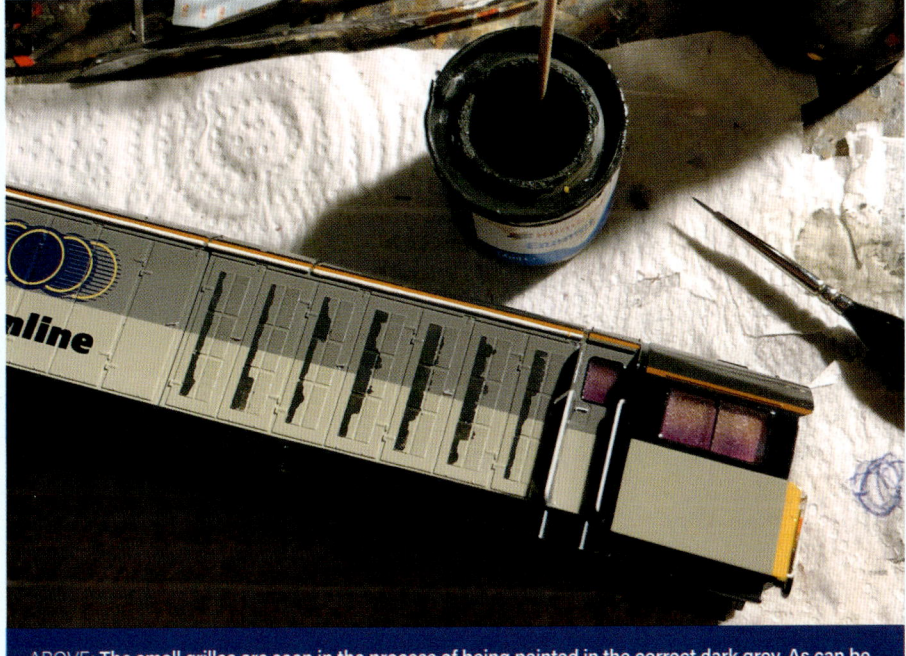

ABOVE: The small grilles are seen in the process of being painted in the correct dark grey. As can be seen, this is a fiddly job that will inevitably require some excess paint to be cleaned off.

doors, which is a style worn by only a few examples. The majority in Mainline blue had the cantrail warning line further down, on the doors themselves.

To alter this is more challenging with each route having its own pitfalls. One method is to use orange warning line transfers, which can be tricky to get straight, or a bow pen, which can take a lot of practice to master successfully. In my case, the method chosen was to mask a fine line using Tamiya tape and then paint the orange on using Humbrol No. 82. Despite careful masking, there was the inevitable paint run under the tape around the odd panel line for the bodyside doors. However, this was carefully removed once tacky by using cocktail sticks and a little enamel thinners, touching in the orange where required. The location of the old, raised orange warning line can then be painted over as required with dark grey paint.

New identities

With all the livery details corrected and the paint dried, it was then time to move on to applying the new numbers and other details to each loco. The transfers were sourced on the main logo, an early batch featuring 'Mainiine' lettering. With some black paint and a fine brush, the unwanted lowercase 'i' can be touched in to the correct 'l'.

Additionally, some batches have appeared with the cab doors and bodyside grilles finished in two-tone grey instead of the correct colours. These can all be painted, using dark grey for the grilles and neat black on the cab doors. It is best to paint the grilles freehand rather than try and mask them as their close proximity makes this hugely laborious and fiddly. Using the 5/0 paintbrush again, each grille was touched in, feathering in the brush on the straight edge and backfilling where needed until each was completed. Given the delicate nature of the detail painting needed, it is highly recommended to do this while the bodyshell is in a gloss-varnished state as any painting slip-ups can easily be wiped off, allowing you to start over.

On the Mainline blue examples, it is important to choose your prototype carefully as there is a variation in the positioning of the orange cantrail warning line. Heljan has modelled this at the top of the bodyside

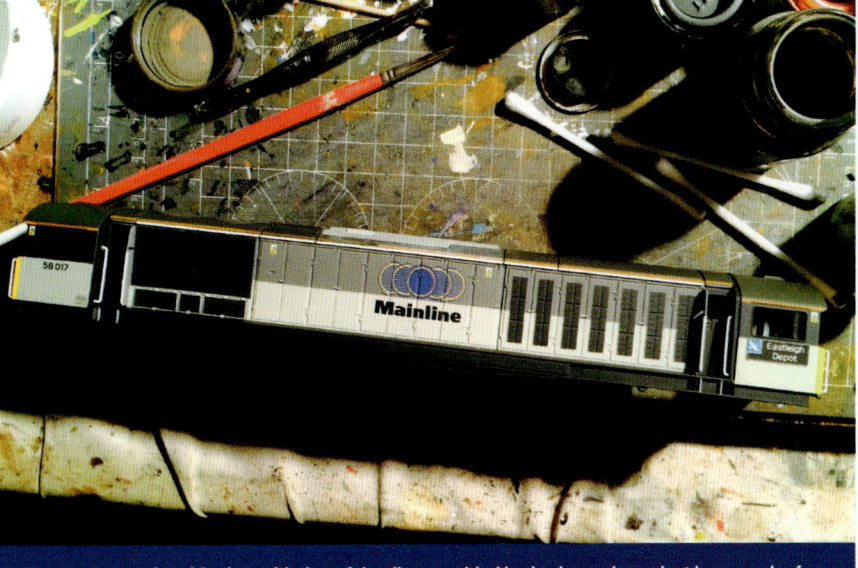

ABOVE: Comparing this shot with that of the disassembled body above shows just how much of an error Heljan made with some triple grey releases. Not only are the small grilles now painted but also the main radiator grilles and the cab doors. The new numbers and nameplates are also in place.

Modelling BR Locomotives of the 1990s   75

Out of the shadows

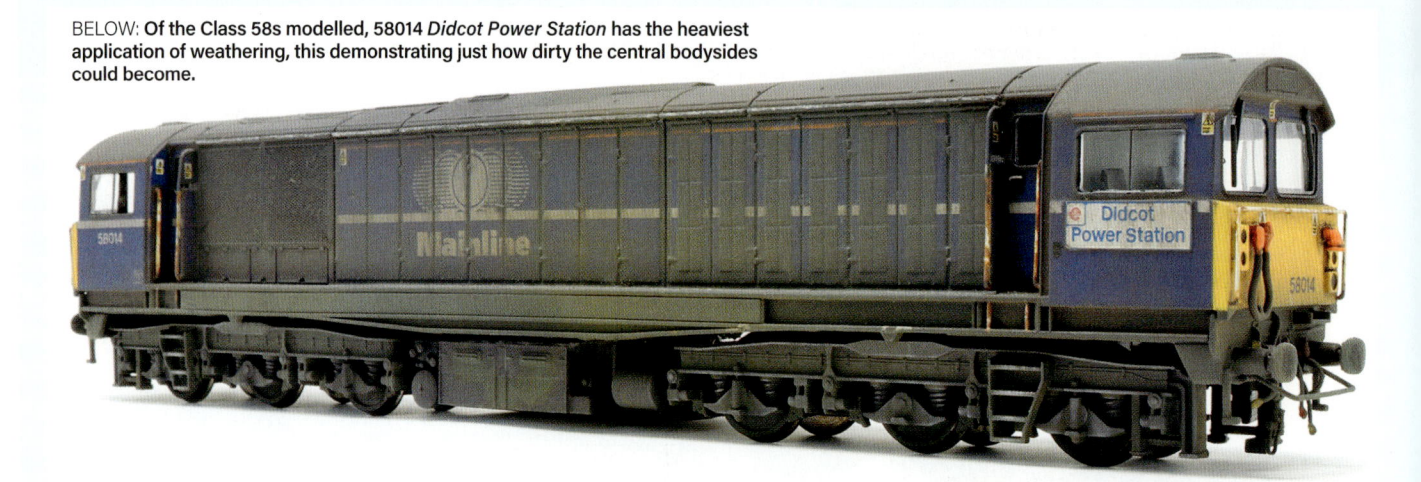

BELOW: **Of the Class 58s modelled, 58014** *Didcot Power Station* **has the heaviest application of weathering, this demonstrating just how dirty the central bodysides could become.**

from a mix of Railtec and Fox with the nameplates coming from the comprehensive selection available from Shawplan. The latter have all been re-drawn in recent years and, as a result, they are of extremely high quality and faithful to the prototype.

The Class 58s had a superb range of powerful and very utilitarian industrial names and, while not always to everyone's taste, this included collieries, depots, and power stations. My chosen selection was 58014 *Didcot Power Station*, 58017 *Eastleigh Depot*, 58034 *Bassetlaw* and 58042 *Petrolea*. In line with all of my models, the favoured approach was to attach the nameplates using varnish, the idea being that the slow drying time gives a great window to ensure the plates are positioned absolutely level. It is important to check prototype photos at this stage as the Class 58 nameplates were mounted in different positions, some sit higher than others on the cabsides and, when it comes to any additional crests, it is not always immediately obvious as to which way up is correct!

Once the nameplates had dried, the locos then received a layer of Railmatch matt varnish. Prior to spraying, it is always worth dusting down the bodyshells and checking that there are no foreign objects attached that can spoil the finish; there is nothing worse than spotting flecks of dust or fibres in your paint finish.

Weathering

Firstly, it is important to spend time observing how the real Class 58s weathered using a range of photos. It is key to model what you actually see, not what you think might be there. Back up every stage of what you are doing by looking at your photos, either by having them printed out or visible on a laptop or iPad during the weathering stages.

As a general theme, the Class 58s tended to accrue heavier weathering on their engine room doors compared to the cabsides due to the recessed bodysides being out of reach of washing plant brushes. The starting point was to apply a range of washes over the bodyshell, dark browns and greys, which were then wiped off with kitchen towel and cotton buds laced in enamel thinners, and working in a vertical motion across each panel on the body. Humbrol colours Nos.186, 113, 251 and 32 were used to build up layers of colour intensity and used to different extents across each locomotive, all the while matching the prototype photos.

Alongside the general grime deposits building up in the recesses, Class 58s could sometimes be seen sporting extensive oil staining that emanated from the bodyside doors around the engine bay and subsequently spilled down onto the solebars. This was replicated by adding dark grey paint and mottling on sparingly with a brush, then dabbing with a cotton bud to remove any excess, along with some dry-brushing of the same colour across the solebars.

When adding oil stains such as this, a deliberate choice was made to only use dark grey rather than black, which can give a very harsh appearance that overpowers the rest of the weathering on the model. Smaller weathering details were then applied, such as

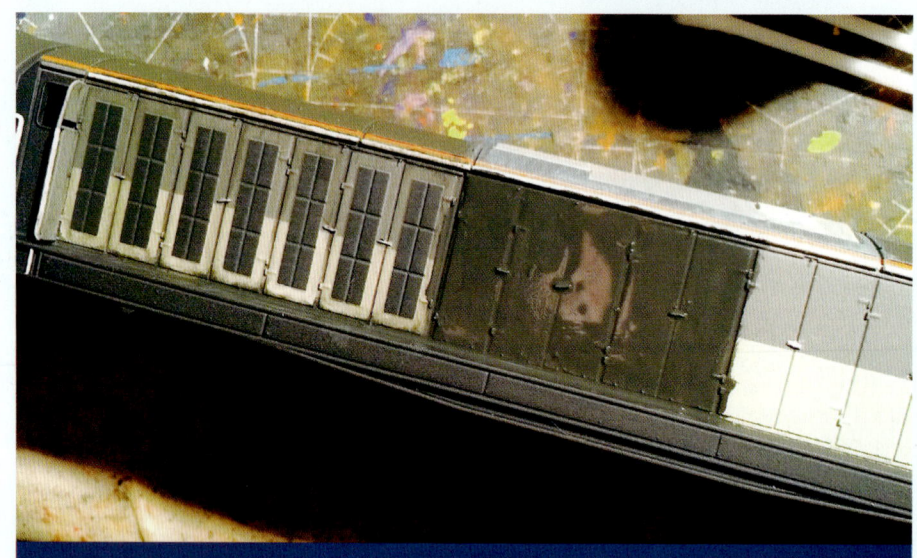

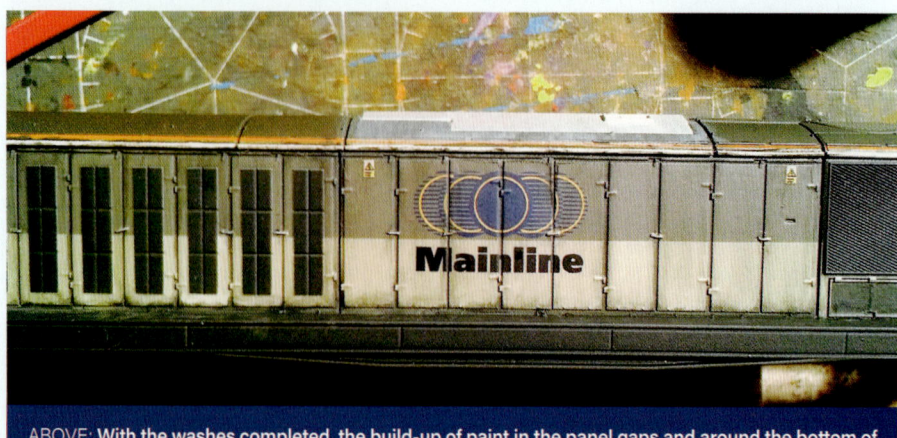

ABOVE: **The first stage of weathering is in progress with a brown wash applied to some of the plain doors. This will mostly be wiped off to give the finish seen on the grilled doors to the left. The handles added earlier to all the access doors can also be seen.**

ABOVE: **With the washes completed, the build-up of paint in the panel gaps and around the bottom of the doors has toned down the factory paintwork and gives a basis on which to build.**

Out of the shadows

BELOW: **One of the earliest recipients of the coloured Mainline logo was 58017 for its naming after** *Eastleigh Depot*. **Unlike many of its sisters, this loco was not exported to France or Spain for use on the construction of new high-speed rail lines and its derelict remains, still in this livery, were scrapped in 2014, ironically at its namesake depot.**

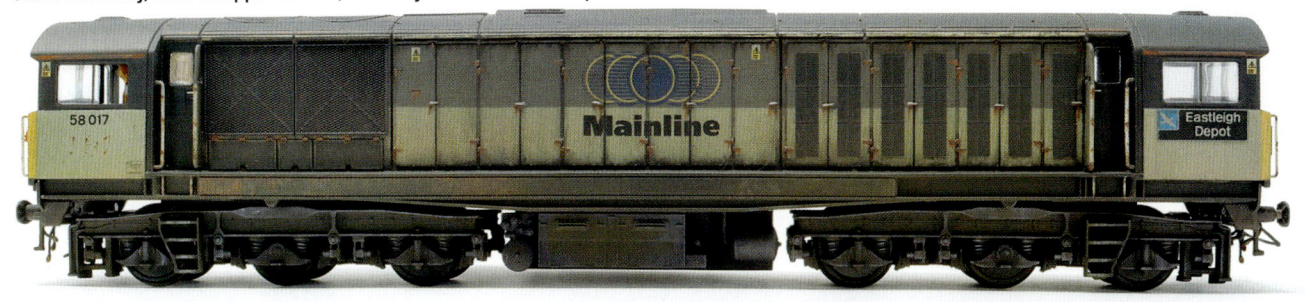

paint chips, damage, and rust patches. A fine 5/0 paintbrush was used, gradually building up variation in the shades used for a realistic look.

Finishing touches

Moving away from the bodyshell, the underframe received a little attention, notably around the ends where air pipes and couplings were added. Many Heljan Class 58s were supplied already fitted with the bufferbeam detailing, however in cases of buying used examples with broken fittings, the pipes were replaced with 0.45mm handrail wire, bent to shape and painted appropriately. Screw couplings came from Smiths, although wire hoops were also added to give compatibility with trains still fitted with tension-lock couplings.

It is important to consider a key detail difference on the Class 58 chassis as later-built examples were fitted with prominent rectangular sandboxes on the corners of each bogie. The bogies later got mixed around between class members, so it is essential to check photos to see which style your chosen locos had.

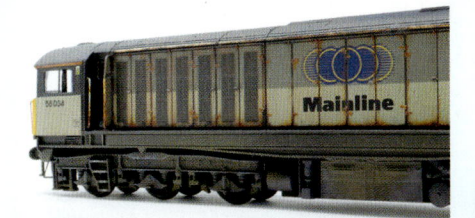

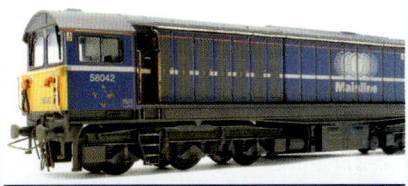

ABOVE: **With the paintwork on the triple grey examples being somewhat older, rust patches were in evidence on areas like the door hinges and bottom edges.**

ABOVE: **Having lost its cabside Toton depot plaque, 58042 shows the diamond-pattern scar from its removal. This is also one of the locos with the lowered cantrail stripe, this running across the top of the bodyside doors. The yellow on white overhead warning notices are also displayed; these became compulsory in 1998 and quickly spread across all stock as required, replacing the previous red on white flashes.**

The underframe was then given an all over coat of Humbrol dark grey (No.32) prior to receiving the regular weathering. At this stage, the models were re-assembled with any masking tape removed from the inside and the Humbrol Maskol taken off the windows. The cab interiors were also painted and weathered at this stage, receiving a black-painted floor to disguise the lack of depth while a driver figure was added at one end.

When it came to the traffic weathering, this consisted of a range of Phoenix Precision colours (brake dust, track dirt, roof dirt and dirty black) being air-brushed across the chassis and roof, carefully matching to photos. Around the exhaust ports, a custom mix of black and dark blue was sprayed to represent the oily exhaust build-up in this area. As a finishing touch, the bogies were dry-brushed with Humbrol Metalcote gunmetal, and footsteps touched in with silver paint to represent wear from drivers clambering up the steps over the years.

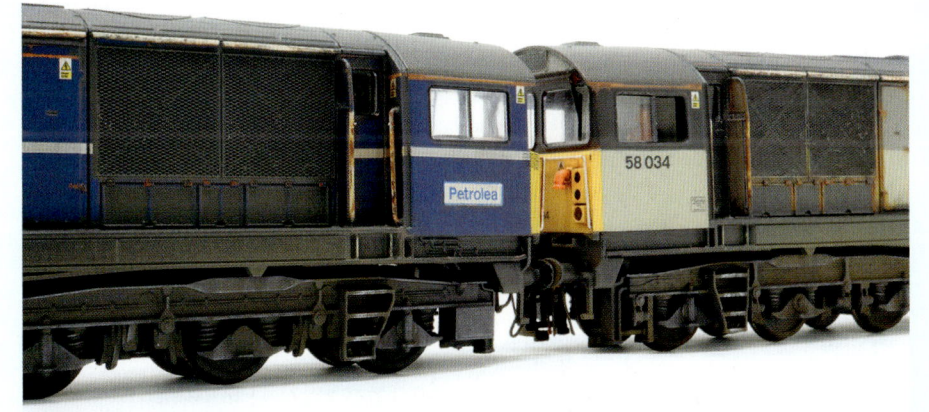

ABOVE: **A comparison between 58042 and 58034 illustrates the difference the sandboxes make to the appearance of the bogie sideframes. Weathering effects of note include the rust on the handrails and the dry-brushing on the bogie steps.**

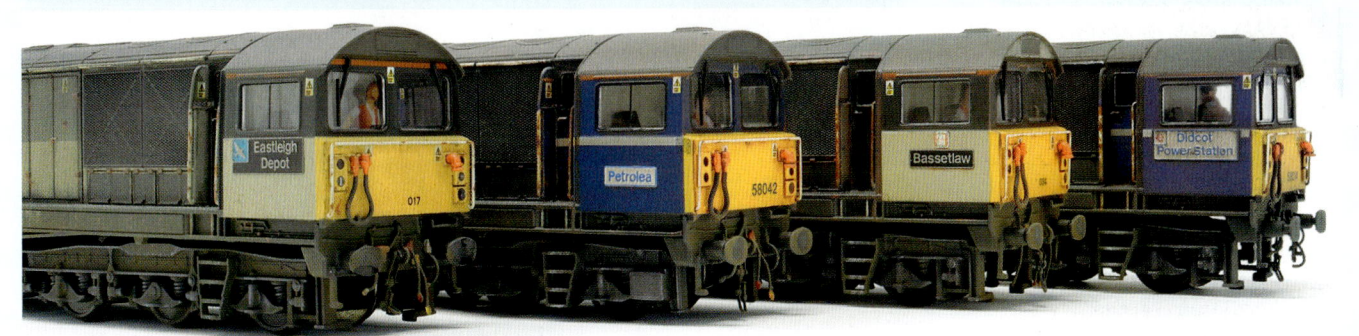

ABOVE: **The four Class 58s pose for an official line-up, all manner of detail and branding variations being apparent on careful study.**

Modelling BR Locomotives of the 1990s 77

Out of the shadows

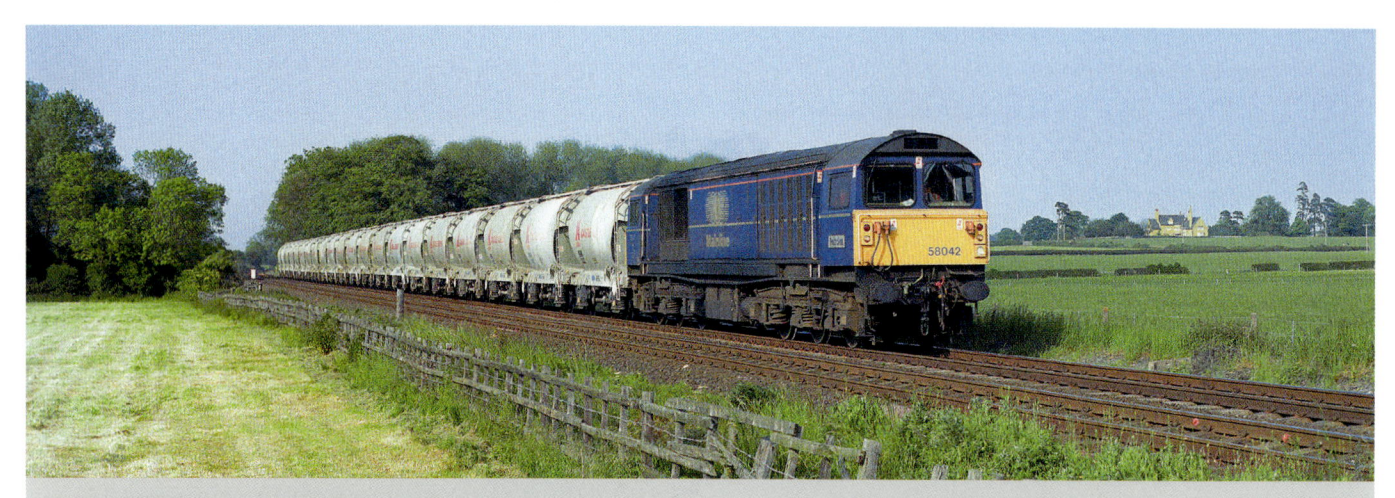

ABOVE: 58042 *Petrolea* illustrates the more diverse duties undertaken by the class in the second half of the 1990s as it passes East Goscote with the 6M93 14.55 King's Cross to Ketton via a reversal at Leicester on June 4 1997. This features a uniform rake of Castle Cement PCA Presflos returning empty and is a flow that still runs today, albeit to a terminal outside St Pancras. High quality models of these PCAs have been produced in N gauge by Realtrack Models and in OO by Accurascale. Bill Atkinson

RIGHT: The class became quite common on the 'Enterprise' workings from Eastleigh under EWS ownership. This wagonload service could turn up a diverse range of commodities and wagon types but china clay slurry originating from Quidhampton, Wiltshire, was a staple. On June 16, 1999, 58020 *Doncaster Works* passes Overthorpe, near Banbury, with the 6S65 15.19 Eastleigh to Mossend. The ICA 'silver bullet' tankers are available in both 2mm and 4mm from Dapol, the factory-weathered examples being particularly impressive. Martin Loader

BELOW: By the time 58013 had its overhaul completed at Doncaster Works in April 1996, Mainline Freight was no more and EWS had taken over. As a result, it was released in unbranded blue and ran in this condition for the remainder of its time in service with EWS. On March 11, 1997, it was heading the 6M63 08.19 Doncaster-Mountsorrel ballast empties as it passes Cossington. The rear of the train features the familiar Seacow ballast hoppers as available in OO gauge from both Bachmann and Hornby while Farish does a 2mm model. The front portion, however, is one of the first sets of autoballasters wagons, this being owned by Tiphook Rail rather than the more familiar vehicles that followed later for Railtrack and Network Rail. A rework and repaint of the Bachmann or Farish JJA wagons could produce these with some effort. Bill Atkinson

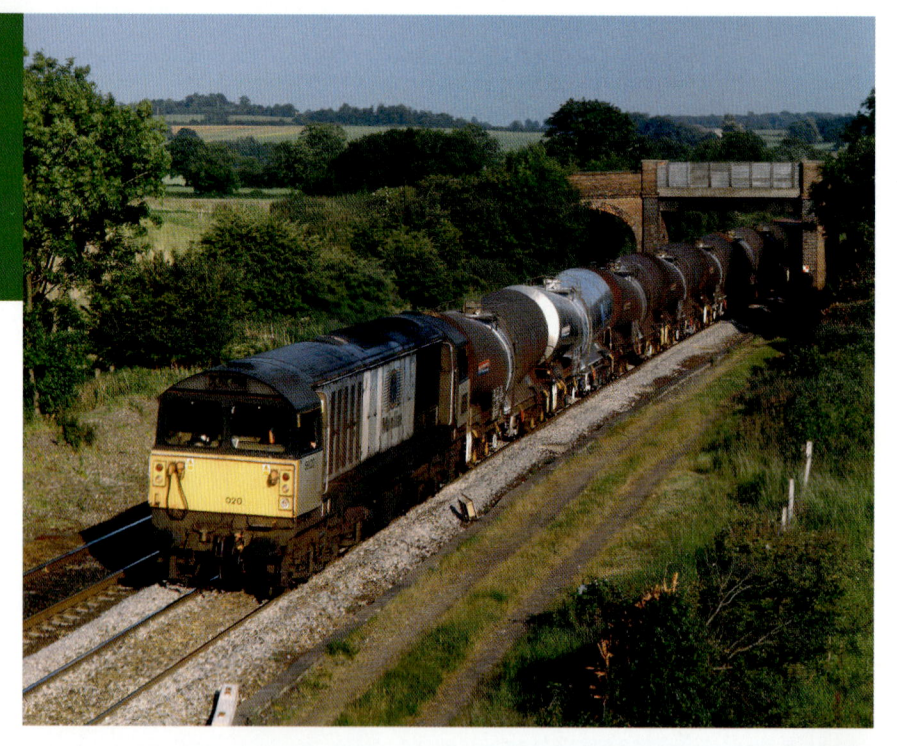

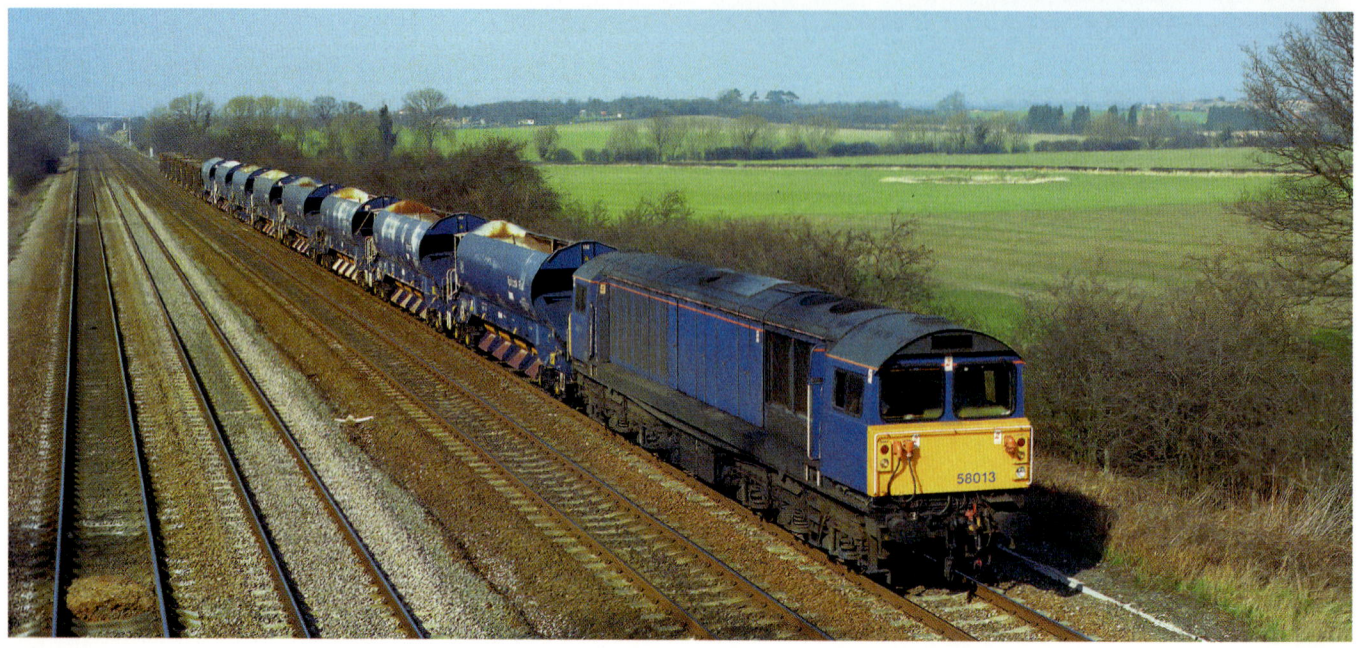

78 www.keymodelworld.com

KEY MODEL WORLD

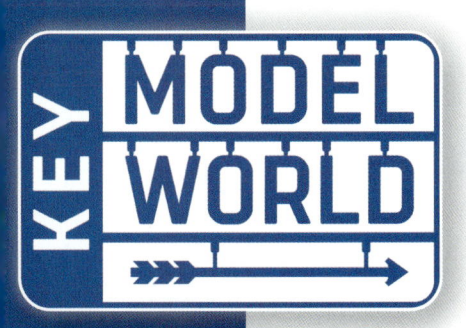

YOUR ONLINE SCALE MODELLING DESTINATION

Featuring **HORNBY** magazine **AIRFIX Model World**

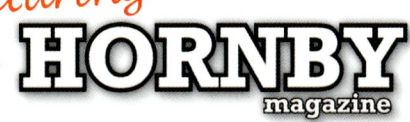

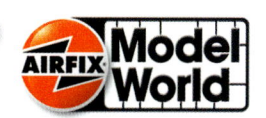

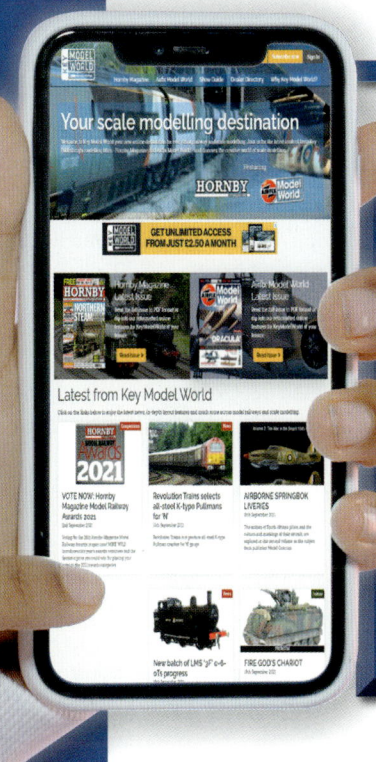

Unmissable modelling inspiration at your finger tips

"A modeller's paradise"
Christopher

"The key that unlocks the world of modelling!"
Graham

- ✓ Get all the **latest news** first
- ✓ **Exclusive** product and layout videos
- ✓ Fresh **inspiration**, tips and tricks every day
- ✓ A fully searchable **back catalogue**
- ✓ Back issues of **Hornby & Airfix Model World magazines**
- ✓ Full access to **Hornby & Airfix Model World magazines** content
- ✓ All available on **any device** - *anywhere, anytime*

Visit: **www.keymodelworld.com**

Out of the shadows

Loadhaul goes large

Introduced in 1994, the black and orange Loadhaul scheme quickly became one of the most popular liveries to ever grace the network and remains so even today. Simon Bendall looks at its development with particular regard to the Class 60s while Alex Carpenter weathers the Hornby model in OO gauge.

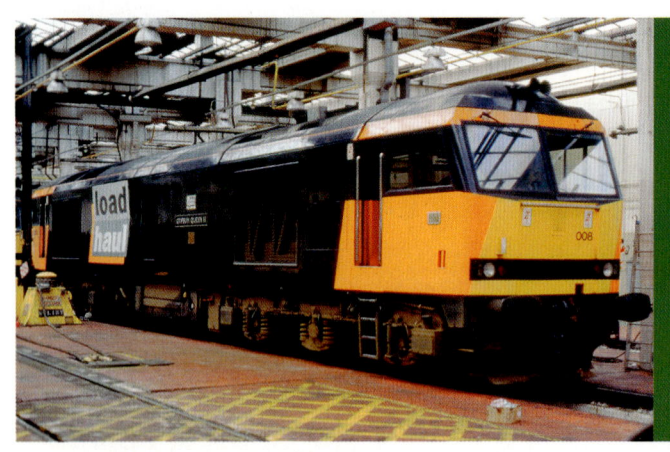

LEFT: Some ten months after its repaint, a still clean 60008 *Gypsum Queen II* receives maintenance inside Thornaby TMD on July 6, 1996. The loco displays the original version of the Loadhaul logo with a light grey background to 'Load' rather than the white that was later adopted. 60038 and 60059 were similarly adorned while 60007 and 60025 had the white version. *Simon Bendall Collection*

The area assigned to Trainload Freight North East upon the segregation of the three regional freight companies in 1994 was the smallest of the lot. However, it encompassed the three busy traffic centres of Humberside, Teesside, and Tyneside, giving the company an extensive portfolio of steel and petroleum workings alongside other commodities.

Trainload Freight North East was also the first of the three to unveil its new identity of Loadhaul that July, it became an independent company three months later. Coupled with the new name was the introduction of a new black and orange colour scheme, this using stock BR colours from the Strathclyde PTE livery. This was also designed to be practical with the black intended to hide oil leaks and exhaust stains as well as disguise bodyside ripples while the orange would help to mask brake dust deposits.

For locos with good quality Railfreight triple grey paintwork, namely the Class 60s, an interim livery was also devised. This envisaged that the main sub-sector emblems would be replaced by Loadhaul logos and that vertical orange triangles positioned by the cab doors would take the place of the sub-sector repeaters.

Yorkshire launch
The first Loadhaul-liveried locos were unveiled at the Doncaster Works open day on July 9, 1994, in the shape of fully-repainted 37713 and 56039 in black and orange while 60050 was finished in the rebranded triple grey version. After a short period of evaluation, the livery was approved, although the parallelogram shaped yellow warning panels used on 37713 and 56039 did not find favour, being changed to a trapezium shape for all subsequent repaints on these two classes.

Repaints of the Class 60s in black and orange did not begin until May 1995 with Brush Traction outshopping 60059 ready for its naming as *Swinden Dalesman* the following month. Marcroft Engineering was also awarded a contract around this time to repaint two '60s' into Loadhaul at its Stoke-on-Trent workshops, 60038 emerging around the same time as 60059 while 60008, the future *Gypsum Queen II*, followed in September the same year. Notably, the Class 60s retained the use of parallelogram-shaped warning panels.

This was a change in policy after the interim idea of simply rebranding triple grey locos failed to gather any momentum. Only two more Class 60s would follow 60050 in gaining new logos while still in grey and 60064 and 60070 did not do so until the autumn of 1995 while receiving attention at Loughborough. Even then, 60064 did not receive the orange triangles by the cab doors, although 60070 did join 60050 in carrying these.

There were certainly no re-brandings done by home depots, in contrast to what was achieved by both Transrail and Mainline Freight facilities. Subsequently, Loadhaul-owned Class 60s passing through Brush were to be treated to a full re-livery but only 60007 and 60025 were completed before repaints were halted in March 1996 on the orders of EWS. Thus, for all its popularity, there were only ever five black and orange Class 60s.

Allocation split
When the Class 60 fleet was divided up between the three regional freight companies in the spring of 1994, a near even split of the 100 locos was made in the interests of fairness, giving each one 33 examples with Trainload Freight West taking the leftover as it had the largest geographical area. In the northeast, the allocation remained divided between Immingham and Thornaby with deployment on petroleum and steel traffic being their main use along with the Immingham to Scunthorpe iron ore circuit.

Apart from the eight rebranded in one variety of Loadhaul or the other, the rest of the fleet largely retained sub-sector badges pertaining to these traffics, including 60002/03/13/14/24/26-28/51/53/54 in Petroleum and 60020-23/30/31/49/52 in Metals. Completing the line-up were the Coal trio of 60004/90/91 while, also once similarly badged, 60067-69 ran in unbranded condition. The latter three were a rare instance of Loadhaul traction losing the previous Railfreight identities.

Among the other loco types, black and orange was not overly common on the Class 37s either with just 37513/16/17, 37698, 37710 and 37884 joining launch loco 37713. Of these, 37516 never received Loadhaul logos, running unbranded to withdrawal. Where Loadhaul colours did make inroads was amongst the Class 56s with 56003/06/21/27/34/35/45/50/55/74/77/83-85/90 and 56100/02/06/07/09-12/16/18/30 all painted during works overhauls. In all, a mere 39 locos received full Loadhaul repaints across the three classes.

RIGHT: Just two weeks after Loadhaul was launched, 60050 *Roseberry Topping* arrives at Newark Northgate on July 25, 1994, with discharged tankers returning north to Lindsey refinery. The train features a mix of 90-tonne GLW TDA and 102-tonne GLW TEA designs mixed together. While a comprehensive range of pre-privatisation bogie tankers remains an aspiration in all scales, the recent release of a further TEA design in OO gauge by Cavalex Models has improved matters, it joining the older 1960s-style produced by both Bachmann and Hornby and, in 2mm, by Farish. *Simon Bendall Collection*

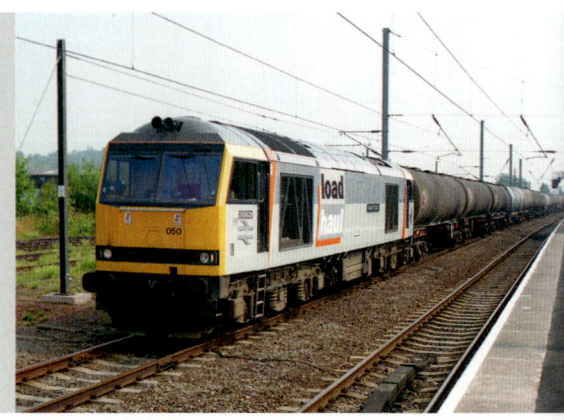

Out of the shadows

The black art of weathering

BELOW: **The Class 60 remains one of Hornby's most impressive diesel models, even more so when the livery application is well-executed. Few would argue that the Loadhaul colours suited the class extremely well.**

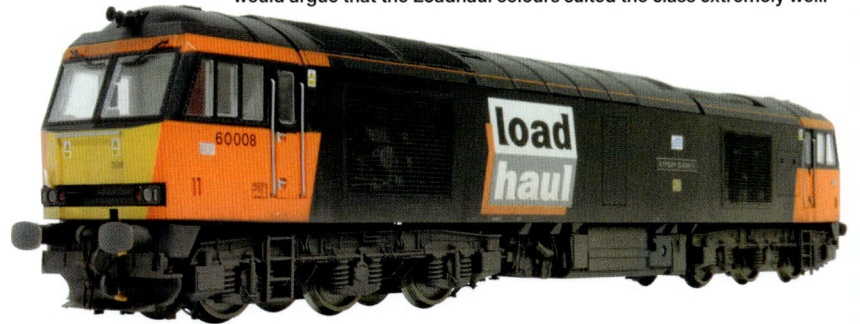

The Loadhaul livery suited the angular lines of the Class 60s very well as shown here by 60008 *Gypsum Queen II*. The loco is modelled as in its earlier years before gaining red-backed nameplates and losing the lower brass plaques. This was a simple renumbering job from the Hornby model of 60007, although I opted to change the entire number rather than just the last digit as the factory printing was not a match to the transfers. The exquisite nameplates came from Shawplan and help to liven up the plain black bodysides no end. These feature a detailed plaque and etched crest overlaid with a colour transfer, making them look superb.

With little in the way of detailing required, the main task was to weather the model, this seeing it taken apart and the body sprayed with satin varnish to get rid of the factory finish, which is not quite matt enough as a starting point. The loco was then given a wash of track dirt colour, which was mostly wiped off. This was done several times until a build-up of different shades appeared. I then used thinners to distress the varnish, this giving it the faded appearance typical of weathered black. This was rubbed on with a cotton bud, streaking up and down to get varying degrees of fading.

Once this was done and fully dry, the final weathering could be done. Much the same method was used for the underframe, paying particular attention to build-up on the lower bodysides and roof panels. Weathering black roofs is tricky as you have to use a slightly grey shade so that the dirt will show up against the black. The same goes for streaks of exhaust dirt washing down from the roof panel gaps, these again being added using a slightly grey/black mix.

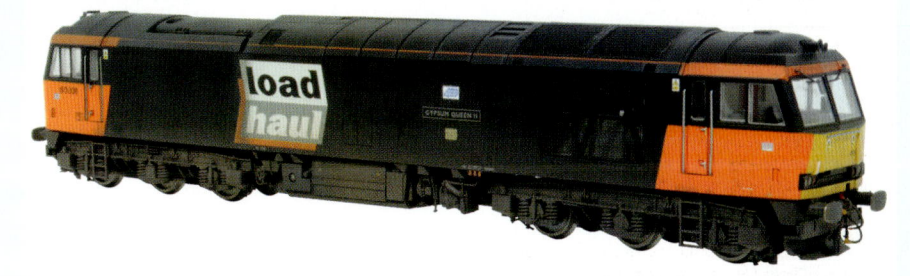

ABOVE: **Hornby has released just one Loadhaul Class 60 to date, this being 60007 in 2006 as part of the initial batch of locos. As a result, the second-hand market usually has to be scoured to find donors to model Loadhaul examples, although they are not particularly hard to come by.**

Model availability

Inevitably, it was Lima that was the first to produce the Class 60s in OO gauge, going on to release a wide variety of models as new colours appeared, including Loadhaul. Following the collapse of the manufacturer and the subsequent acquisition of its assets by Hornby, the model was not one of those to re-appear in a red box. Instead, Hornby released its own highly-detailed Class 60 at the end of 2005, and this has since gone on to appear in most of the liveries carried over the last 34 years. While there has been no black and orange Loadhaul example for 16 years, a more recent release has been 60070 in triple grey with Loadhaul brandings.

In N gauge, Graham Farish offers a nice recreation of the Class 60s that has similarly appeared in many liveries, although it lags behind its 4mm cousin slightly in this regard. The Loadhaul release here, again from some years ago, was 60059 *Swinden Dalesman*. Not to be outdone, Heljan holds sway in O gauge with its sizeable recreation of the Brush Type 5s. A second batch of models has recently swelled the number of liveries available considerably, this bringing a second Loadhaul release that is fully finished, again as 60059. The original un-numbered Loadhaul model from several years ago is best avoided as it features a livery error that sees the orange angled in the wrong direction by two of the cab doors, Heljan acknowledging the error at the time but doing nothing else to rectify the mistake.

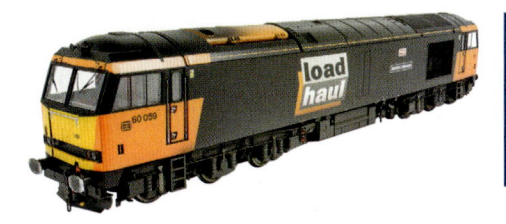

LEFT: **Heljan's second Loadhaul release in O gauge was 60008 *Gypsum Queen II*, this being fully finished with name and numbers after the initial un-numbered model.** Image courtesy Kernow Model Rail Centre

BELOW: **A relatively recent release in OO gauge from Hornby, 60070 *John Loudon McAdam* carries the Loadhaul logos and orange triangles by the cab doors that also featured on 60050. The third of the rebranded trio, 60064, just had the main logos.** Image courtesy Kernow Model Rail Centre

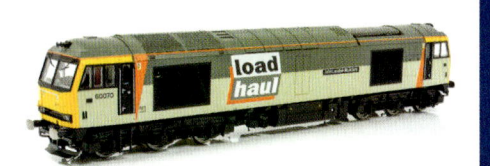

ABOVE: **The Graham Farish release in N gauge depicts the first of the class to be repainted, 60059 *Swinden Dalesman*. The naming marked Loadhaul's relationship with construction company Tilcon, its principal quarry being at Swinden, near Skipton.**

Modelling BR Locomotives of the 1990s

Out of the shadows

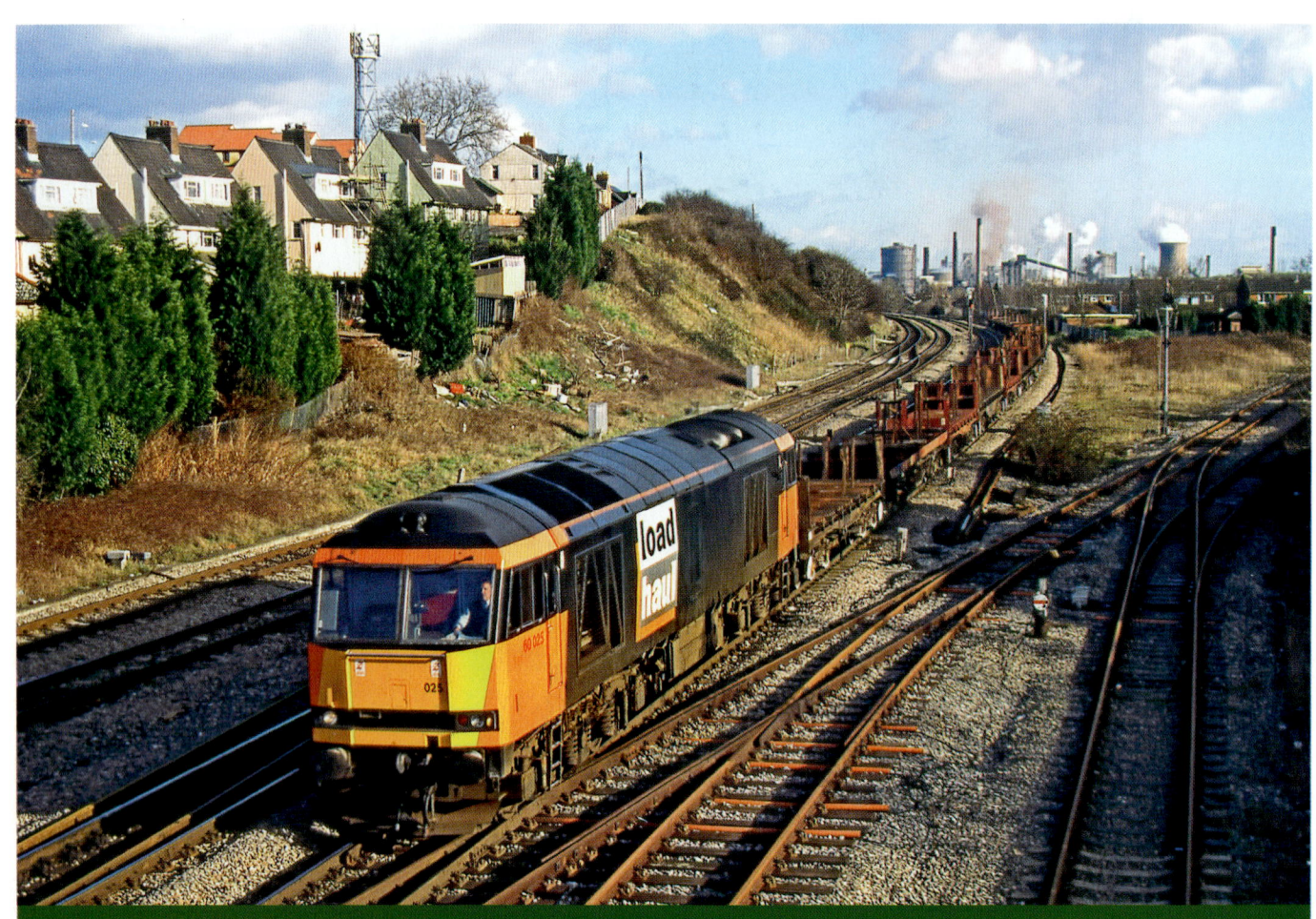

ABOVE: With Llanwern in the background, 60025 passes East Usk on February 7, 1998, with the 6V75 09.02 Dee Marsh to Margam. The consist is mostly empty BAA and BBA steel flats with a solitary BDA bogie bolster second in the formation; two of the BAAs being in relatively fresh EWS maroon. In 4mm, Bachmann does the BAA and BDA with Cavalex offering the BBA, while Graham Farish produces the first two wagons in 2mm. *John Chalcraft/Rail Photoprints*

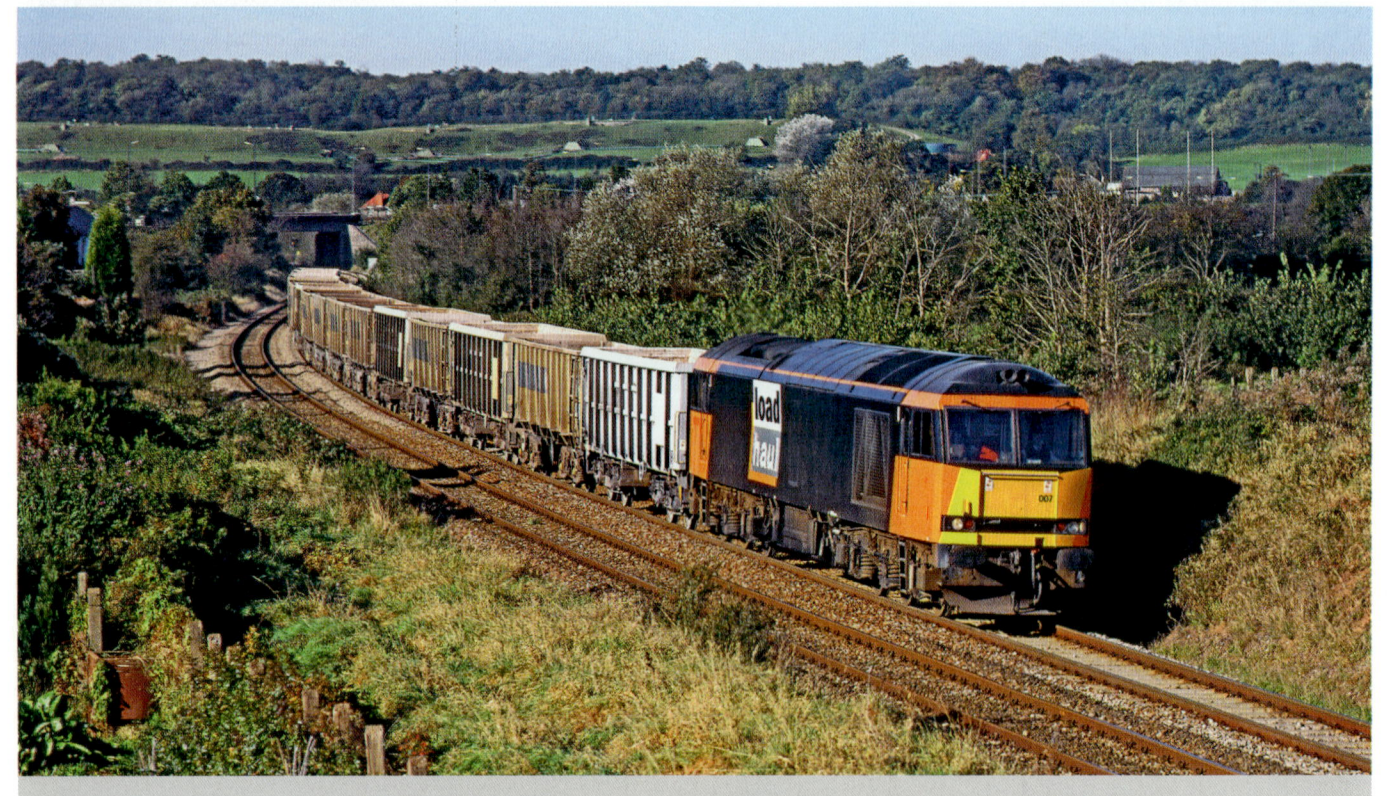

ABOVE: Following the EWS takeover of the three freight companies, the Class 60s became a countrywide common user fleet, bringing the Loadhaul colours to new areas. On October 28, 1997, 60007 was continuing the long association of the class with the Mendip stone traffic as it powers the 10.30 Avonmouth to Whatley empties past Brentry, on the outskirts of Bristol. The box wagons are a mix of Foster Yeoman JYA and JTA/JUA, the latter being more numerous in the train and available in 4mm scale from Accurascale and as a 2mm scale kit from the N Gauge Society. No RTR model yet exists of the JYA, but S Kits does a resin kit in 4mm. *John Chalcraft/Rail Photoprints*

Out of the shadows

RIGHT: On an unrecorded date in 2005, 60059 *Swinden Dalesman* stands at Goole glassworks while its train of WBB Minerals PAA sand hoppers are discharged, the traffic having originated from Middleton Towers, near King's Lynn. The two-axle PAAs were similar in design to the PGA aggregate hoppers but with top doors to protect the load from the elements and originally carried the white and yellow livery of British Industrial Sand. No accurate RTR model currently exists in any scale unfortunately. Simon Bendall Collection

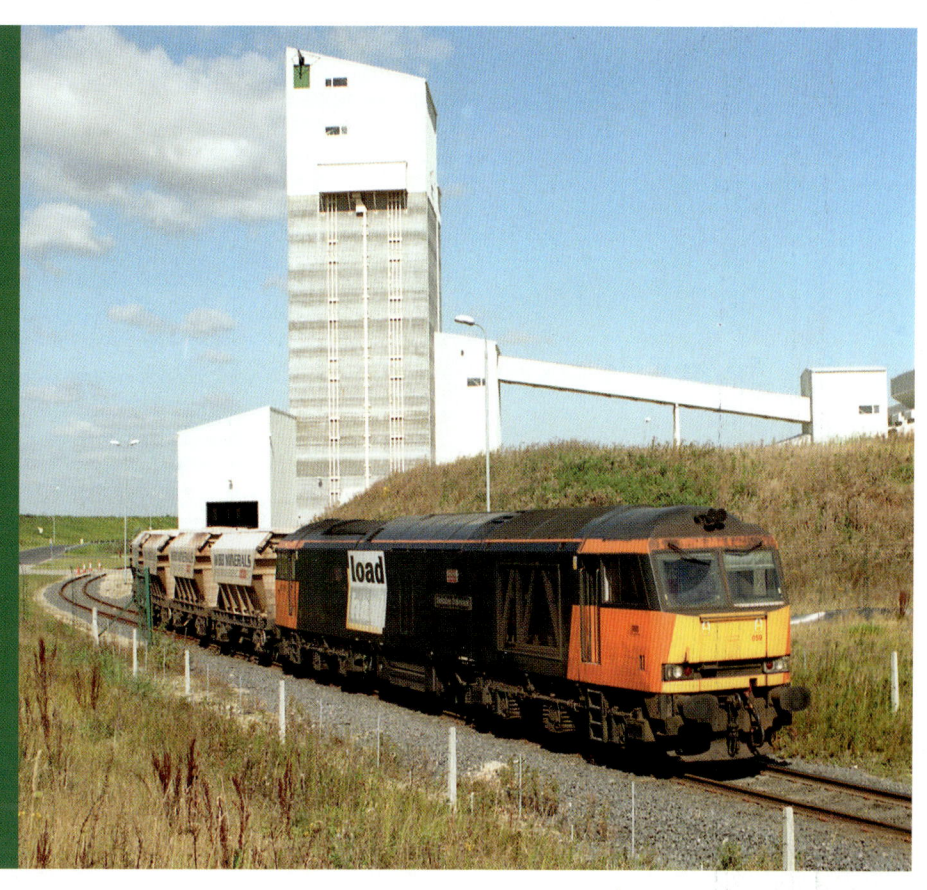

RIGHT: The iron ore traffic between Immingham and the steelworks at Scunthorpe has been a feature of north Humberside for 50 years, the Class 60s having seen considerable involvement for around half of this time. In August 2000, 60008 *Gypsum Queen II* heads west at Knabbs Bridge, Melton Ross, with a loaded train of ore. These JTA/JUA tipplers have been in use throughout this time, although being BREL-built they have a number of differences compared to those later constructed by Redpath Dorman Long for the other main steelworks. Lima produced a dimensionally-compressed model of the BREL batch in 4mm, the tooling for which now resides with Hornby. Simon Bendall Collection

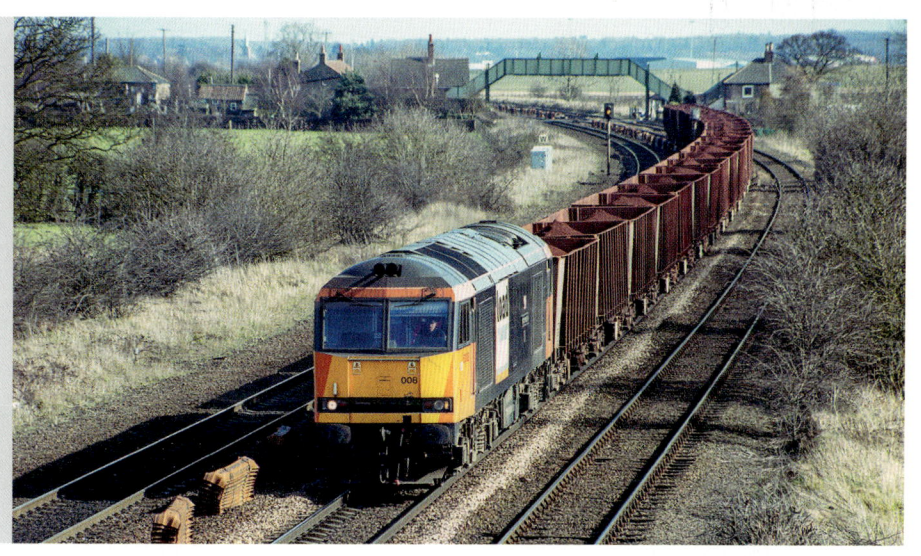

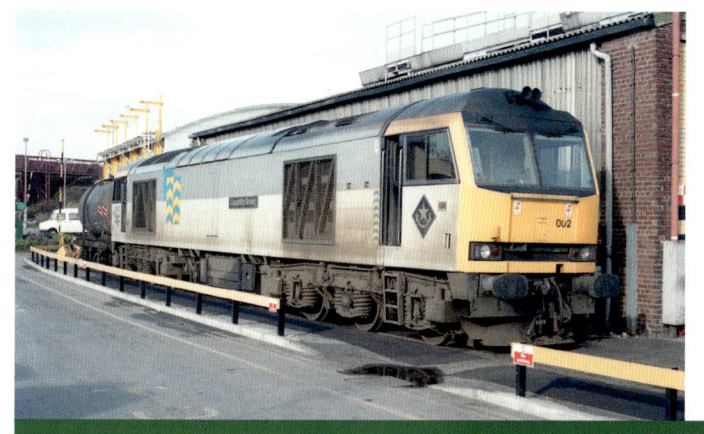

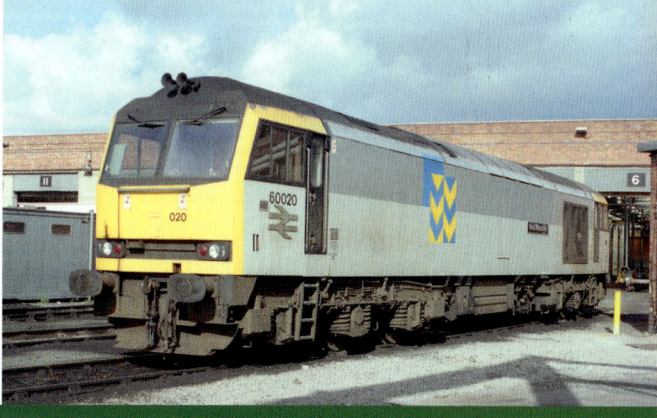

ABOVE LEFT AND ABOVE RIGHT: As mentioned, the majority of Class 60s under Loadhaul ownership retained their sub-sector badges throughout their time with the company and on into the EWS era. 60002 *Capability Brown* is seen at Knottingley on January 15, 1995, still in Petroleum and displaying the scroll and star plaque of its home depot Immingham. Meanwhile, Metals-branded 60020 *Great Whernside* was stabled at its home depot of Thornaby on April 4, 1996. Simon Bendall Collection

Modelling BR Locomotives of the 1990s 83

Out of the shadows

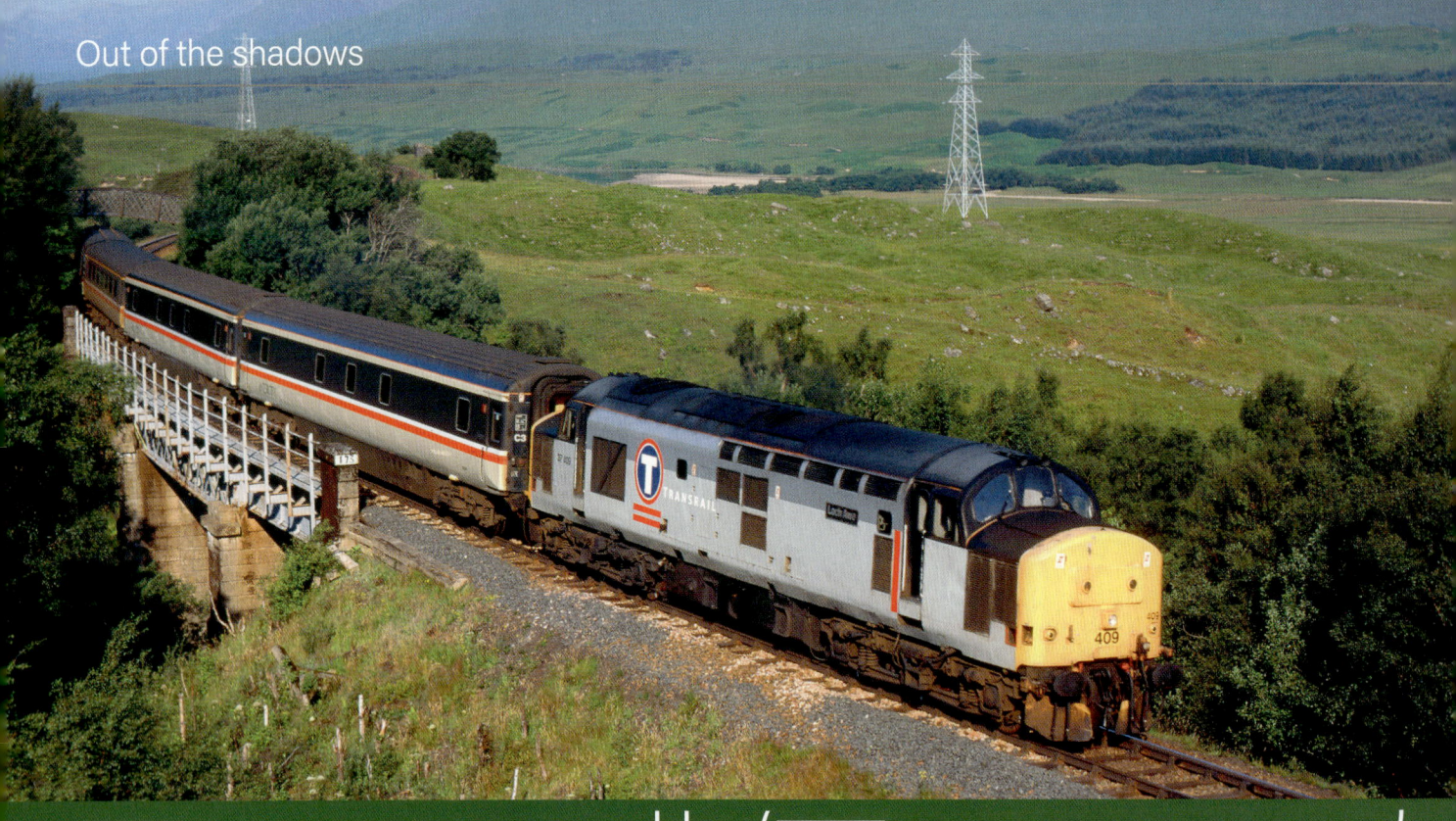

Transrail 'Tractors'

Transrail was the only one of the three regional freight companies to have examples of all the Class 37 sub-classes on its books, ranging from the as-built '37/0s' to the re-engined '37/9s'. Simon Bendall looks at the development of the Western freight identity, particularly on the Type 3s, while Timara Easter models a pair of Scottish examples.

Of the three regional freight organisations, Trainload Freight West was the largest, with services stretching from Cornwall to the Scottish Highlands. From October 1994, the company became independent from the British Rail structure and was christened Transrail, the new name reflecting the company's primary purpose of transporting goods by rail.

The bold logo, soon nicknamed the 'Big T', consisted of a wheel above rails motif and was finished in the national colours to present a nationwide image. Where bodyside space permitted, the Transrail name was also added in white upper-case lettering. Unlike Loadhaul and Mainline Freight, Transrail refrained from creating a totally new livery, instead opting to continue with the Railfreight triple-grey scheme, a decision no doubt aided by the fact that the colours already adorned a high proportion of its fleet so most locos would simply require a change of logo.

The Transrail identity first appeared on the side of a loco on July 14, 1994, when 60015 was rolled out from Cardiff Canton for inspection and official photographs. For several weeks, the Class 60 remained the sole loco in the new identity while design work continued for other classes and consideration was given to alterations, such as finishing nameplate and depot plaque backgrounds in house colours as well as adding smaller 'T' logos to the cab fronts; neither idea coming to fruition.

September 5 marked the official launch of the company to customers and the media, the event taking place at Warrington Yard where 60015 was joined by rebranded 37509, 56099 and a selection of wagons in showing off the new identity. With events also taking place around the country to make staff aware of the changes in the weeks prior to and after the launch, the opportunity was taken to rebrand a selection of locos with Transrail logos. For the Class 37s, this encompassed 37410, 37412, 37695 and 37889 by mid-September along with 56044/72/73, 60037/96/97 and a fully-repainted 31105.

In the west

Transrail's most westerly allocation of Class 37s was unsurprisingly in Cornwall for the still relatively buoyant china clay traffic. While Class 60s would soon arrive in the south west to handle the long distance workings to Cliffe Vale (Stoke) and Irvine, there were enough local trip workings, mostly to Fowey Docks, to keep the Type 3s employed. These continued to be maintained at St Blazey, although Canton was their notional home depot.

A snapshot allocation as of May 1995 included most of the former Railfreight Distribution Class 37/5 fleet in 37669-74, all of which would come to gain the 'Big T' logos as would 37413, 37668 and 37696 alongside the aforementioned 37695. Proving that not everything was rebranded, 37229 and 37521 clung resolutely to their respective Trainload Coal and Metals sub-sector emblems throughout Transrail's existence while 37416 retained its BR-era Mainline livery.

As the company's primary depot, Canton was home to four further pools of Class 37s, including Mirrlees-engined 37901-04 and the Ruston-powered pair of 37905 and 37906. Only the first and last of the soon to be cult-followed sub-class would go Transrail, the others remaining in Metals as they went about their heavy freight work in and around South Wales. Also retained at Cardiff for the same purpose were 15 of the refurbished

ABOVE: **One of the key duties for Transrail Class 37/4s based at Motherwell was to power the Edinburgh to Fort William and return sleeper portion, the service having survived political interference and attempts to withdraw it. By July 22, 1997, 37409** *Loch Awe* **was in EWS ownership but still displaying its previous allegiance as it passes through Achallader with the 1Y11 05.05 sleeper, which had departed from Euston at 21.30 the previous evening. The lightweight load of four coaches features two Mk.3a sleepers, a Mk.2f lounge car conversion and a Mk.1 Full Brake (BG), all in InterCity colours despite this now being a ScotRail operation. The sleepers are available in OO gauge from Hornby (ex-Lima) and Dapol in N gauge while Bachmann and Graham Farish have produced an appropriately-liveried BG. The lounge car would require modification from a Mk.2f FO as also made by Bachmann and Farish.** Martin Loader

84 www.keymodelworld.com

Out of the shadows

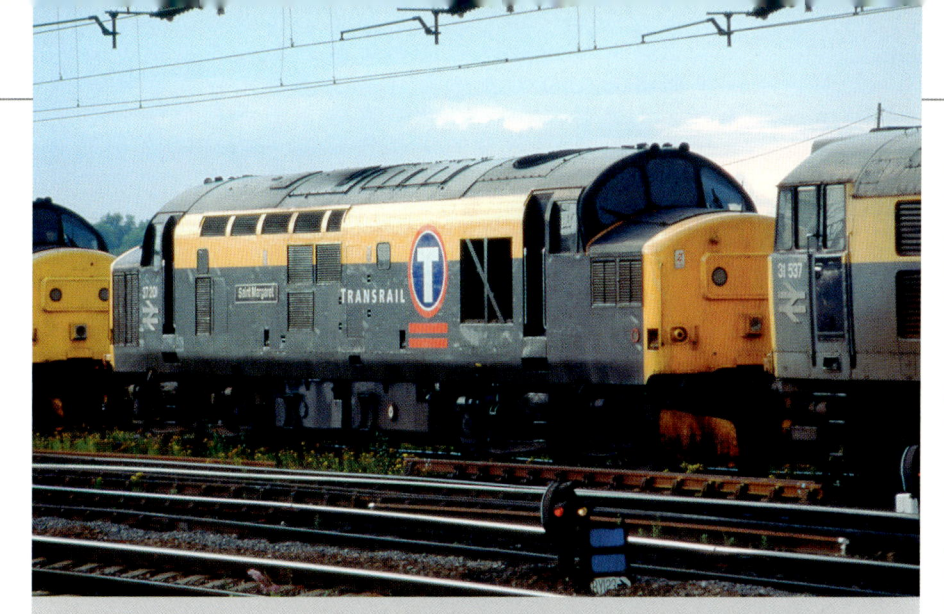

ABOVE: The 'Dutch' version of the Transrail livery made for an attractive sight with its pleasing combination of colours. By now based at Bescot, 37201 *Saint Margaret* shows off its new look while stabled at Rugby in the company of 31537 on July 28, 1995. The loco was an early casualty of the EWS reign, having just 14 months left in traffic, although it was not scrapped until 2009. Simon Bendall Collection

Class 37/7s, these all being former Trainload Coal machines. Of these, 37701/02/99 and 37802/87/96/97/98 would join early launch loco 37889 in receiving the new logos, but 37704/96/97 and 37894/95/99 retained their existing 'black diamonds' through to the EWS era.

Also in the Canton stable were two smaller groups of mostly Class 37/0s that were nominally for infrastructure duties. Of these, 'Dutch'-liveried 37197, 37230, 37254 and 37258 along with Trainload Coal 37213 had received a hopper in the former boiler compartment and dispensing equipment so they could lay sandite on the rails during the autumn leaf fall period. Further members of the class would also be modified for the same purpose later on. The rest of the infrastructure allocation involved 37141/46/58 and 37263, all in 'Dutch', and debranded triple grey 37178.

Also in this pool were Transrail-branded 37411 and 37413, which were most commonly found powering passenger trains to the likes of Weymouth for the newly-formed South Wales and West train company. This operation would also encompass workings to Birmingham New Street and Manchester Piccadilly from Cardiff and ran until September 1999, by when EWS was in control and numerous Class 37/4s had made appearances.

Through the Midlands

Heading north to Birmingham, around 20 Class 37s were allocated to Bescot by May 1995 for mostly infrastructure duties, this including a number of examples that had been based in Scotland for years but moved south a few months earlier to replace Class 31s. Most notable where the 'celebrity' duo of BR large logo 37025 *Inverness TMD* and BR standard blue 37275 *Oor Wullie*. During 1996, both were stripped of their BR arrows as a condition of privatisation, this being rather more obvious on 37025 given their size!

The rest of the allocation featured 'Dutch'-liveried 37071/87/99, 37142/84/88/91, and 37201/07/11/40/55 in addition to Transrail-badged 37111, 37154 and 37212 while 37261 stayed in faded Railfreight Distribution. The final Bescot-based Type 3 was 37116, which in 1995 was still in BR large logo blue with the Tinsley name of *Comet* and with its bufferbeam cowls resolutely in place.

February 1996 saw 37116 emerge from overhaul at Doncaster Works as a transformed loco. Now finished in BR blue with 'Big T' logos, this had included the removal of its split headcode boxes and the fitting of flush marker lights in their place while the bufferbeam cowls were also gone. Named *Sister Dora* shortly afterwards, the loco became an instant 'celebrity' which continued through its time in EWS ownership.

The Class 37/4s based at Crewe for North Wales passenger duties have already been covered but, of these, 37407 would be suitable branded by Transrail. The other Transrail Class 37s to be found in the northwest of England were based at Wigan Springs Branch, the mixed bunch covering infrastructure and freight traffic, including out of Peak Forest. Aside from 37509, the 'Big T' was conspicuously absent here with a mix of Railfreight triple grey and Mainline liveries dominating. The latter included 37405/15/19/20/26 while the sub-sector badges encompassed 37026 and 37107 in Distribution, 37518 and 37520 in Metals and unbranded 37108 and 37417. Matters were completed by the 'Dutch' duo of 37066 and 37133.

North of the border

In Scotland, the use of no-heat Class 37s on the Inverness and Aberdeen portions of the sleeper services to Edinburgh and onwards to London Euston came to an end in May 1995, these having latterly come under Transrail control and were based at Motherwell. Their use on these trains had commenced three years earlier with generator vans provided to supply power to the coaches. Power for the West Highland portion to Fort William continued to be an ETS-fitted Class 37/4 and this remained the case for another 11 years.

Motherwell therefore had a sizeable number of the Type 3s on its books, the general fleet absorbing the former sleeper locos, which included 37152, 37221/51, 37505/10 and 37683/85 in their InterCity Swallow colours. Of these, 37221, 37505 and 37683 would be fully repainted in Transrail triple grey but the remaining quartet carried InterCity until withdrawn or sold by EWS. Also in this pool, 37156 was another to receive a full Transrail repaint, having previously been in 'Dutch', while 37073, 37100 and 37214/50 would be variously re-badged from Distribution, Construction or Metals.

Completing matters in this particular Motherwell pool were a number of 'Dutch' examples, namely 37043/69/88, 37153/65/70/75/96 and 37232/94, along with Departmental grey survivor 37262. The Scottish depot duly became the main proponent of the 'Dutch' Transrail scheme where locos in the grey and yellow had Transrail logos and lettering added to their existing paintwork. First seen in May 1995, 37043/88, 37153/65/70, 37232 and 37351 would be so adorned as were Canton's 37197 and 37230 along with 37201 from the Bescot allocation. The only other Transrail locos to sport this look were 31112 and 56036/47/49.

The Transrail brand was quite widely applied to the Scottish-based Class 37/4s, partly because some were already in triple grey and it was a simple rebrand, such as 37401/06/23/28, while others fell due for overhaul and were repainted as part of the work, namely 37404/09/10/24/30. Also in this pool, which was largely retained for West Highland freight work alongside the sleepers, were BR green 37403, Regional Railways 37427 and Mainline 37431, the latter two having been released from their previous ScotRail passenger duties.

Lastly from the Motherwell fleet were seven refurbished Class 37s retained for freight work, such as coal and petroleum traffic. These were 37675/92/93, 37712/14 and 37801/93, of which 37675/93 and 37893 came to be Transrail branded with the others retaining their sub-sector logos. Also in this pool was 'Dutch' Transrail-liveried 37351 on account of it having the same re-geared CP7 bogies, even though it was not refurbished. All of the Transrail Class 37s across the country would pass to EWS ownership in 1996, bringing further allocation changes.

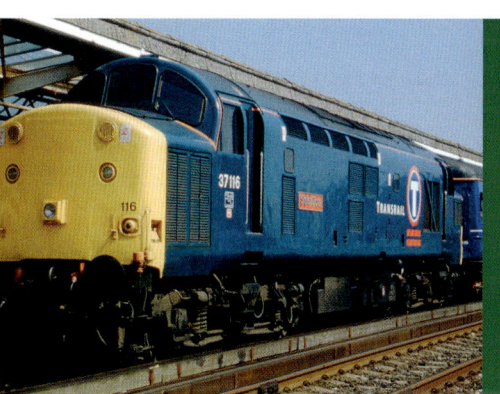

LEFT: The appearance of 37116 *Sister Dora* in BR blue at the end of Transrail's existence was a surprise, as was the removal of the split headcode boxes in favour of marker lights. The South Wales & West loco-hauled services to Weymouth provided much gainful employment for Cardiff-based Class 37s in the mid-1990s and the newly-created 'celebrity' is seen taking its turn at Weymouth in June 1996 as it waits to depart back to Bristol. Just visible is one of the TOC's blue-liveried Mk.2b coaches, a livery that will hopefully feature on a future batch of OO gauge models from Accurascale. Simon Bendall Collection

Modelling BR Locomotives of the 1990s 85

Out of the shadows

'Big Ts' in Scotland

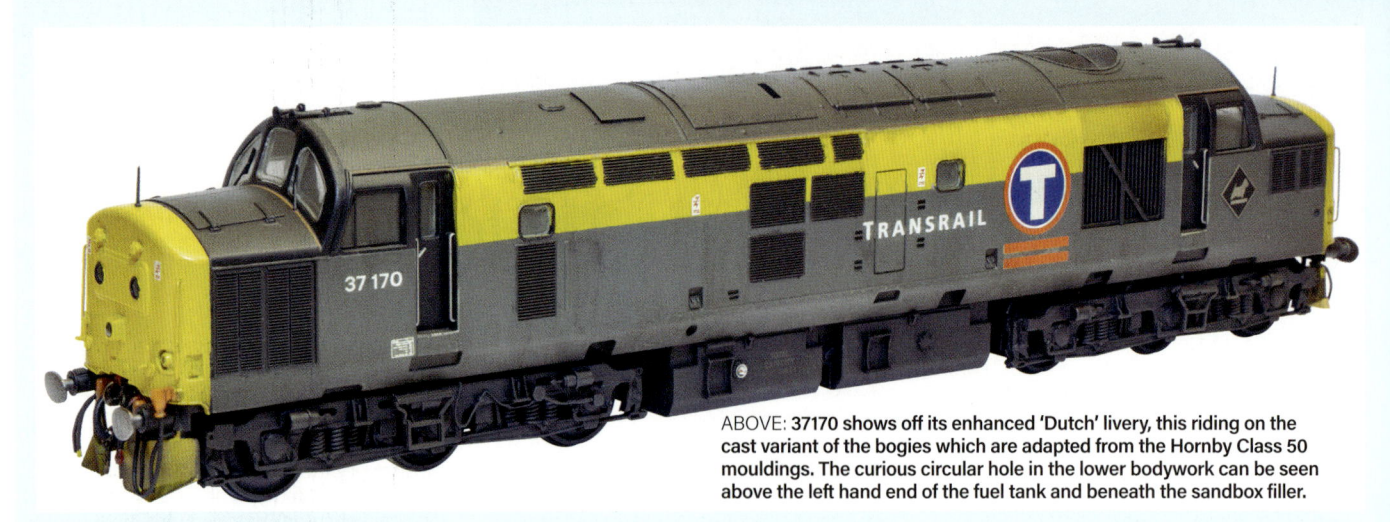

ABOVE: 37170 shows off its enhanced 'Dutch' livery, this riding on the cast variant of the bogies which are adapted from the Hornby Class 50 mouldings. The curious circular hole in the lower bodywork can be seen above the left hand end of the fuel tank and beneath the sandbox filler.

To some, the Transrail livery was a bit uninspiring, given its use of the existing triple grey or 'Dutch' liveries and just adding a new logo over it. From a personal perspective, it added something to the original livery. For many years, one of my main modelling interests has been the Scottish scene in the mid-1990s. As such, many of my fleet are in Transrail colours and these two locos reflect this. At the time, there was a large fleet of Class 37s allocated to Motherwell, which were divided into distinct pools such as LGHM for West Highland Line '37/4s' and LGBM for more general use examples.

I regard 37170 as a truly quintessential Scottish Class 37, given it spent more than a decade in Scotland; it being transferred to Eastfield in 1987. Five years later in 1992, it was repainted into 'Dutch' as it had become part of the InterCity-sponsored fleet of infrastructure locos. Transrail logos were added in early 1996, although the cast cabside BR arrows were removed not long afterwards, and it is this condition in which the model is portrayed.

My starting point was Bachmann's OO gauge model of 37239 in Trainload Coal. All the un-necessary decoration was removed and then work could start on the body modifications. There were one or two areas that needed filling in, such as the additional footstep in the lower bodyside and a strange cut-out that I am pretty sure no loco ever carried. Once the filler had hardened and been smoothed back, a hole was drilled in the appropriate place on one side, which was unique to this particular loco.

'Dutch' paint

The next stage was painting. At the time I started this model, I was keen to retain elements of the original paintwork that were common to both liveries, such as the roof grey, so the areas being retained were masked off before primer and then the 'Dutch' colours were sprayed on, the latter employing Railmatch Departmental grey and warning panel yellow. Nowadays, I would just strip the body to bare plastic and do a full repaint now my painting skills have improved.

This loco ran on a pair of bogies with cast sideframes rather than the more common fabricated style. Bachmann does not produce these, so the originals had to be replaced. The sideframes were carefully cut off the retaining plate and replacement spares from Hornby's Class 50 were fitted in their place. These needed modifying into the earlier type of cast frame, which entailed the removal of elements of the end stretchers and restoration of some spring detail hidden by the original moulded-on footsteps.

A new etched towing plate on the leading ends came from the Shawplan Extreme Etchings range as this type of bogie was usually found under the Class 55 'Deltics' until the withdrawal of the class; after which the bogies found their way into the Class 37 spares pool. A scratchbuilt speedometer and associated cable were added to the No.2 bogie using various bits of rod, wire and even a small handrail knob! I chose to retain the original Bachmann footsteps for the time being as these are, after all, very much 'layout locos' so need some robustness.

Adding heat

I have long been a fan of Class 37/4s and 37410 is one of my favourites, maybe second after 37403. This is not my first recreation

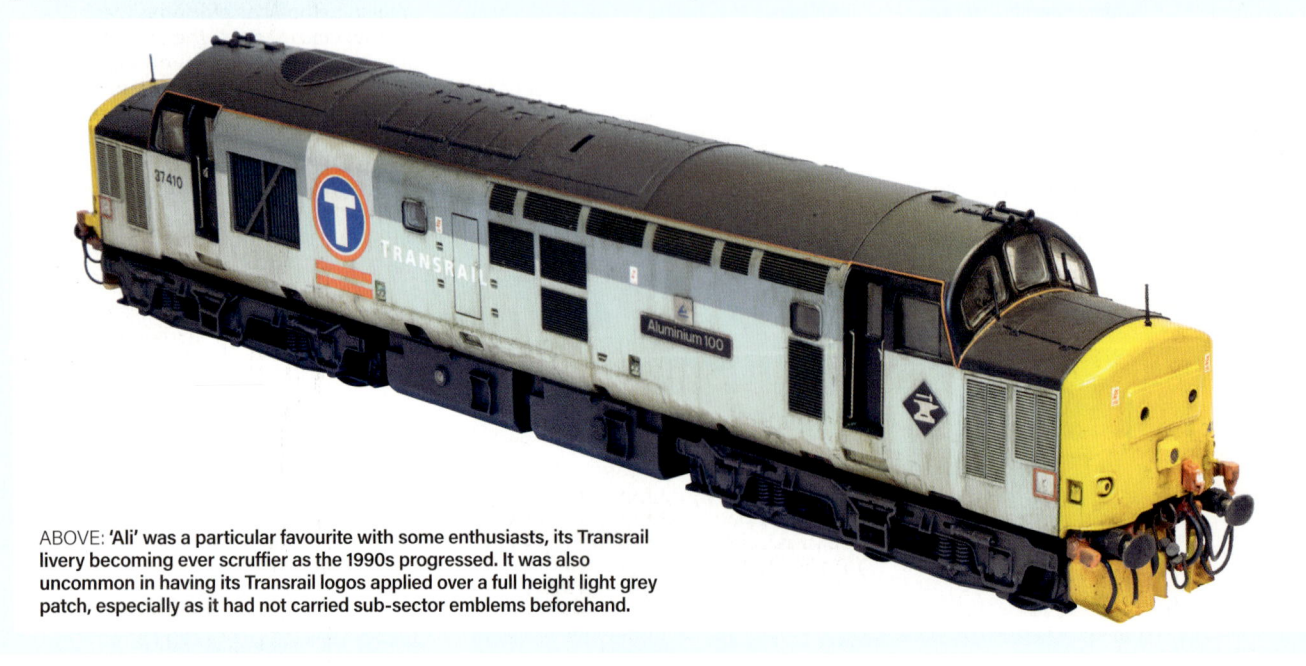

ABOVE: 'Ali' was a particular favourite with some enthusiasts, its Transrail livery becoming ever scruffier as the 1990s progressed. It was also uncommon in having its Transrail logos applied over a full height light grey patch, especially as it had not carried sub-sector emblems beforehand.

Out of the shadows

of it though as the loco had a body change when more recent models appeared with better shades of grey. My starting point for this second one was a Trainload Petroleum donor, where I carefully removed the squadron markings with a home-brew scraper-cum-chisel before the remainder came off with some T-Cut on a cotton bud.

The result was a blemish-free triple grey bodyshell upon which the Transrail logos could then be applied. 37410 was unusual in having a lighter patch of grey under the upper half of the logo, which was replicated by carefully masking off, priming, and then matching to the lower grey using Phoenix Precision Railfreight silver-grey. The transfers from Fox could then be applied. To make the ETS pipework, the socket on the secondman's side of the bufferbeams came from Heljan Class 47 spares and that under the driver's side was scratchbuilt from plastic section.

Both locos received EM gauge wheelsets from Kean Maygib, these using the original Bachmann gears and bearings. Detailing common to both locos included Shawplan etched roof grilles, Hornby Class 31 buffers and Heljan three-piece miniature snowploughs. Also added were vacuum pipes, Roco air pipes and Smiths screw couplings with the remainder of the bufferbeam pipes made from thin black coated wire. The air horns and multiple working sockets were modified in the same way as described for 37429 on page 47.

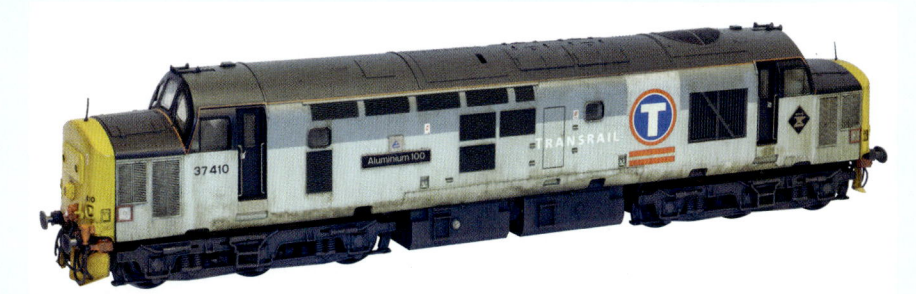

ABOVE: 37410 was one of the Class 37/4s that enjoyed a long association with Scotland, it being comparatively rare for it to come south of the border for any length of time. Thus, when it arrived at Didcot for a period of local workings around 2002, it was much pursued by photographers as an EWS repaint would soon follow.

The weathering of both locos was matched to prototype photos taken during the period modelled, this being 1996. This again followed the same method as described for their Regional Railways classmate, airbrushing on lighter and then darker colours, and removing much of each application with a white spirit-dipped brush.

Model availability

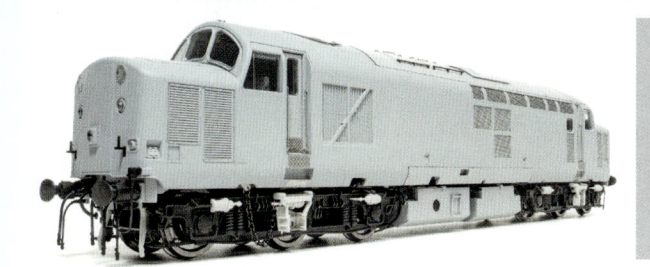

LEFT: The new Accurascale model is seen in pre-production form as a Class 37/7, this having a bodyside window removed on each side to allow for the fitting of ballast weights, which in turned increased tractive effort.

In OO gauge, the Class 37 has seen progressive development over the decades from the original Tri-ang toy through the flawed Lima model of the 1980s and 1990s, which now resides in the Hornby range, to the various incarnations produced from the start of this century by Bachmann. The latter has undergone two significant re-tools over its life and various smaller upgrades, albeit not always with the best results, but the sheer number of liveries now available means it has been the model of choice for many years. There was also the short-lived ViTrains offering in the 2000s, but this rather failed to capture the cab shape correctly.

However, a new 4mm model is on the way from Accurascale, which promises to be a step change in the level of options and detail available. This not only includes sub-classes previously unseen in model form, beginning with the Class 37/6s, but also a choice of running numbers across the same liveries. Currently also announced are the '37/0s' and '37/4s' from particular eras along with the Class 37/7 'Heavyweights'.

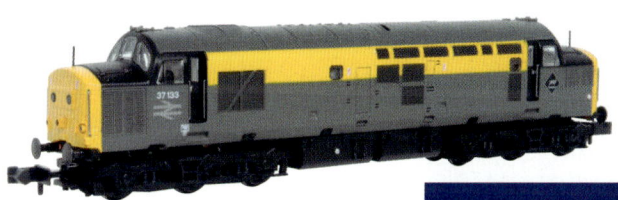

The current Graham Farish Class 37 has seen development over the years so that most significant sub-classes are now covered across the various periods. In O gauge, Heljan has also progressed from just having an as-built split box model with bufferbeam cowls to examples with centre headcodes and no cowls while the Class 37/4s have also appeared. While the number of liveries available is now considerable, the company has unfortunately not addressed some fundamental dimensional errors.

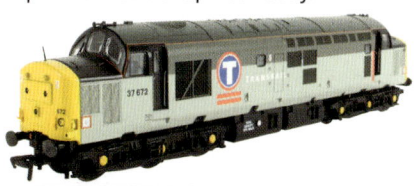

ABOVE: Transrail has never featured particularly strongly on RTR releases. One useful release though was Cornish favourite 37672 from Bachmann quite some years ago.

RIGHT: Heljan has produced its O gauge Class 37/4 in both un-numbered and fully finished forms, this being the Railfreight triple grey release which could easily become a Transrail example with suitable transfers. A factory-finished model in Transrail colours but without numbers was commissioned by Blackpool retailer Tower Models in 2021. Image courtesy Kernow Model Rail Centre

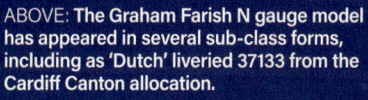

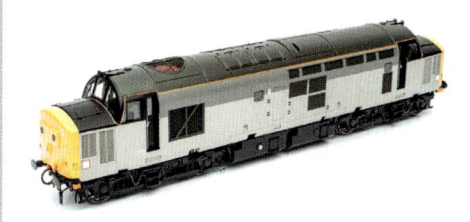

ABOVE: The Graham Farish N gauge model has appeared in several sub-class forms, including as 'Dutch' liveried 37133 from the Cardiff Canton allocation.

Modelling BR Locomotives of the 1990s 87

Out of the shadows

RIGHT: **Some five months into EWS ownership, the now Crewe-based 37509 and 37413 *Loch Eil Outward Bound* power through Ashley with the 7F48 07.30 Tunstead-Oakleigh on July 20, 1996.** These limestone workings out of Peak Forest fell under Transrail's remit during its short existence, a wide variety of Class 37s being recorded atop the vintage former ICI hoppers, something which continued under EWS until replacement air-braked wagons could be introduced. Coded JGV at this point, a RTR model of the hoppers finally appeared in OO gauge a few years ago, being exclusively available from Hattons. These are currently sold out though with N gauge having yet to see a manufacturer take up the baton.
Martin Loader

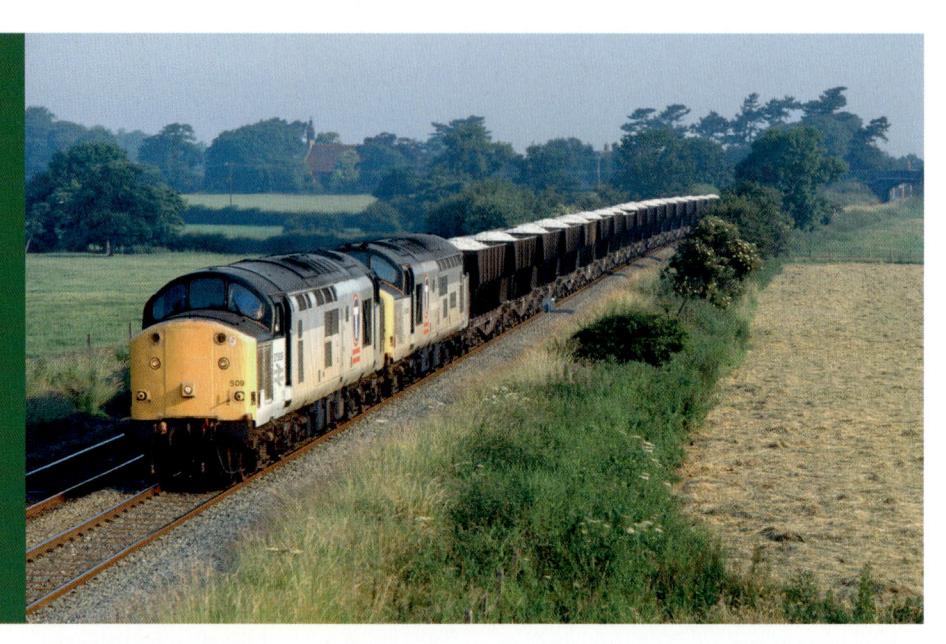

RIGHT: **Proving that you do not need lots of space to model merry-go-round coal train operations, 37701 patiently waits at Pontycymer on June 25, 1996, while a single mechanical shovel loads the HAA hoppers.** Once completed, the doyen of the Class 37/7 sub-class would depart for Aberthaw Power Station. Such a scene would perhaps be best suited to N gauge where Farish and Peco offer the wagons while Accurascale, Cavalex and Hornby all do likewise in 4mm and Dapol in O gauge. The Type 3 would be withdrawn in the final month of the decade. Brian Robbins/Rail Photoprints

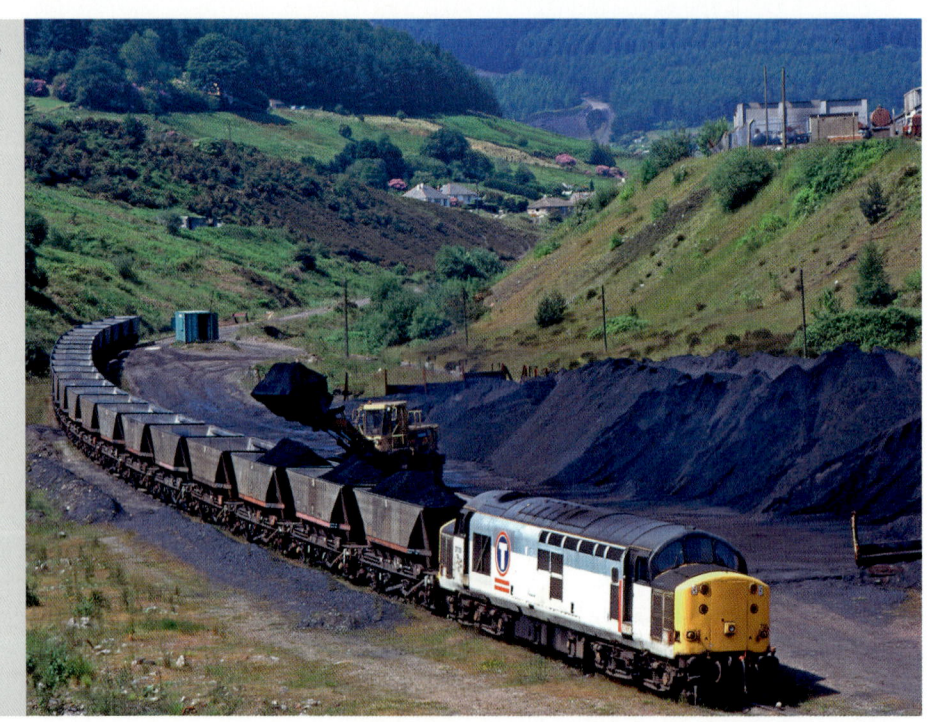

RIGHT: **The re-engined Class 37/9 sub-class would become quite celebrated as they neared the end of their careers working in and around South Wales. Ruston-powered 37906 growls along at Marshfield on August 27, 1998, with the 6Z52 11.05 Cardiff Docks to Llanwern empties.** The rake of MEA box wagons had earlier transferred blast furnace slag from the steelworks for use in the construction of the Cardiff Bay Barrage, this short-term flow being diagrammed for the re-engined locos due to the weight of the train. The Class 37/9s were largely dispensed with at the end of that year but 37906 would out-last its sisters, going on to become part of the EWS heritage fleet and later be preserved. In OO gauge, 37905 and 37906 were produced with appropriate tooling alterations for their later years by Bachmann in 2011 as an exclusive commission for Kernow Model Rail Centre but the more extensively modified 37901-04 have yet to be seen in RTR form. As for the MEAs, these have long been a staple of the Bachmann and Farish ranges, although it is worth seeking out more recent releases of the OO gauge model as these have a retooled and much improved underframe.
Martin Loader

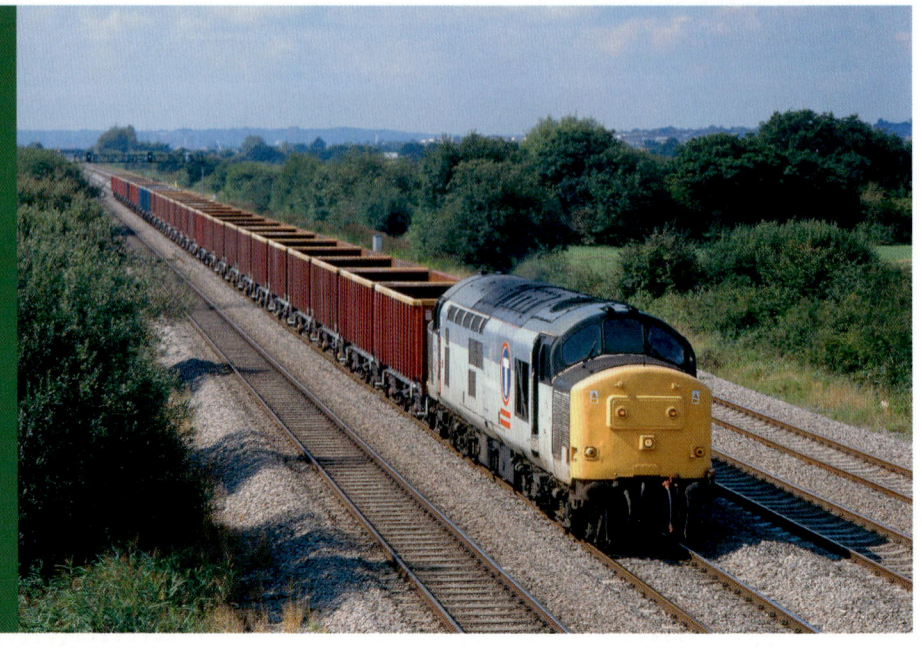

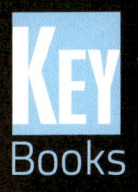

MAIL ORDER
Key Books

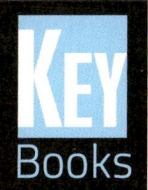

CLASS 66/0

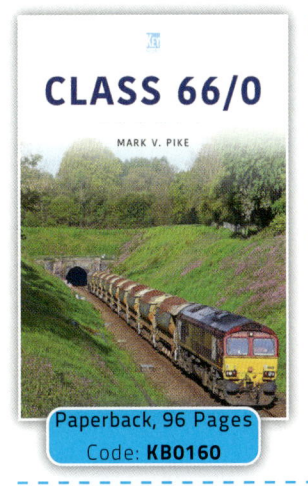

Britain's Railways Series, Vol.32
This volume covers the Class 66/0s from their early days up to the present at various locations around the UK.

ONLY £15.99

Paperback, 96 Pages
Code: KB0160

Subscribers call for your £2 discount

HSTs: AROUND BRITAIN, 1990 TO THE PRESENT DAY

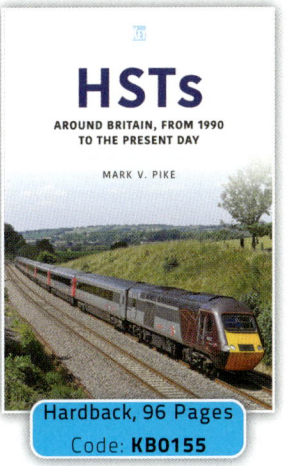

NEW

Following on from HSTs: The Western Region
Illustrated with over 230 images, this book shows HSTs over the past 20 - 30 years, in numerous UK locations, highlighting why they have served so long and why they should be saved.

ONLY £15.99

Hardback, 96 Pages
Code: KB0155

Subscribers call for your £2 discount

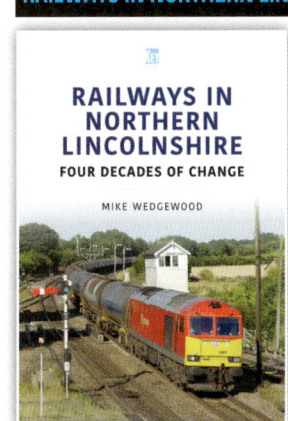

RAILWAYS IN NORTHERN LINCOLNSHIRE: FOUR DECADES OF CHANGE

Britain's Railways Series, Vol 29
Set against the contrasting rural and industrial scenery of northern Lincolnshire, this book illustrates the area's fascinating passenger and freight trains, railway infrastructure, stations and signalling over a 40-year period.

ONLY £15.99

Paperback, 96 Pages
Code: KB0138

Subscribers call for your £2 discount

BRITAIN'S PRESERVED RAILWAYS

Lavishly illustrated with colour photographs showing some of the best locations for lineside and station photography, this book is a vital guidebook for anyone looking to explore Britain's preserved railways.

ONLY £16.99

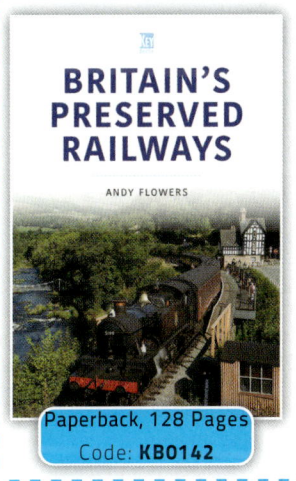

Paperback, 128 Pages
Code: KB0142

Subscribers call for your £2 discount

GRAND CENTRAL

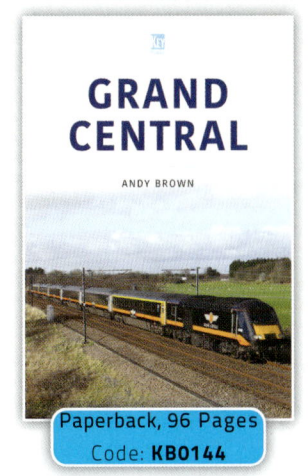

Britain's Railways Series, Vol 31
This book illustrates the wonderful landscapes of Grand Central's routes, the types of trains operated, including the iconic HSTs, and some rare behind-the-scenes locations not often seen by the public.

ONLY £15.99

Paperback, 96 Pages
Code: KB0144

Subscribers call for your £2 discount

CLASS 67s

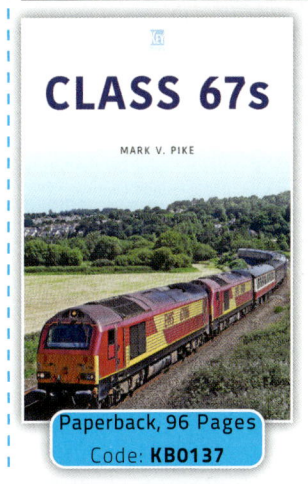

Britain's Railways Series, Vol 30;
Containing 220 images, this book illustrates all 30 locos in the class during their first two decades in service. During the 20 years that they have been in service, Class 67s have been very reliable with only occasional failures.

ONLY £15.99

Paperback, 96 Pages
Code: KB0137

Subscribers call for your £2 discount

shop.keypublishing.com/books

Or call UK: 01780 480404 - Overseas: +44 1780 480404

Monday to Friday 9am-5:30pm GMT. Free 2nd class P&P on all UK & BFPO orders. Overseas charges apply.
All publication dates subject to change

TO VIEW OUR FULL RANGE OF BOOKS, VISIT OUR SHOP

The railway reborn

The railway reborn

With the railway restructured ready for privatisation, a three-year period saw all of the freight companies sold into private ownership while the passenger operations were similarly let under the franchise system. A handful of new firms also appeared on the scene with the intention of taking a slice of the freight or locomotive hire market, as Simon Bendall explains.

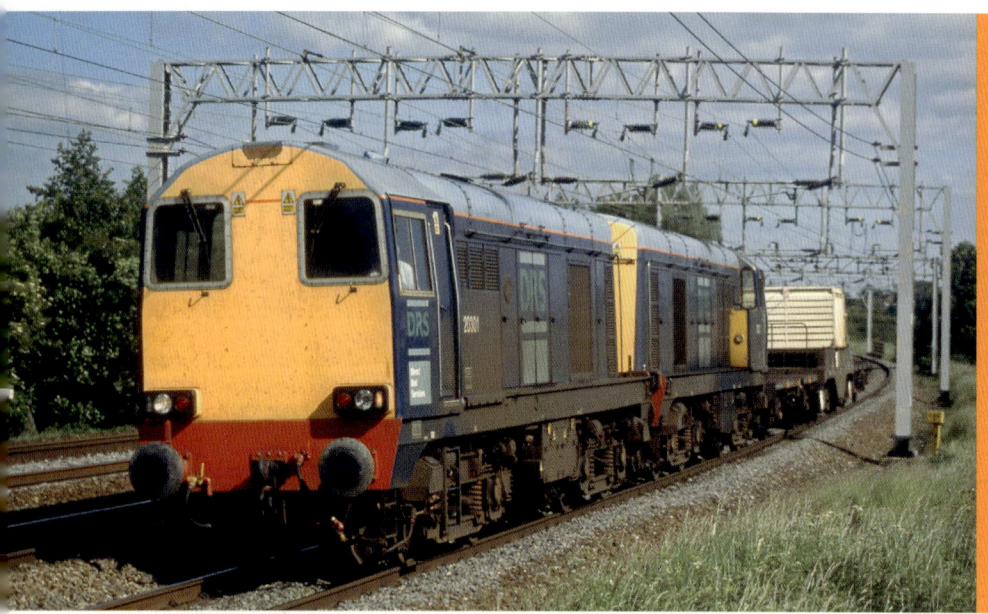

LEFT: Direct Rail Services finally commenced the movement of irradiated fuel from nuclear power stations during 1999 as the contracts held by EWS came to an end. On June 9 that year, 20301 and 20303 pass Heamies Farm atop the 7M56 13.10 Berkley to Crewe Basford Hall. For OO gauge modellers, 2021 finally brought the release of ready-to-run Class 20/3s thanks to Bachmann, these depicting the 20306-15 batch rather than the initial five machines; there being a number of differences between the two. In N gauge though, the wait goes on but, on the wagon side, the FNA flask is available from both Bachmann and Farish. At this time, barrier wagons were still required, these being PFAs converted from the underframes of OBA open wagons and a simple rebuild using a Cambrian kit in 4mm for example. Paul Robertson

The sell-off of the freight and parcels companies began at the end of 1995 with American operator Wisconsin Central announced as the winner in the bidding process for Rail Express Systems, it took control of the mail operation from that December, this including all of its locos, coaches, staff, maintenance facilities and other assets. This was followed just three months later by the acquisition of Mainline Freight, Loadhaul and Transrail, the three regional freight companies being reunited under a single owner and immediately making Wisconsin a dominant force in the UK rail freight market.

Soon operating under the new name of English Welsh & Scottish Railway (EWS), the company had not finished its acquisitions either, it eventually adding Railfreight Distribution to its portfolio late in 1997. This was a slightly reluctant acquisition as RfD was losing £1 million a week at this point but it gave EWS access to the Channel Tunnel while restructuring of the business, including sharing maintenance depots, was predicted to bring considerable savings.

April 1998 also saw EWS complete the acquisition of National Power's rail division, this including the transfer of the six Class 59/2s, 106 hopper wagons and the maintenance depot at Ferrybridge. EWS had long coveted the operation while National Power was now happy to divest itself from a non-core activity following the stabilisation of the rail industry after privatisation.

EWS was already employing Class 59s at this point, having reached a hire agreement with Mendip Rail to deploy two Class 59s on the Port Talbot to Llanwern iron ore workings from March 1997. The locos were available for redeployment following a significant downturn in aggregates traffic, the agreement lasting until the start of 1999 when demand picked up again. To replace them, two of the now EWS-liveried Class 59/2s were moved to South Wales from February 1999, this arrangement lasting for six months with Class 60s then returning.

In the event, the six former National Power machines would be moved away from their Yorkshire duties early in 2000, heading to the southeast for aggregates work in particular.

GM dominance

Almost as soon as EWS was created in 1996, it placed an order with General Motors for 250 freight locos, the Class 66s, as they soon became, being based on the Class 59s to speed acceptance procedures but geared for 75mph operation rather than 60mph. This made them suitable for most freight work,

BELOW: Of the three rolling stock leasing companies, Porterbrook was the most publicity conscious, a policy that was startlingly reinforced in April 1996 when 47817 was rolled out from Crewe Diesel TMD, fully re-liveried in the company's new corporate colours. With one cab and bodyside being predominately white and the other cab and bodyside finished largely in purple, the effect was certainly radical. The livery was intended for application to Class 47s assigned to spot-hire and 'Thunderbird' rescue purposes rather than those on long-term lease to train operators and would also be applied to 47807 four months later. On May 24, 1997, 47817 is seen after arrival at Paignton with the 09.30 from Glasgow Central; it would gain Virgin red/grey the following year. Simon Bendall Collection

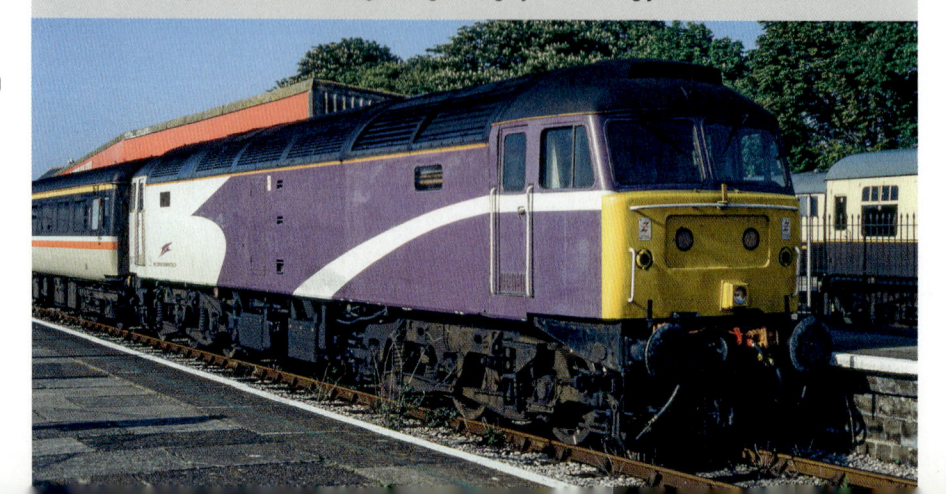

The railway reborn

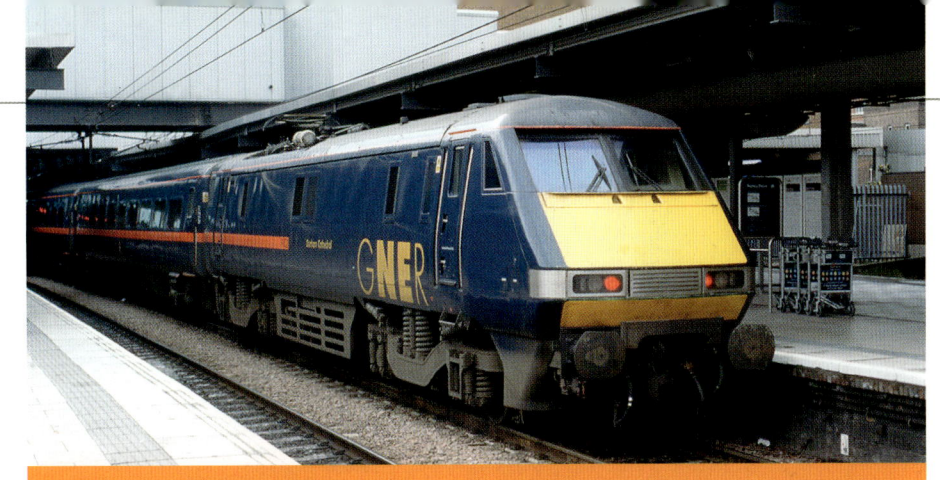

ABOVE: The stylish GNER livery was launched in April 1996 upon Sea Containers taking control of the former InterCity services on the East Coast Main Line. The logo went through three versions, initially being gold, then white and finally a golden-yellow, as seen on 91102 *Durham Cathedral* at Leeds in January 2003. By this time, the loco had been refurbished in order to cure the reliability issues afflicting the class, this including the addition of extra bodyside grilles to improve ventilation. Hornby does both versions of the class in OO gauge thanks to its new model while the locos have previously also featured in the N gauge Farish range in as-built condition. Simon Bendall Collection

The competition

With EWS' near clean sweep of the former BR freight businesses, this just left Freightliner as the only company not under its control. Following the management buyout in 1996, over £20 million was invested in the company in its first two years, this including the Class 57 re-engineering project, investment in wagons and terminals, such as new container cranes, and staff expansion. By May 1998, Freightliner was transporting an average of 2,000 containers per day as global shipping continued to expand and took delivery of its first five Class 66s, 66501-05, in the summer of 1999. Moves were also afoot to diversify into other freight commodities in order to grow the business, a contract with Blue Circle Cement being an early breakthrough during 2000.

Meanwhile, February 1995 had seen the creation of Direct Rail Services by parent company British Nuclear Fuels as it sort to ensure continuity of transport for all the materials associated with nuclear fuel reprocessing. By the end of that year, it had received its initial batch of five refurbished Class 20/3s and would run its first trains in late January 1996 following the belated granting of approval by Railtrack. A further ten modernised Class 20s would follow in 1998, a year after the company had invested in its first Class 37s by purchasing 37607-12 from European Passenger Services. It was not until 1999 though that DRS could commence transporting irradiated fuel from power stations as EWS' contracts expired.

GB Railfreight was also founded during 1999, although it would be the following year before it was awarded its first contract, this being for infrastructure duties with Railtrack, with its first Class 66s arriving in March 2001.

Although not a freight operator, mention should also be made of Fragonset Railways, which was formed in 1997 as a locomotive hire company, its first acquisitions being some of the Class 47/7s from the defunct Waterman Railways. These soon found use with Virgin CrossCountry to bolster its own fleet of Type 4s while 1998 saw Fragonset reactivate its first Class 31s, these having been acquired from EWS. The Type 2s allowed a mini-renaissance of loco-hauled services in some areas, train operators hiring the locos and accompanying coaches to cover for a shortage of multiple units.

Passenger operators

The transfer of the train operating units to private control began in February 1996, one of the first being the Stagecoach-controlled South West Trains. This still had 73109 on its books for use on stock transfers and rescue duties and the loco would duly receive the Stagecoach-inspired livery in 1997.

Of the former InterCity routes still operating locomotives, GB Railways took over Anglia Railways from January 1997, National Express was given control of Gatwick Express from April 1996 and Sea Containers launched GNER the same month. Great Western Trains was another early transfer to private hands with Great Western Holdings commencing operations in February 1996 while Virgin Trains acquired CrossCountry in January 1997 and West Coast two months later. Naturally, this brought a raft of new liveries as each company looked to put its own stamp on their train services.

although they lacked the tractive effort to haul the heaviest petroleum and stone trains effectively for which some of the Class 60s were retained.

Class pioneer 66001 was delivered in April 1998 for initial testing and training with production deliveries commencing four months later with 66003-05. Thereafter, there were regular deliveries to Newport Docks and by the end of 1999, 66002 and 666006-189 were all in the UK. While the locos initially helped to drive traffic growth, it was inevitable that the former BR fleet was under severe threat as well from the modern replacements. Initial targets included the Railfreight Distribution Class 47s as well as the remaining Class 31s, Class 33s, and un-refurbished Class 37s.

At the same time as the Class 66s were ordered, EWS was also seeking a fleet of 30 locos that would be 125mph capable and with electric train supply for use on the Royal Mail services that had been acquired with Rail Express Systems. While initial thoughts were for a Class 66 variant, extensive design work showed the concept was technically challenging, especially after the company failed to reach agreement with Brush Traction for the use of the only proven 125mph-capable three-axle bogie suitable for UK use, as employed under the Class 89 prototype.

The project was instead reconceptualised as a Bo-Bo design and by the summer of 1997, EWS and General Motors had reached agreement with GEC-Alstom to construct 30 locos, designated Class 67, at the latter's Valencia plant in Spain. Not only did GEC-Alstom have a suitable high-speed bogie available, but it also had experience of building General Motors locos under licence. However, the use of two-axle bogies did have a drawback as the 90-tonne locos would have an axleload right on the maximum limit of 22.5 tonnes each and therefore be restricted as to where they could operate.

In the event, only 67003 would be delivered to the UK before the end of the decade, arriving at Newport Docks in October 1999. Even then, it was found to be slightly over-weight, resulting in the rest of the class being held back in Spain while modifications were devised. Initial testing and training were allowed to begin though, the loco running with only a partial load of fuel to bring the weight down to an acceptable level.

Once all of the Class 67s were delivered in 2000, that was largely it for the Rail Express Systems Class 47s, although some were retained for charter train work. However, with the early 2000s bringing a change in EWS policy and increasing competition from rivals, decimation of the remaining ex BR types soon followed.

BELOW: For its Anglia Railways franchise, GB Railways introduced an attractive turquoise livery to replace the InterCity colours on its Class 86/2 fleet along with the predominately Mk.2e/f coach sets. On August 22, 2000, 86217 *City University* awaits departure from Norwich with a service to Liverpool Street. Heljan has previously produced the livery on its OO gauge Class 86/2, although it has yet to grace the current re-tooled model, while the same is true for Dapol's N gauge version. Similarly, Hornby has offered both its ex Dapol Mk.2d coaches in turquoise in the past along with a Mk.3a buffet while the all-important Mk.2f DBSO is due in 2022 from Bachmann. Gareth Bayer

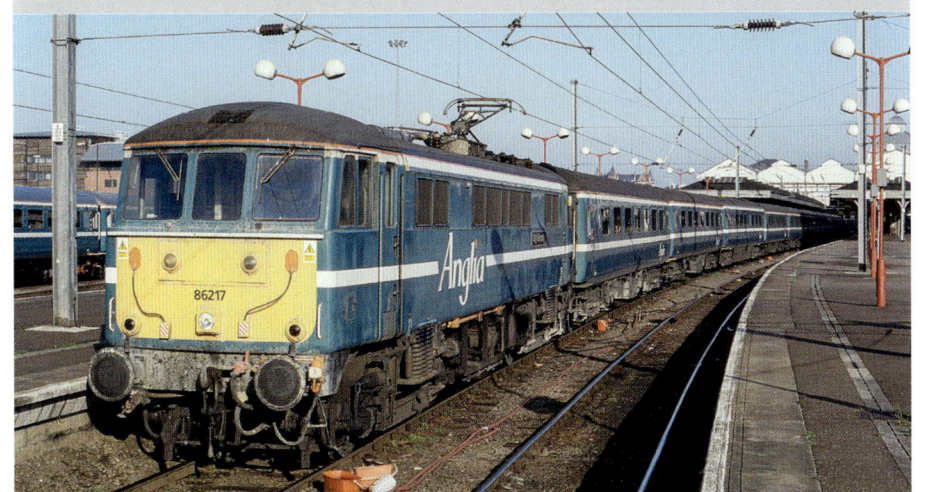

Modelling BR Locomotives of the 1990s **91**

The railway reborn

RIGHT: **The Class 66 invasion began in 1998 with the arrival of the first EWS examples while Freightliner also had its initial machines before the decade was out. The 'Sheds' quickly spread across the country on all manner of freight workings, ranging from coal and steel to infrastructure workings. On May 24, 1999, 66060 passes Plean in charge of the 6D46 13.30 Inverness to Mossend 'Enterprise' service, this conveying VGA vans and FIA 'Multifrets' loaded with Safeway refrigerated containers returning from Georgemas Junction. Both wagon types are available in 4mm from Bachmann and 2mm from Graham Farish, although the Safeway containers are not currently produced. The third VGA is carrying Lovatt Spring mineral water logos, and this has previously been released by Bachmann. Meanwhile, there is much competition on the Class 66 front with Bachmann, Hattons and Hornby all offering 4mm models while Dapol and Farish do likewise in 2mm. Dapol also has a 7mm Class 66 under development, which promises to be an interesting addition to the larger scale.** Martin Loader

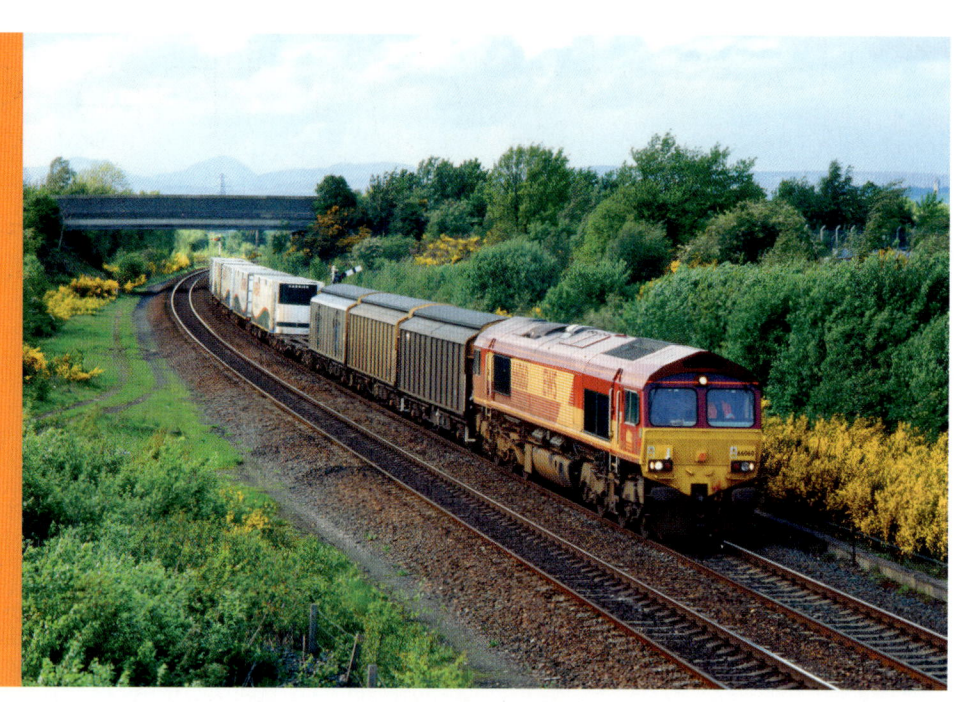

RIGHT: **The Class 67s just about qualify for inclusion in this volume thanks to the arrival of 67003 in the UK in October 1999. Almost a year later, it tops 67014 on the 14.05 Low Fell-Plymouth mail working at Plawsworth on September 22, 2000. Hornby has a monopoly on the class in OO gauge while Dapol has likewise in N. The train is formed of two Super BGs either end of three Super GUVs and can be replicated in 4mm using the respective models from Bachmann and Hornby (ex-Lima). It is a more difficult proposition in 2mm as while the Super BG can be found in the Graham Farish range, the Super GUV remains a notable omission in the scale.** Bob Lumley

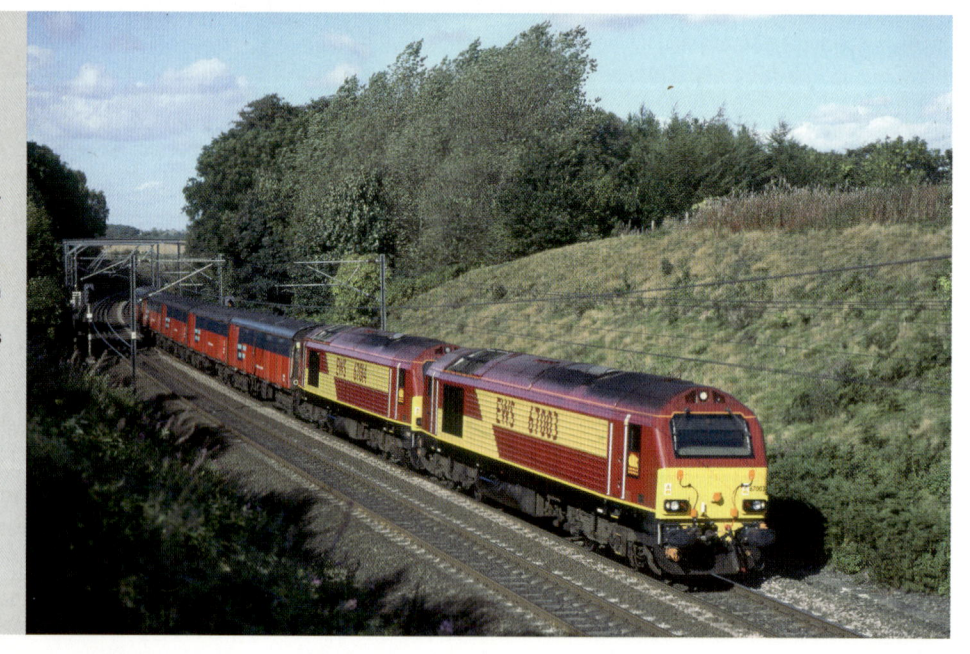

RIGHT: **The arrival of Fragonset on the scene brought loco-hauled workings to several routes long devoid of such excitement. One of the first train operators to avail itself was Silverlink, which hired two Class 31s and a pair of coaches to work between Bedford and Bletchley for periods in 1998/99 due to poor availability of its Class 117 and Class 121 DMUs. On October 12, 1998, 31452** *Minotaur* **heads the modeller-friendly formation at Kempston while working the 09.46 Bedford to Bletchley with 31468** *Hydra* **on the rear. The Mk.2a coaches were on hire from Forward Trust and carry its dark blue and cream livery. Hornby has previously produced its Class 31 in Fragonset livery as has Graham Farish, although this was using the old and now-replaced tooling.** Martin Loader

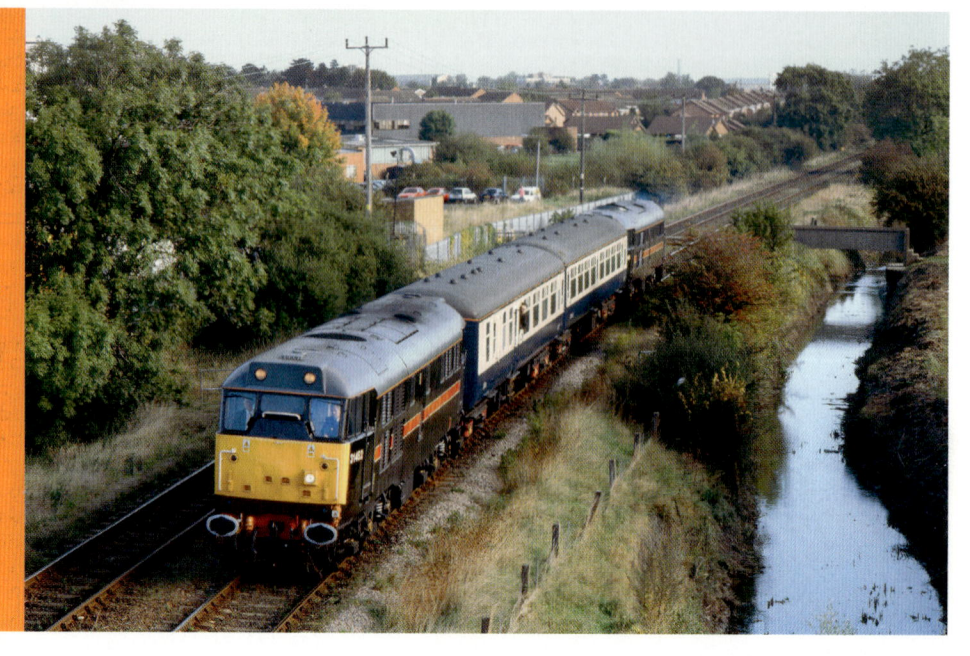

The railway reborn

Ghosts on the system

Following the acquisition of the three regional freight companies by Wisconsin Central, there was a short transitional period while the EWS brand was created. As a result, several locos appeared in traffic in undercoat while awaiting the new colours. Simon Bendall **details their history while** Alex Carpenter **models the solitary Class 60.**

Following the sale of Mainline Freight, Loadhaul, and Transrail in February 1996, instructions were soon issued by new owner Wisconsin Central to workshops and depots to cease all repaints into any of the three liveries. This was partly to prevent the further application of what were now redundant brands, but also to save money, incoming EWS chairman Ed Burkhardt later bemoaning the thousands of pounds that had been spent on creating and applying the new colours for such a short existence.

At the time though, a number of locos were in the process of being overhauled, particularly at Doncaster Works but also Brush Traction, while the odd depot repaint was underway. As a result, these were outshopped in undercoat with numbers, data panels, orange cantrail stripe, overhead warning flashes and all other details applied over the top pending a decision on what the new livery would be.

Most of the locos that were completed in this condition came from Doncaster, the works using an off-white undercoat, which soon lead to the affected locos being dubbed 'ghosts'. In some cases, the locos ran in this condition just for their main line test outings, this including the solitary Class 58, 58033, along with 56096. They were then retained at the works for the few weeks it took to choose maroon and gold, develop the specification and put them through the paintshop.

Out haunting

In contrast, those locos that received undercoat earlier in the painting hiatus were released back to their depots and returned to traffic. Notably, it was former Loadhaul traction that was the most significantly affected as 37682, 37717, 37885, 56041 and 56068 were returned to Immingham and 60022 to Thornaby all in off-white when, just a couple of months earlier, they would have been in black and orange. Some attempt was made to keep them on local workings close to their depots, but this was not always possible.

In contrast, just one former Transrail loco received the 'ghost' treatment, 37893 being returned to Motherwell from Doncaster and finding itself back on the Ayrshire coal circuits among other duties. Of the former Mainline Freight machines, 37174 was in line for a coat of blue at Stewarts Lane when the stop order came through, it carried a much darker shade of undercoat when put back in traffic that was more akin to Departmental grey. At Toton, 37051 and 37057 both escaped this fate, their overhauls taking long enough to see them become the first locos in EWS colours.

In some cases, the 'ghosts' were recalled for final painting before the end of 1996 but the likes of 56068 and 60022 were longer-lived, the Class 60 lasting for a year while 56068 made it to the autumn of 1997. Inevitably, given the impracticality of the colour, both were filthy by the time they were finally sent for completion.

White night

One further main line loco would appear in undercoat in July 1996, this being Porterbrook-owned 47846 *Thor*. Much like the EWS machines, this was done following overhaul at Crewe Works in advance of going on lease to Great Western Trains for use on Night Riviera sleeper trains. With the train operator introducing a new livery, the Class 47 was finished in a base coat of gloss white to allow easy repainting rather than give it a fresh application of InterCity Swallow. In the event, the loco would run like this for the best part of two years before receiving the all-green Great Western scheme with Merlin logo.

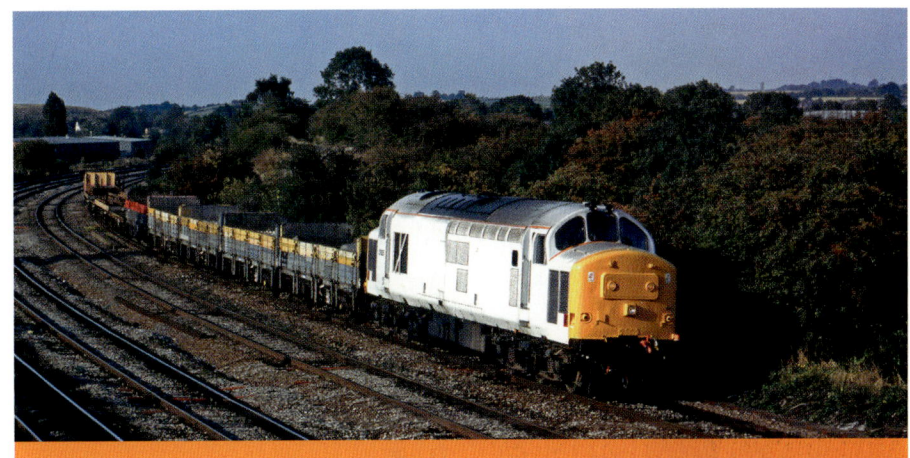

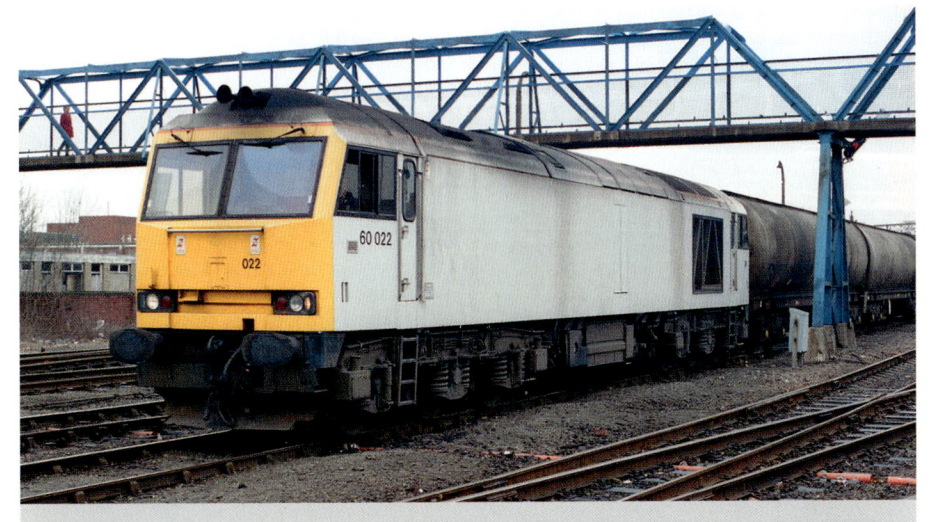

ABOVE: The state of 37885's roof clearly shows the disadvantage of the undercoat finish as the former Loadhaul-owned machine nears its destination at Stapleford with the 6M22 13.47 Castleton-Toton. Taken on September 17, 1996, the Type 3 would be in the EW&S-lettered version of maroon and gold by the following February. The consist is mostly ZDA Bass, which were in the process of being recoded back to OBA, along with two YAA Brill (ex BDA) loaded with overhanging switch and crossing assemblies and separated by runner wagons. The BDA and OBA are available RTR from Bachmann in 4mm and Graham Farish in 2mm. Paul Robertson

ABOVE: Only one Class 60 was finished in undercoat, 60022 carrying the increasingly work-stained off-white for around 12 months. On February 27, 1997, the Type 5 passes through Lincoln with the returning 6E50 Langley to Lindsey, the leading two TEAs being of the same design now produced in 4mm by Cavalex Models. Simon Bendall Collection

Modelling BR Locomotives of the 1990s 93

The railway reborn

A ghostly apparition

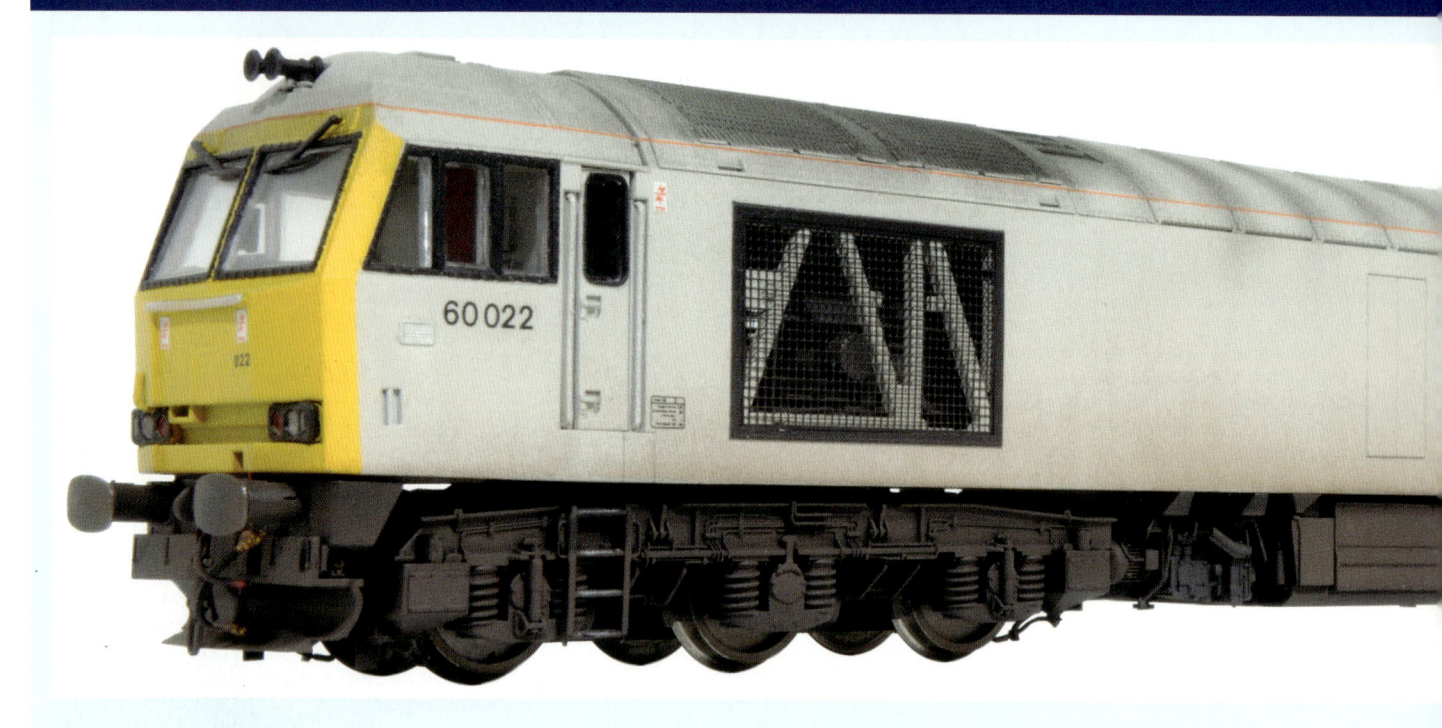

In 4mm scale, the Hornby Class 60 was the only place to start but for a project such as this, it is preferable to choose a plain livery as a donor. This makes life easier in the stripping department as the existing livery has to be removed to avoid it showing through beneath the paint. The bodyshell first needed to be stripped down as much as possible. The cab interiors are sometimes fixed in place with what appears to be adhesive from a glue gun, but this is easily broken away, allowing the interior and lighting board to pull out as one. It is best to leave the light lenses in place as they are too much trouble to remove and are easily masked off.

The glazing came out be exerting gentle pressure from the outside and pushing inwards; be careful as some will need a lot more persuasion than others as the amount of factory glue varies a lot. If a window is being stubborn, gentle fettling from behind with a scalpel will help to free it. Take your time as Hornby glazing is hard to come by as spare parts. However, if you do damage any, Shawplan's Laserglaze is a simple option if you were not already planning the upgrade. The only tweak when using Laserglaze is that the cab radio phone detail on the Hornby model is attached to the glazing; this can be simply transferred onto the central pillar instead. The cab door assemblies should be left alone, unless you are planning to glue them shut.

60022 was unusual in having black bodyside grilles applied over body coloured framework, so this can only be replicated by removing the etched grilles and refitting after painting the body. The etches are held in place by tabs, so these have to be bent straight from behind with a scalpel and the grilles carefully teased out by pushing on the tab from behind while lifting with a scalpel from the front. Be careful as these are very fragile, and the etched tabs will snap easily, and the grilles will distort.

Currently there are no etched replacements either! The last thing to take off is the silencer, this is simply removed by pushing out the four locating pins from underneath with the corner of a flat screwdriver; the glue will give under pressure and the silencer will pop up and out with a little persuasion.

Preparation
The donor model will dictate the amount of stripping required. In this case, the EWS donor needed the gold band removing, which was done with fine wet and dry paper used wet, constantly rinsing off and cleaning any excess with a toothbrush so you can see what still needs to come off. Basically, keep going until you are left with a plain maroon body. A tricky area is the bodyside access panel as overzealous use of the wet and dry here will remove the rivet detail, so a remnant of the yellow band will usually be left over if you look closely under the paint.

The cantrail line does not need removing but the solebar reflective stripe does along with the cab front numbers. All were done in the same fashion as above. Once removed, the body was thoroughly washed in warm water, working out all of the dust and debris with a toothbrush and allowed to dry.

A coat of Halfords grey primer was then applied and left to dry. This will highlight any areas that require further attention. Seeing as the loco was going to be white, I applied an overall coat of Railmatch matt white to give a good basis.

Which white is right?
The undercoat colour was cause for much deliberation and after looking at numerous pictures of 60022 in various lighting conditions, it was still a struggle to decide. First thoughts were that it could be similar to Rail grey but a picture of the loco stabled next to a triple grey sister put paid to this theory.

A phone call later and a new colour was considered, this being silver-white, as used for the lower bodysides of the InterCity Swallow livery. So, a jar of Railmatch No. 240 was duly purchased and applied to the model; first impressions were good although it was difficult to gauge exactly with only one colour in place. Nevertheless, I decided it was probably as near as I was going to get and looked the part when I replicated the triple grey comparison in model form. Getting good coverage from white is harder than you might imagine and about four coats were needed, despite the use of a white basecoat.

Once dry, the unusual full yellow ends were masked off. As these went all the way up and around the cab windscreens following the contours of the body, this made masking easy. The final colour to be sprayed was the black around the bodyside grille surrounds. As these are part of the body moulding rather than the etch, they have to be masked off and painted. Take your time to mask off the framework exactly as touching up white over black is not easy if you make a mistake. A little finishing touch was to pick out the

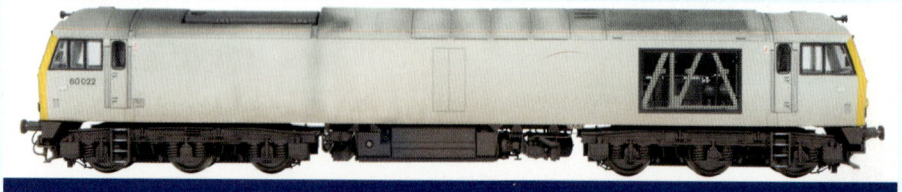

ABOVE: Weathering touches on the underframe include black staining around the fuel filler and silver tread wear on the bogie steps. This is in addition to the build-up of dirt across the whole chassis.

94 www.keymodelworld.com

The railway reborn

BELOW: The Hornby Class 60 looks very much the part finished in undercoat as 60022, the full yellow cab fronts and off-white grille struts being unusual aspects of its appearance.

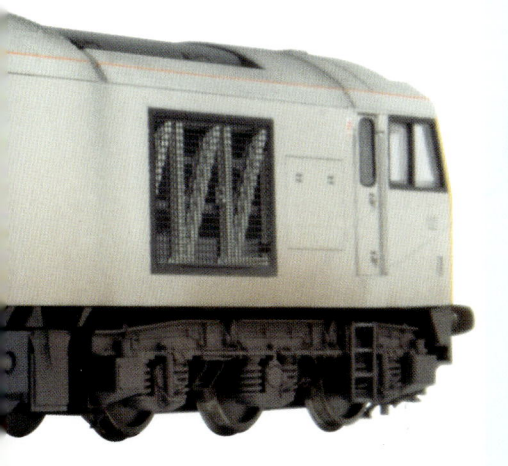

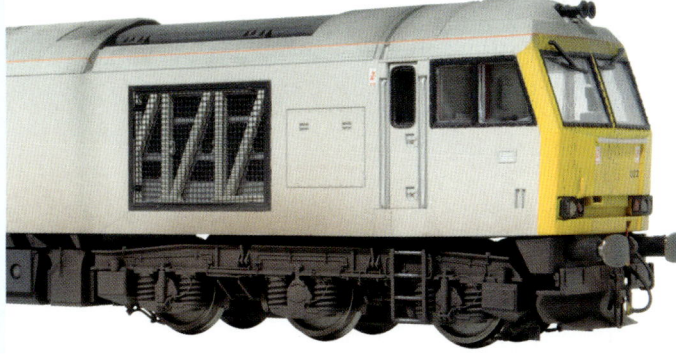

LEFT: Painting the baffle plate behind the No.2 end grille improves its appearance as does weathering the silencer, the factory-finish of the latter having originally being uniform rust or silver on more recent models.

cabside vents in silver. Once happy with the paint finish, the whole body was coated with Railmatch gloss varnish and allowed to dry prior to applying transfers.

Finishing
The transfers required were simple, amounting to black TOPS numbers and front repeaters, black data panels, overhead warning flashes and orange cantrail lining. Once the numbers and overhead flashes were applied, the hardest part was the cantrail lining. I used the Replica Railways product; this being immersed in warm water for around 30 seconds before positioning on one end of the model and carefully sliding off the backing paper along the entire length of the roof. Once it was roughly in place, it was coaxed into the correct position with a cocktail stick.

It is well worth getting the cantrail stripe spot on, especially on a model like this where it will show up any errors. Once pressed into position with a lint free cloth, the excess was trimmed off before moving onto the next strip, ensuring they all lined up on the cab roof corners. Once dry, a generous coat of satin varnish sealed everything in.

Turning to the chassis, the supplied screw couplings, ploughs, and air pipes were all fitted in place, the pipes having first had the taps repainted in more appropriate shades. The only other thing I do is paint the baffle plate behind the bodyside grille, which considerably enhances its appearance by highlighting the detail. This is easily done by prising it off and cleaning up the glue, so it is a snug fit when refitted. I used Humbrol aluminium acrylic spray for this as it is fast-drying and gives a visible contrast from behind the etched grille. The baffle plate vents were hand-painted in matt black, which is rather time consuming but well worth the extra effort. Also at this stage, the exhaust silencer can be painted as desired and refitted, while the GPS aerial bracket over one set of air horns also needed to be removed as this is out of period. The model was then reassembled.

Weathering
Unsurprisingly, 60022 got quite dirty in traffic so the model was given a medium weathering to give it a well-used look. Employing the usual Railmatch acrylic sleeper grime and roof dirt, the standard method of spraying on and then taking it off was used, but more care than usual had to be taken as every single stroke of the airbrush was going to show up on this livery.

Sleeper grime was built up in layers on the underframe and lower bodysides, gently working it upwards with a cotton bud dipped in acrylic thinners. This helps to even out and distribute the weathering colour, otherwise you would have a dirty lower bodyside and a totally mint condition upper bodyside. I made a point of building up the track colour around the No.2 end of the air intake as dirt always got deposited here.

On the roof, I chose not to use the usual method of spraying everything and wiping it off, instead opting to apply the dirt directly where it was needed and then blending it all in. Particular emphasis was given to the engine roof panels; simply working along all the panel gaps with the airbrush and leaving it 'as is'. The same technique was used for the radiator grilles as these got quite dirty.

The exhaust recess was quite tricky as, with the model being white, the dirt had to be worked into every visible recess, which would usually be un-noticeable on a different livery. Exhaust dirt was then added, working around and away from the port down the length of the roof in either direction. The No.2 end cab roof got particularly mucky, and dirt spread down the cab front too. Finally, light streaks of roof dirt were added down both bodysides, coming from the exhaust recess gutters. The buffer heads and fuel filler areas were given a dose of black too. A final finishing touch was tread wear on the cab steps, added with a little silver paint.

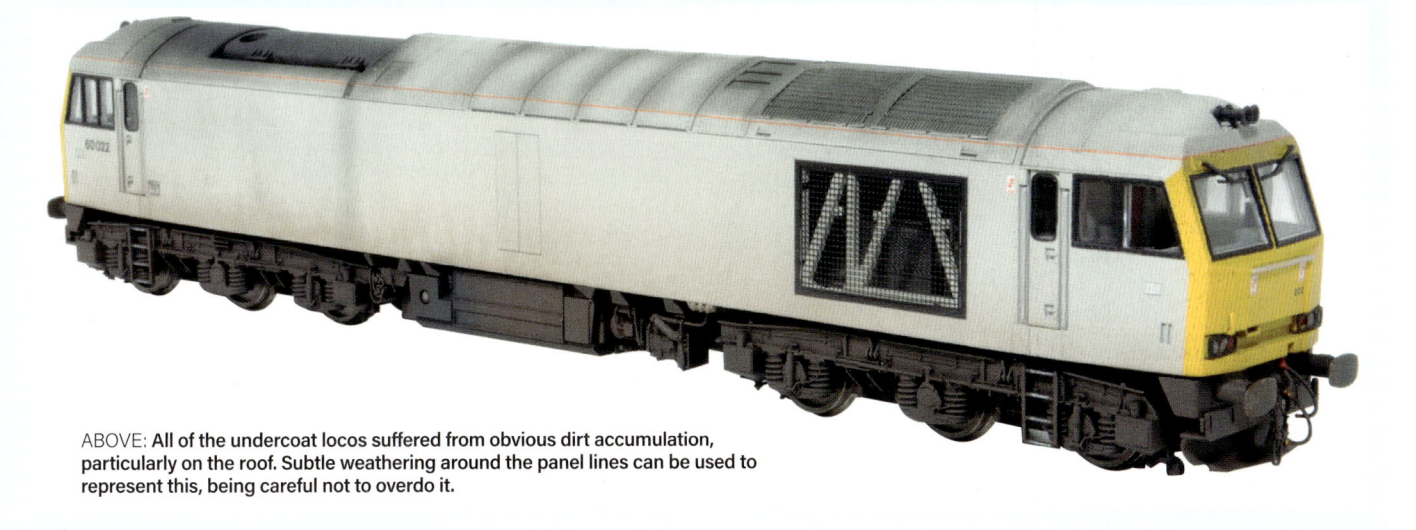

ABOVE: All of the undercoat locos suffered from obvious dirt accumulation, particularly on the roof. Subtle weathering around the panel lines can be used to represent this, being careful not to overdo it.

Modelling BR Locomotives of the 1990s

The railway reborn

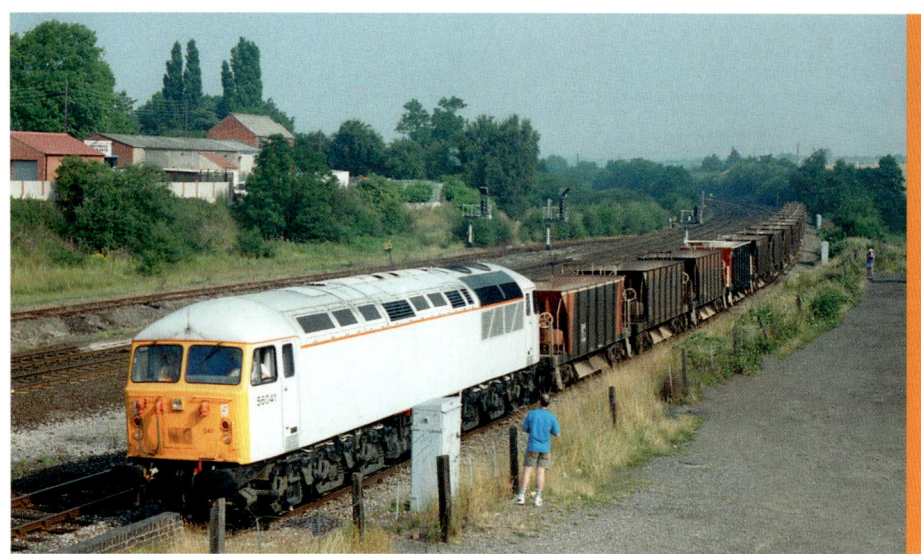

LEFT: Still to gather much dirt, 56041 rolls through Clay Cross in July 1996 with a rake of 16 or so empty Seacow/Sealion ballast hoppers. This was one of three Class 56s given a series of modifications at Brush Traction for Loadhaul at the beginning of the year, the most obvious sign of this being the five replacement cantrail grilles. Altered in the same manner were 56068 and 56102, EWS later implementing a scaled-back package of alterations on other class members. Two of the hoppers are finished in Loadhaul colours, the remainder in dirty engineers' grey/yellow, while the leading examples are all of the riveted design, as produced in 4mm by Bachmann and Hornby (ex-Lima) and 2mm by Farish. Simon Bendall Collection

RIGHT: Seen almost a year later than its classmate, a similarly-modified 56068 was resting at Knottingley on May 10, 1997, and would become the last of the 'ghosts', remaining in traffic until that autumn. The loco displays previous alterations as well, the original round headlight and adjacent single-piece handrail having given way to a standard square fitting and with the central handrail section cut away. Simon Bendall Collection

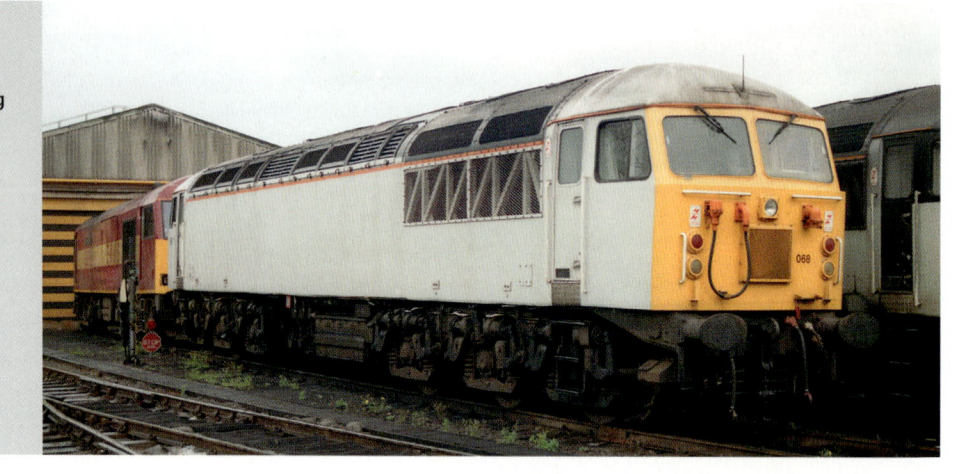

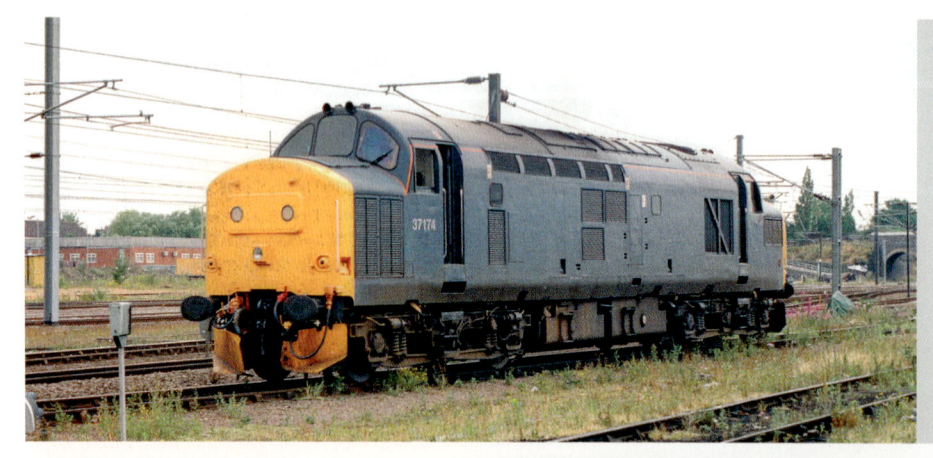

LEFT: Denied Mainline Freight blue, 37174 was the odd one out of the EWS undercoat locos, carrying a shade of grey that resembled Departmental grey. Seen at Peterborough in June 1996, the miniature snowploughs bring some enhancement and would be retained when EWS was applied early in 1997. Simon Bendall Collection

RIGHT: With its gloss finish reflecting the lights of Plymouth station, 47846 *Thor* waits time on August 8, 1996, with the Penzance to Paddington sleeper. The loco had only been released from overhaul at Crewe Works the previous month and was newly on-lease with Great Western Trains. At this time, the sleeper stock was still in InterCity colours with a Mk.1 Full Brake leading the Mk.3 stock. Simon Bendall Collection

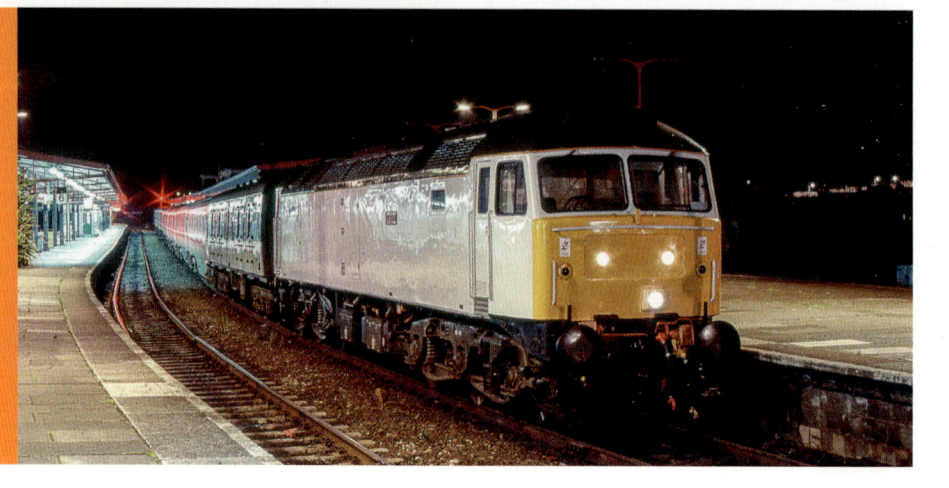

The railway reborn

'Grids' reunited

With EWS purchasing both Transrail and Loadhaul, the Class 56s again became one fleet but with a much expanded scope of operation. **Simon Bendall** takes a look at their maroon years while **James Makin** improves the OO gauge Hornby model.

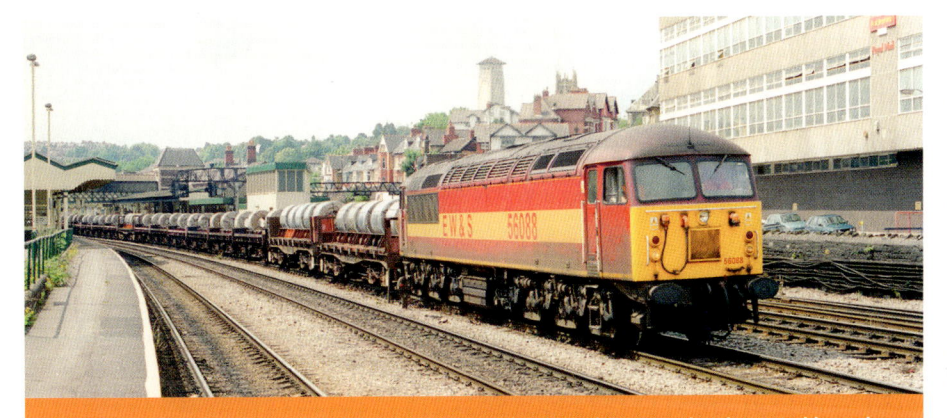

ABOVE: Carrying the original EW&S livery, 56088 rumbles through Newport in July 1999 with a train of imported steel coil bound for the Avesta Steel plant at Panteg. It is also displaying the much-reduced version of the cantrail grille modifications with just the nearest pair over the electrical cubicle compartment having been changed to a new style. The train is made up of three BZA (ex BAA) bogie wagons and at least a dozen two-axle SCA, all carrying plastic-wrapped coils. The SCA, initially coded SKA, were converted in 1997 from SPA steel plate wagons, these seeing the sides removed in favour of low side rails, called curb rails, and the fitting of three coil cradles to the floor, these coming from BZAs. In OO gauge, Bachmann does the BZA in ready-to-run form while the SCA would have to be modified from either the SPA marketed by EFE Rail/Kernow Model Rail Centre or the plastic kit of the same wagon from Cambrian. The latter would be the easier and more accurate option with cradles coming either in etched brass from the Stenson Models range or spares from the Bachmann BZA. Graham Farish does both the BZA and the standard SPA in N gauge. *Simon Bendall Collection*

Of the 135 Class 56s constructed, an operational fleet of some 116 examples was taken on by what soon became EWS during February 1996. The deficit was largely made up of Romanian-built examples that were either stored or withdrawn early.

Of the former Transrail allocation, these were divided between Motherwell and Cardiff Canton, the latter's fleet featuring locos assigned to traffic originating in South Wales and others for use on workings in the Midlands and northwest. Similarly, the erstwhile Loadhaul machines were split between Thornaby and Immingham, some of those based at the Humberside depot covering duties of a local origin while others worked around Yorkshire, particularly on power station coal trains.

By the end of 1996, the Class 56 fleet had been reorganised with Thornaby's allocation removed completely and the previous regional divisions broken down. Immingham was now the principal home of the 'Grids' with its considerable allocation encompassing Romania examples 56003/04/06/07/11/21/22/25/27/29, Doncaster-built 56031/33-39/41/43/45-51/54/55/59/61-63/65-71/74/75/77/78/80-99 and 56100-02/05-12/14, and from the Crewe Works batch 56116-18/20/25-27/30-35. This was essentially an England-wide pool that covered all the type's traditional areas of employment and more besides.

In contrast, those allocated to Cardiff Canton were now much reduced, namely 56010/18/32/40/44/52/53/60/64/73/76 and 56103/13/15/19/21, while the remaining operational examples were still based at Motherwell in the form of 56056-58/72/79 and 56104/23/24/28/29. Liveries at this time were a complete mixture with Loadhaul and Transrail triple grey intermingled with classmates that still carried their Railfreight sub-sector emblems and others that were in debranded triple grey. In addition, 56031/46/48 retained Civil Engineers 'Dutch' grey/yellow as did 56036/47/49 but with the addition of Transrail logos while 56004 was still running in BR blue.

EWS makeover

The application of maroon and gold to the Class 56s was underway by the early summer of 1996 with 56089 the first to be completed and which was quite rapidly followed by 56041/51/57/58/88/96 and 56105/14/20, these all having the original EW&S lettering. Thereafter, the livery was updated to remove the ampersand and add the EWS 'three beasties' logo to the secondman's cabsides, this version duly appearing on 56011/18/32/37/38/59/60/62/65/67-69/71/81/87/91/94/95 and 56103/13/15/17/19 over the following couple of years before the company largely ceased repaints on its inherited and increasingly doomed ex BR fleet.

The modification programme implemented by Loadhaul to improve the internal airflow as well as provide cleaner air via new filters was continued by EWS. However, rather than fit the five new cantrail grilles per side given to 56041, 56068 and 56102, it was cut back to just two per side, these being at the No.2 end above the electrical cubicle. Recipients of this revised arrangement were 56003/04/06/07/10/11/18/21/22/25/27/29/31-40/43-60/62-67/69-96/98/99 and 56100/01/03-21/24/26-35. All other Class 56s were withdrawn without this modification.

September 1997 saw all of the Class 56s concentrated on Immingham with Canton and Motherwell losing their allocations while tatty Railfreight Red Stripe-liveried 56019 was also reinstated to traffic around the same time after more than a year in store. Later repaints saw 56063 receive a unique inverted version of triple grey around 1999 following a graffiti attack on both sides while 56006 was repainted into BR blue in 2000 and became part of the EWS heritage fleet.

With the introduction of the Class 66s, the inevitable rundown of the class began in 1999 with several of the Romanian examples being culled. The process accelerated through the first four years of the new century with 56078 and 56115 bringing down the curtain on EWS' operation of the type at the end of March 2004. For the last six months of its EWS career, 56078 carried BR large logo blue, having been repainted as a farewell tribute to the class.

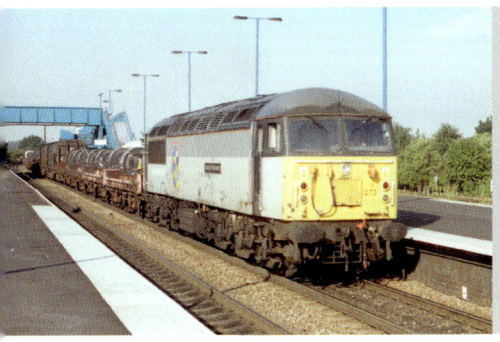

LEFT: One of the scruffier members of EWS' Class 56 fleet was 56073 *Tremorfa Steelworks*, its appearance not being helped by the partially removed Transrail logo on one side that revealed the Trainload Metals badge beneath, it remained like this to withdrawal in 2002. With 11 months left in traffic, the 'Grid' passes through Barnetby with the 6M99 Immingham to Wolverhampton Steel Terminal on July 21, 2001, this conveying imported steel coils. The wagons are again mostly two-axle SCA/SKA but with two of the bogie BHA prototypes built in 1990 also included, these running without their distinctive red hoods at this point. *Simon Bendall Collection*

Modelling BR Locomotives of the 1990s **97**

The railway reborn

Last years of the 'Grids'

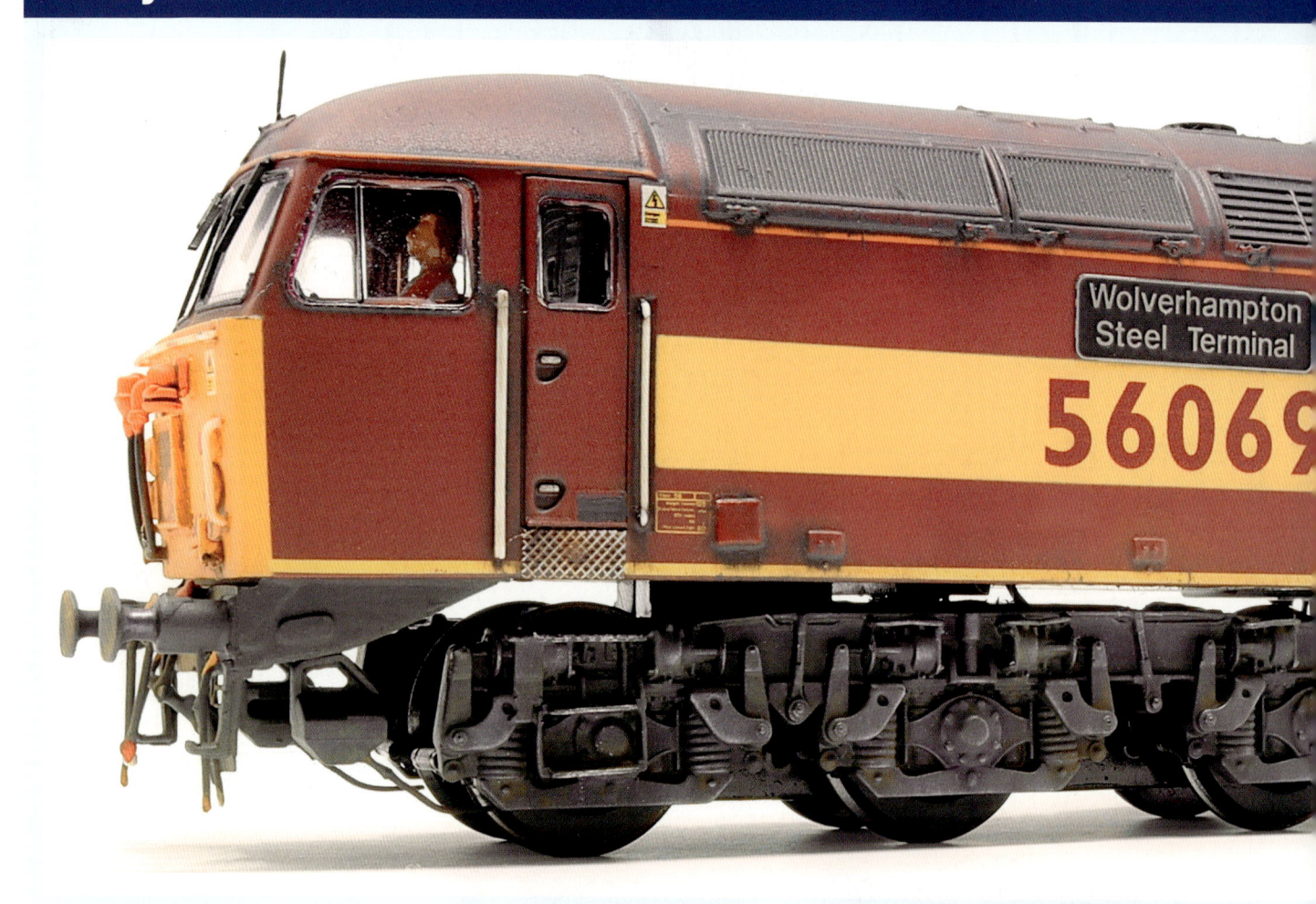

Prior to the big EWS 'switch off' of early 2004, the freight giant had a healthy number of the well-loved Class 56s going about the network during the late 1990s and early 2000s, hauling both heavier freight flows and also lighter duties like 'Enterprise' workings. Seeking to recreate my teenage spotting years at Didcot, this meant modelling a few of the class that were diagrammed on the Welsh steel traffic flows and, by the late 1990s, a fair number of the class had been repainted into the fresh new colours of EWS.

At the time, a very inspirational VHS video was released, this going behind the scenes at EWS' Toton depot. This included following the overhaul and repaint of 56094 from tatty Trainload Coal livery into the shining maroon and gold colours of the day, and this video stuck in my mind sufficiently to later form the basis behind the models tackled here.

This project was undertaken prior to the announcement of the upcoming Cavalex Class 56, so makes use of the current Hornby model, which is ripe for further detailing and makes for a relatively straightforward project.

Plan of action

Before starting work, the first point was to plan what aspects would and would not be tackled. As modellers, we are spoilt for choice with the Extreme Etchings range produced by Shawplan to the extent that

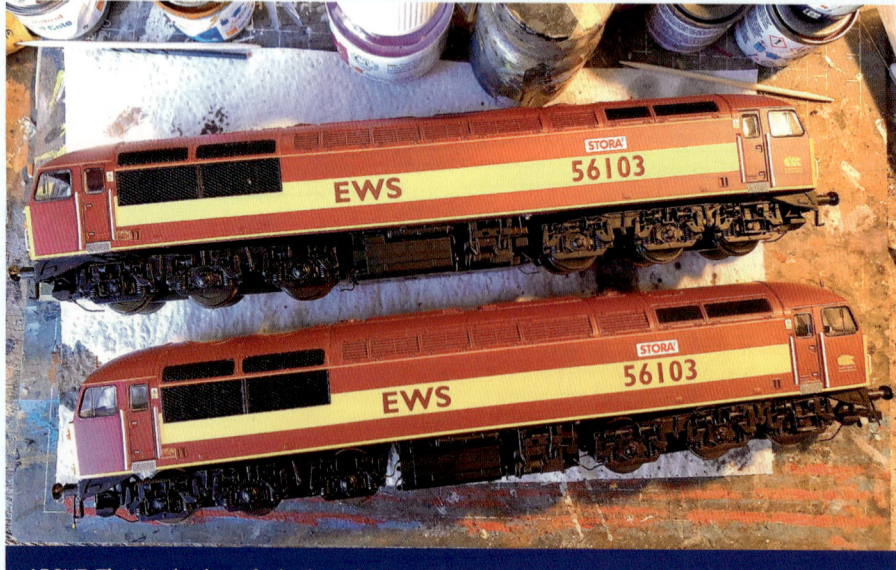

ABOVE: The Hornby donor for both models was 56103 *Stora*, this having all the features of an EWS-era Doncaster-built machine, including the modified cantrail grilles.

one has to decide just how far to go with the detailing. Next, it is key to decide upon the identity of the locos before going further as it impacts upon the detailing parts required, especially with the key differences between the batches built in Romania, at Doncaster and later Crewe.

The first choice to be modelled had to be the aforementioned 56094 *Eggborough Power Station*, which was then joined by 56069 *Wolverhampton Steel Terminal*. The latter appealed as it featured in my trainspotting notes from the time and the very industrial-sounding name simply tickled my fancy! As it happened, I already had a few EWS-liveried Class 56s in the collection so two of these were dug out and stripped down ready for reworking.

The railway reborn

BELOW: **The Hornby Class 56 can be upgraded in a number of areas, some being largely essential to improve its accuracy while others are more optional. Fitting new fan grilles and plating over the lifting points are in the former category.**

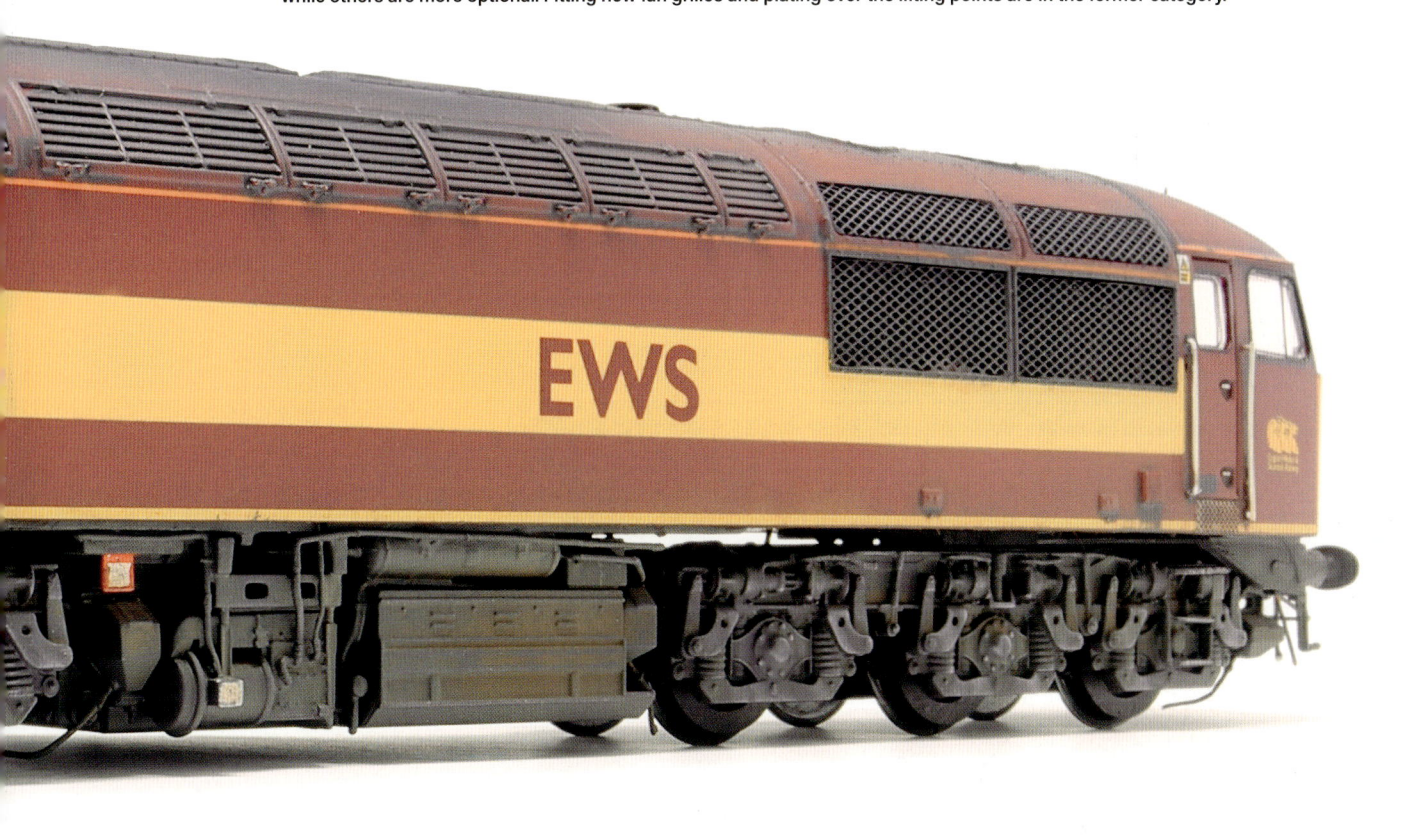

Both of the chosen locos were late-build Doncaster machines so very similar to the Hornby donor models. The areas that needed attention would be the roof grilles, the bodyside lifting point covers and around the cab ends. Each model would additionally need finishing with new decals and nameplates, together with some light weathering to reflect the condition of the prototypes at the very end of the 1990s.

Getting started

Once taken apart, the most noticeable area requiring improvement on the Hornby bodyshell is the roof fans and grilles. The latter are too deeply recessed and the mesh no match to the finesse of the Extreme Etchings replacements. The existing Hornby roof grilles were pushed out of the body by hand and the circular plastic shroud attached to each metal grille was carefully separated. The two shroud mouldings were then glued back down into the fan recesses and filed down ready for attaching

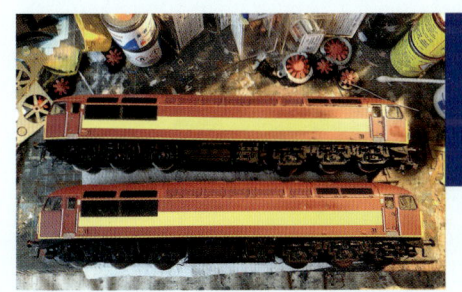

LEFT: **Both locos have seen much of their printing removed, it being necessary to delete and replace the EWS lettering so that there is a colour match with the new number transfers. Removing the 'beasties' also allows transfers with more colour density to be applied.**

the Shawplan grilles on top with contact adhesive.

As the Shawplan mesh is so fine, it is easy to put a thumb, file, or paintbrush through it during the modelling stages, so a great way to get around this is to apply some low-tack Tamiya masking tape to the inside of the body and across the top of the grilles to keep them safe until the painting commences. Sitting underneath

BELOW: **The revised cantrail grilles fitted at the No.2 end of both locos are shown to advantage, these being designed to improve internal airflow. Hornby's tooling allows for both this style and the original.**

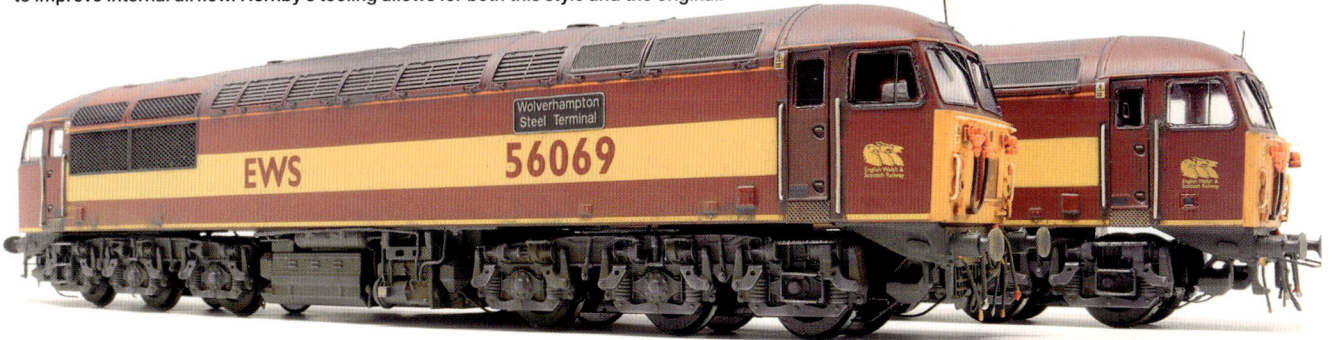

Modelling BR Locomotives of the 1990s

The railway reborn

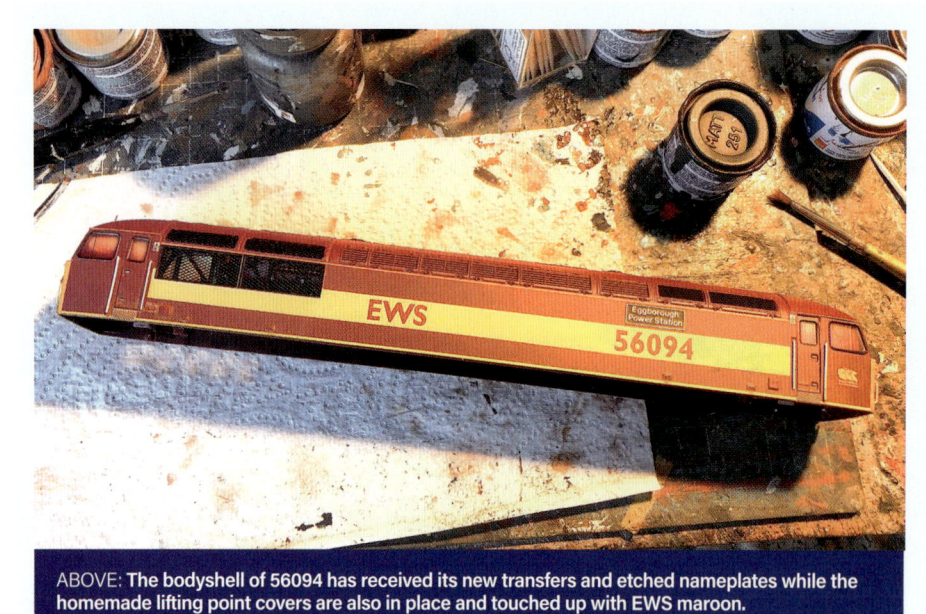

ABOVE: The bodyshell of 56094 has received its new transfers and etched nameplates while the homemade lifting point covers are also in place and touched up with EWS maroon.

the roof grilles is Hornby's rotating roof fan unit, which runs on a belt connected to the flywheels. On some examples, it has been noted to impair performance, so I elected to cut through the rubber band driving the fans and leave them for visual appearance only.

Moving down to the bodysides, one notable mistake with Hornby's Class 56 is that it is modelled with the lifting point covers missing, two per side. Shawplan produces a simple blanking plate etch for these or, alternatively as I did, you can cut a small sliver of card to represent each one and glue these to the sides with PVA for a very low-cost modification.

As luck had it, both Hornby models were already portrayed with the revised cantrail grilles at the No.2 end. If your donor has the original style and needs updating, Shawplan produces etched brass replacements that can be fitted once the original moulding has been filed smooth. This is another reason why research before starting a project is important as it allows the right tooling to be chosen and saves a tricky job.

Cab detailing
The cab shape and details vary considerably on the Class 56s, this being one of the main distinguishing areas

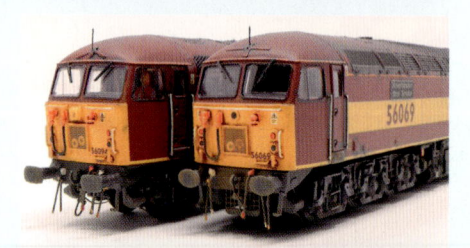

ABOVE: The Class 56s were a complex class with many detail differences, sometimes at opposite ends of the same loco. Although 56069 and 56094 were both late-build Doncaster examples, variations include aerial bracket style, headlight and handrail arrangement, buffer type and the presence or not of the coupling banger plate.

between the respective batches built in Romania, at Doncaster or Crewe. With both of these being Doncaster-built locos, there were relatively few changes required to the donor models but there were small variations between 56069 and 56094 that, without prototype pictures being used throughout, could have slipped through the net.

56094 was fitted with a replacement square headlight at both ends so a Replica Railways plastic moulding was added in place of the original round version on both cabs. A circular piece of clear plastic was used to extend the light guide at each end to enable the Hornby lights to project out from the new moulding.

The fitting of the new headlight also typically required the centre section of the horizontal handrail above to be removed, this leaving just the outer parts in place. This alteration was carefully made to the Hornby model using a sharp scalpel to cut the handrail section away.

There are further options to enhance some of the front end detail using Shawplan parts, such as the air horn grilles and light clusters. However, given that these particular models were already well-finished in the correct livery, a decision was made to retain the existing arrangements on this occasion. Hornby's model is also supplied with opening cab doors but the drawback of these is that if left open, you can see the door mechanism and overscale springs, so instead each door was secured in the closed position with PVA glue.

On the cab roofs, the aerial mounting bracket was changed on 56094, this example having the 'V' style at the No.1 end, which was different to the 'T' version on the Hornby model. Small pieces of styrene strip were cut and fixed to the roof for this but there are also Shawplan etches available for both types.

Bufferbeam attention
The Class 56s also had notable differences around the bufferbeams, the original cowlings used on the Romanian batch giving way to partial and then complete removal on the later Doncaster and Crewe-built examples. Buffers also varied throughout the type's career, ranging from round Oleo types through to ovals and the later rectangular style as fitted to Class 60s.

My two EWS versions had the more common oval buffers fitted, except at the No.1 end of 56094 where it had the newer rectangular style. On the model, the Hornby oval buffers and shanks were removed with pliers to be replaced with a set of cast whitemetal Class 60 buffers from Shawplan. Screw couplings were added using those supplied by Hornby alongside the bufferbeam pipework in the detailing pack. Once again, homemade pipes crafted from 0.45mm handrail wire were employed where the originals had been misplaced.

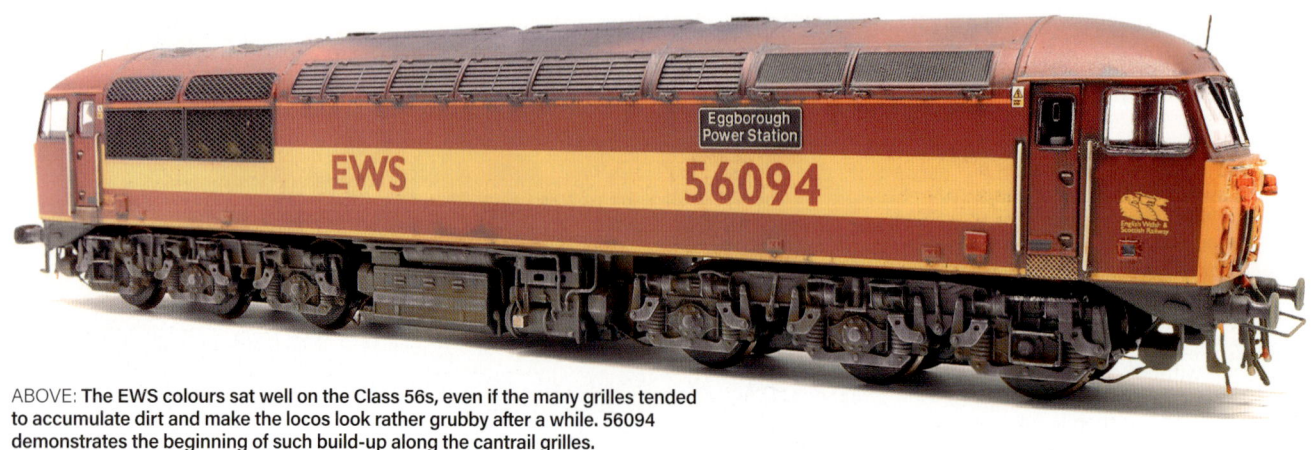

ABOVE: The EWS colours sat well on the Class 56s, even if the many grilles tended to accumulate dirt and make the locos look rather grubby after a while. 56094 demonstrates the beginning of such build-up along the cantrail grilles.

The railway reborn

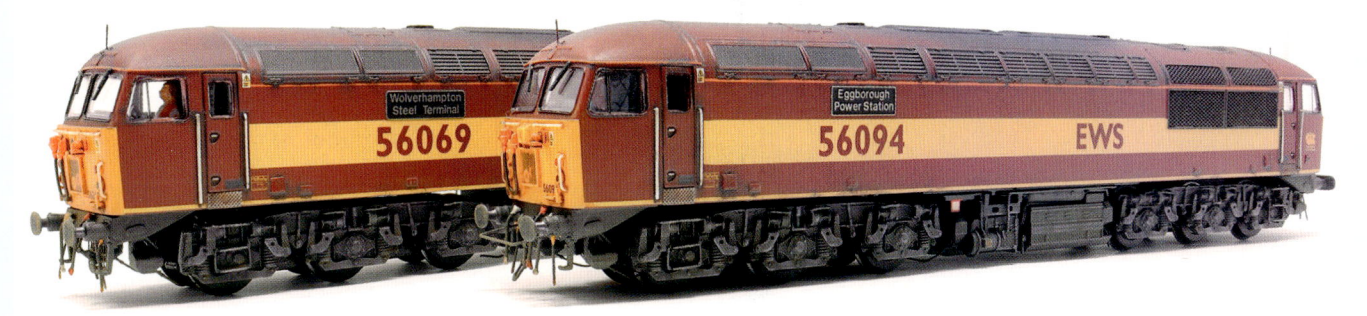

ABOVE: Both of these 'Grids' carry the revised version of maroon and gold with the ampersand removed from the EWS lettering and the 'three beasties' logo on the secondman's cabsides. It was very rare for any loco with the original EW&S lettering to be updated to the later style, irrespective of class.

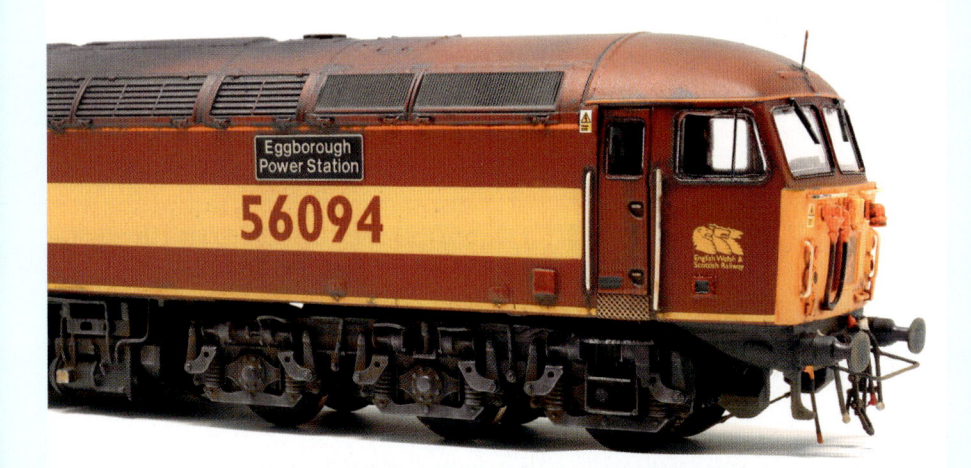

ABOVE: Another difference between the pair is the cabside ventilator beneath the EWS 'beasties' on 56094, this modification appearing on the secondman's cabsides from 56091 onwards through to 56135. This is again scratchbuilt, but Shawplan also offers an etch.

Below the bufferbeam and behind the coupler, many Class 56s had a grid-like banger plate at each end to stop the screw coupling swinging back and hitting equipment behind. Hornby supplies these as solid plastic parts in the detailing pack but the Shawplan etched brass replacements are both finer and see-through. These were fitted on 56069 but are absent on 56094 as per the real thing.

Branding

As each loco was already in EWS livery and the main elements were correct, the plan was to retain the livery but just patch paint any new items such as the roof grilles, aerial brackets and lifting point covers in Phoenix Precision's EWS maroon. When it comes to removing the old printing, such as the lettering, numbering and nameplates, some models are easier than others.

On these '56s', I started by gently scraping away at the shiny top layer of the Hornby printing with a fresh curved-bladed scalpel. This helped to remove the top glossy layer to reveal a more matt finish below. Next, a cotton bud was dipped in enamel thinners and rubbed over the Hornby printing, which gently lifted from the surface without damaging the yellow paint beneath.

The next stage was then to apply an all-over coat of Railmatch gloss varnish to give a good base for the new transfers to sit on. Railtec's EWS decals were applied to each loco, its pre-made numbersets arriving all lined-up and matched to the prototype, this saving a lot of time in the modelling process. New etched nameplates were added, these coming from the Fox Transfers range and glued in place using matt varnish. Finally, a coat of the same Railmatch varnish was applied and the model left for a month to allow the varnish to harden

Weathering

Both locos were in a reasonably clean condition during my late 1990s period, the duo having been recently outshopped in their new EWS colours so, going by prototype photos, there was only a small amount of weathering to be added. Firstly, washes of Humbrol dark brown (No.251) and dark grey (No.32) were painted on and wiped away with kitchen towel, working in a vertical motion on the bodyshell, before being wiped down further with cotton buds dipped in enamel thinners. This paint on and wipe-off process helps to build the grime in the recesses, while the rest of the bodyshell is left in a clean condition.

Further down on the chassis, this was painted all over in dark grey prior to replacing the bodyshell on the chassis and then airbrushing on the traffic grime, consisting of Phoenix Precision's brake dust, track dirt, roof dirt and dirty black. Around the immediate exhaust areas, a bespoke mix of neat black with dark blue was applied to represent the oily exhaust deposits found in this area. Final touches included dry-brushing Humbrol Metalcote gunmetal across the bogies and cantrail grilles to highlight the raised edges, and a further dry-brushing of silver on the bogie footsteps.

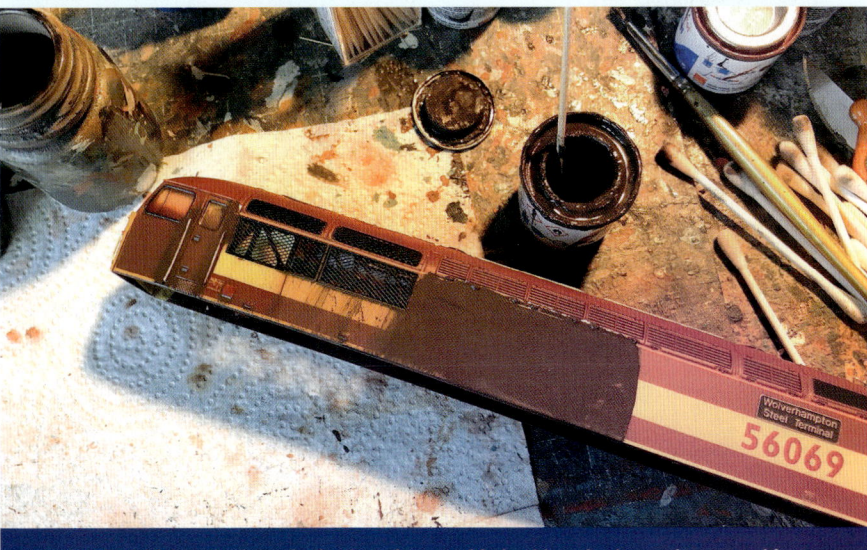

ABOVE: The initial wash of weathering is underway with the thinned paint partly removed from around the cab but with final cleaning still to be done.

Modelling BR Locomotives of the 1990s **101**

The railway reborn

RIGHT: No longer an undercoat 'ghost', 56041 passes Scunthorpe with the 6M05 Roxby Gullet to Northenden empty 'binliner' on October 6, 1999. Mirroring the operation seen in London to some extent, the refuse of Greater Manchester was at this time collected from three terminals around the city and sent across the Pennines to be disposed of. These workings employed KFA container flats owned by the city council. Just ten Class 56s received the initial EW&S-lettered version of the livery. Simon Bendall Collection

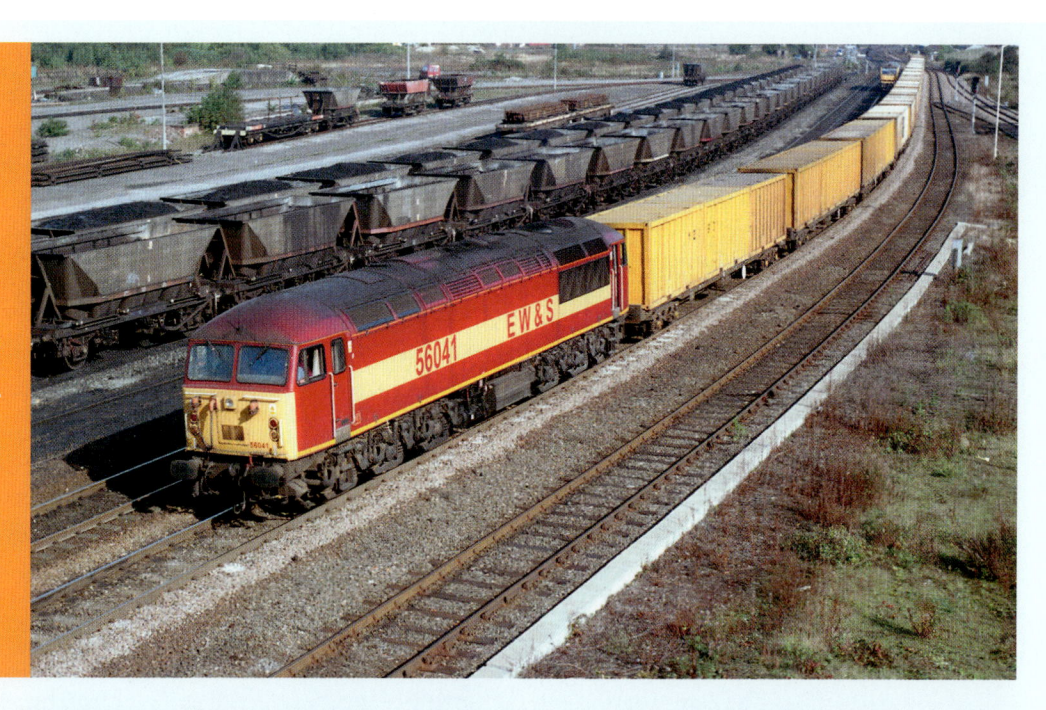

RIGHT: The new era of EWS operations is represented not by 56061 in its scruffy Trainload Metals livery but rather the rake of maroon-liveried BYA covered steel wagons forming the 6E02 11.54 Toton-Boston Docks empties at Ancaster on April 29, 1999. These were the first of the Thrall-built wagons to roll out of York Works at the end of the decade and continue to serve successor DB Cargo to this day. Spoiling the rake is a solitary BBA modified with a sliding roof, this being either a BIA, BWA or BXA depending on the internal cradle arrangement. Bachmann has long produced the BYA in both 4mm and 2mm under its Farish brand while Cavalex has the BIA/BWA/BXA under development in 4mm. Bill Atkinson

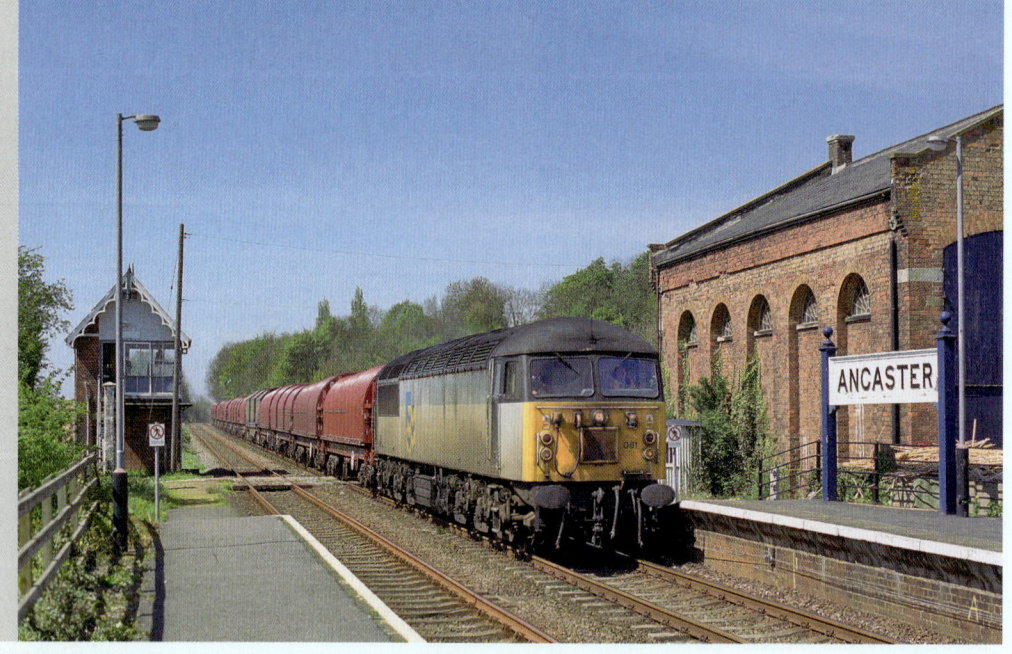

RIGHT: An early traffic success for EWS was the movement of imported paper reels from Immingham Docks to Ripple Lane in East London for use by the newspaper industry. This brought the sight of Class 56s powering along the East Coast Main Line for a time, like on August 28, 1998, as 56018 brings the 6L71 06.55 loaded working south to the capital at Marston, near Grantham. The trains were formed of a long rake of Cargowaggon IZA twin-vans, these being a pair of two-axle vans semi-permanently coupled together. Modelling this working is straightforward as Kernow Model Rail Centre offers an OO gauge model while Revolution Trains has done the same in N gauge. Bill Atkinson

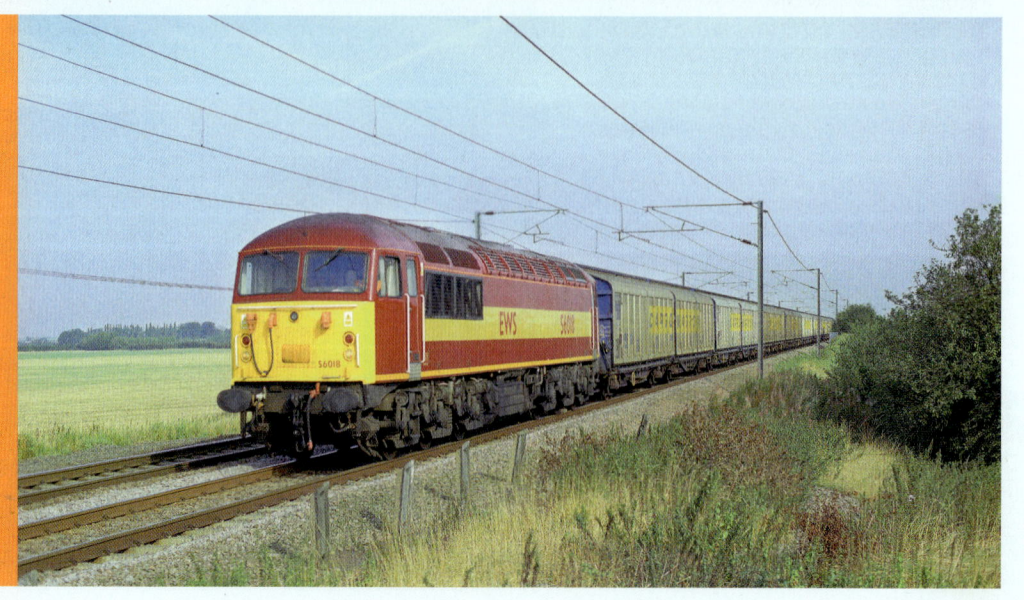

102 www.keymodelworld.com

The railway reborn

RIGHT: Some four years after it launched the Loadhaul livery at Doncaster, 56039 powers north on the West Coast Main Line at Chelmscote with the 6S75 11.10 Sheerness to Mossend 'Enterprise' service on September 21, 1998. Once named *ABP Port of Hull*, the nameplates had been surrendered to classmate 56087 the previous year. This is another formation that can now be modelled in its entirety in both 2mm and 4mm scales with the IWA Cargowaggon 'hold-all' vans being available from Revolution Trains and the ICA clay slurry 'silver bullets' on the rear from Dapol. Meanwhile, the SPA opens carrying coiled wire in the centre of the train can be found in 4mm from EFE Rail and Kernow Model Rail Centre with the 2mm version covered by Graham Farish. Bill Atkinson

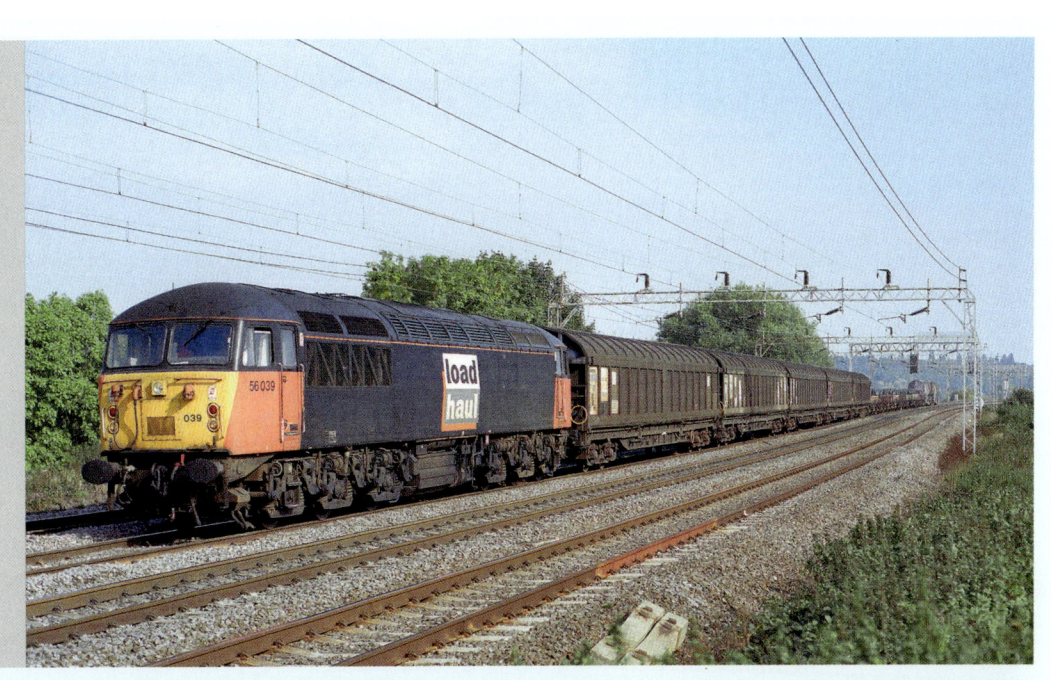

Model availability

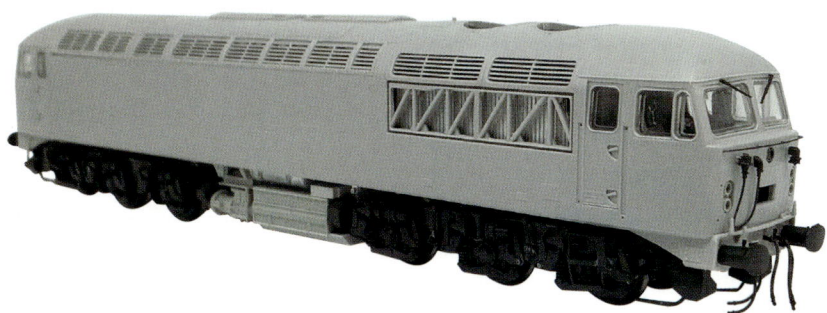

ABOVE: The forthcoming OO gauge Cavalex Class 56 is seen in early pre-production form, this being a hand-assembled prototype that is subject to all manner of improvements. Nevertheless, it shows the potential of the model, this being the Romanian-built version. Cavalex Models

ABOVE: Hornby's high-end Class 56 has appeared in several variants of triple grey, included Construction-badged 56037 *Richard Trevithick*.

ABOVE: Dapol's N gauge releases have included Railfreight Red Stripe survivor 56019, which lasted long enough to work for EWS in these colours.

An OO gauge Class 56 has been available for almost as long as the class has existed thanks to the Mainline model of the early 1980s, this being widely lauded at the time for its fine detailing. The tooling later passed to Dapol and then into Hornby ownership, where it was widely used to produce a range of liveries around the early 2000s. It was subsequently retired upon the arrival of Hornby's own modern rendering, this catering for Romanian, early Doncaster, and late Doncaster/Crewe builds, although the proportions produced of each has been variable along with the liveries.

Now in development is a rival 4mm offering from Cavalex Models, which promises to have an extensive tooling suite to allow almost any variant to be catered for, including locos with different cabs at each end. The initial tooling sample arrived as this publication was being written with the first batch of models expected to be released in the first half of 2023.

In N gauge, Dapol is the current provider of a Class 56 with an assortment of build variations catered for, this having thankfully consigned the misshapen Graham Farish model of the 1990s to history. In O gauge, the Class 56 in late-build Doncaster form is the most recent addition to Heljan's roster of heavyweight models, this initially appearing in all the key BR era liveries as well as Loadhaul.

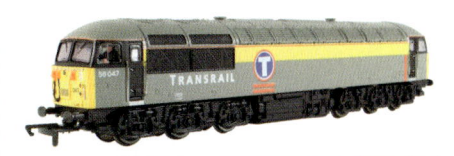

ABOVE: The OO gauge Mainline Class 56 tooling passed to Dapol and then Hornby, the latter's release of 56047 in Dutch Transrail being a colourful addition.

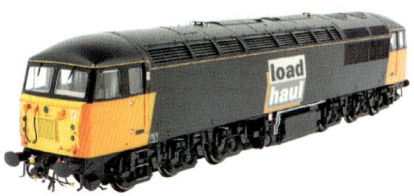

ABOVE: Heljan's recent O gauge model largely focussed on BR liveries for its first batch but did include an un-numbered Loadhaul example. Image courtesy Kernow Model Rail Centre

Modelling BR Locomotives of the 1990s 103

The railway reborn

Enter the 'Bodysnatchers'

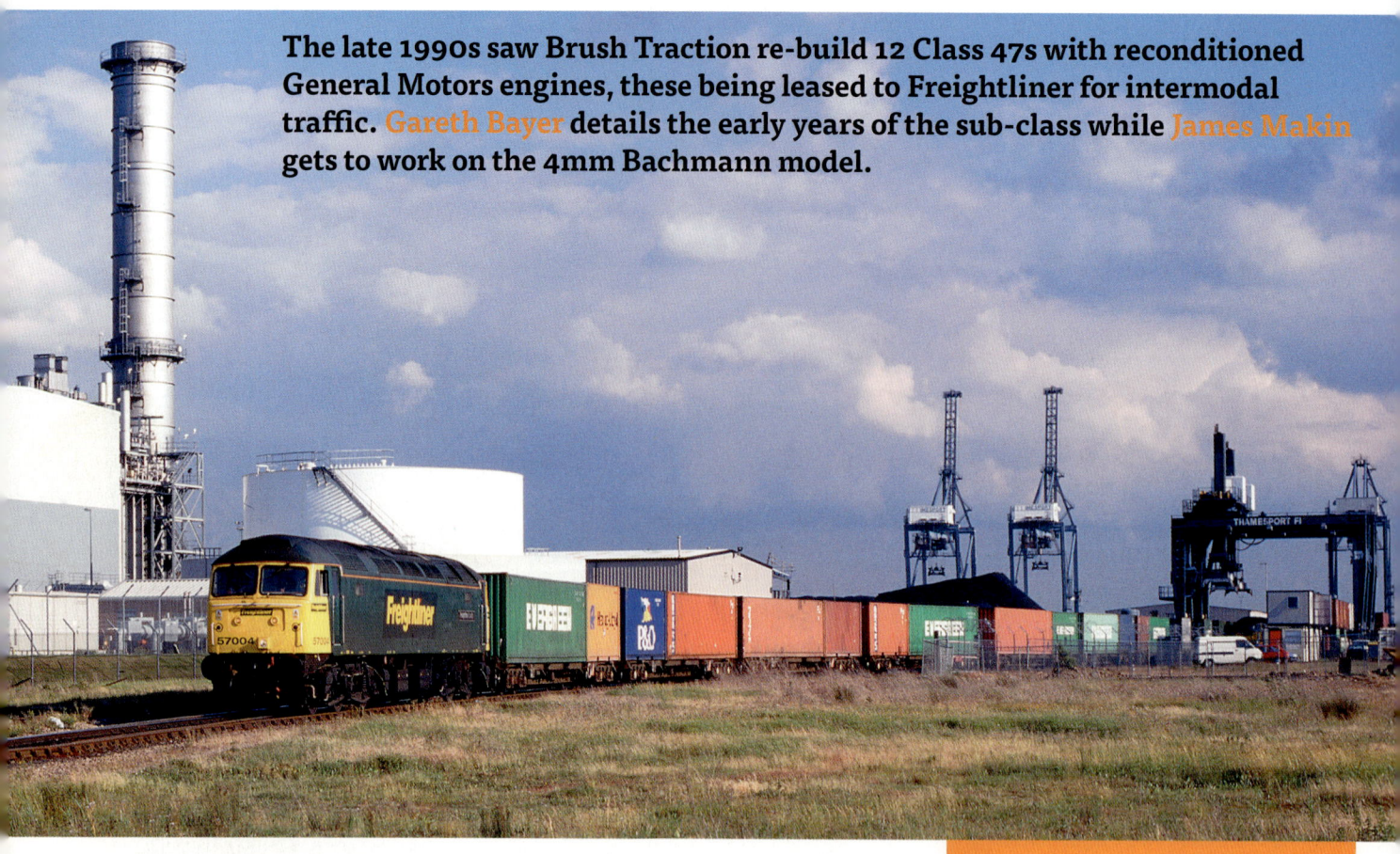

The late 1990s saw Brush Traction re-build 12 Class 47s with reconditioned General Motors engines, these being leased to Freightliner for intermodal traffic. Gareth Bayer **details the early years of the sub-class while** James Makin **gets to work on the 4mm Bachmann model.**

Following the management buy-out of Freightliner in the spring of 1996, the company soon identified a pressing need for replacements for its hard-worked Class 47 fleet. Mainly inherited from Railfreight Distribution, the intermodal operator got the short end of the stick, with many of the locos that it took over having not received an overhaul for many years.

The urgency of the requirement and the costs of introducing a new loco type were seen to be prohibitive, especially with the Railtrack rolling stock acceptance regime then in place, so Freightliner took the bold decision to re-engine 12 of its Class 47s with a General Motors power plant, which would be combined with a refurbished Class 56 alternator. While the intention to order new Class 66s from General Motors was also in place, the first of these would not arrive until 1999 as the EWS order had to be largely processed first.

Brush Traction of Loughborough was contracted to upgrade the locos, which would see the Sulzer 12LDA28C replaced with a secondhand but reconditioned GM-EMD 12-cylinder 2,500hp 645E3. The test bed for the programme was 47356, which was admitted to Brush's Falcon Works in early 1998, with its new power unit being lifted into place on March 16th, at which point the loco became 57001. When released to Freightliner, it was finished in a new green and yellow livery, this replacing the previous triple grey as the company's brand going forward.

The programme also saw the Class 57/0s gain refurbished cab interiors with modified control desks and improved sound insulation, an early plan for entirely new cabs being shelved due to cost. The locos also featured sanding gear on the bogies and Brush's wheelslip detection system to improve traction. The benchmark was that the locos should be able to lift a 1,600-tonne train up a 1 in 77 gradient in poor weather conditions and then be able to maintain a maximum speed of 75mph on the main line. Externally, the only other significant changes were the prominent angled silencer panel on the roof and the toughened window frames on the cab fronts.

It had originally been intended for more Class 57/0s to be cycled through Brush but the increasing cost of the GM engine and the lack of second-hand alternators on the market eventually saw the end of the programme once 57012 was rolled out. There were also issues with the donor Class 47s where, due to the number of modifications undertaken over the years, each conversion was almost a bespoke job.

Green means Heinz

The original pool code for the Class 57/0s was DFHZ, the HZ part of the code allegedly being a reference to Heinz of '57 varieties' fame. 57001 *Freightliner Pioneer* was sent to the Toton open weekend over the August 1998 bank holiday, where it showed off Freightliner's new look to enthusiasts. It was then sent to Ipswich for crew training,

ABOVE: On a bright autumn day in 1999, 57004 *Freightliner Quality* stands at Thamesport some six months after conversion. The green and yellow livery was certainly a bold departure from the previous triple grey colours and helped give Freightliner a bold new identity in the privatised world as it sought to expand beyond its intermodal roots into heavy freight commodities. The visible wagons are once again quad sets of FSA-FTA-FTA-FSA, which at this time were the dominant container wagon type, most of the earlier FFA/FGA having been withdrawn as life-expired.
Simon Bendall Collection

which saw it employed most nights on the 4E50 Ipswich to Leeds and 4L83 return until 57006 *Freightliner Reliance* replaced it. The latter machine was the first of the class to be fitted with the then new TPWS equipment and was extensively used on trials of the system at Haughley Junction, just north of Ipswich.

The second Class 57/0 to be released, 57002 *Freightliner Phoenix*, was originally sent to Crewe, while 57003 *Freightliner Evolution* started off its career at Southampton. The other locos were not specifically deployed anywhere after release and once the programme had reached the halfway point, the locos could be seen on almost any Freightliner workings, including the then fledgling Heavy Haul services. 57007, named *Freightliner Bond*, was the first of the second batch of conversions to be completed and rather than use long-term stored machines as had been the case

The railway reborn

| Freightliner Class 57/0s at a glance |||||||
Number	Name	Previously	Released	No.1 end	No.2 end	Underframe tanks
57001	*Freightliner Pioneer*	47356	07.98	Flush	Standard	1 (4)
57002	*Freightliner Phoenix*	47322	11.98	Standard	Standard	1 (4)
57003	*Freightliner Evolution*	47317	01.99	Standard	Standard	1 (4)
57004	*Freightliner Quality*	47347	02.99	Flush	Standard	2 (3)
57005	*Freightliner Excellence*	47350	03.99	Standard	Standard	1 (4)
57006	*Freightliner Reliance*	47187	04.99	Standard	Standard	1 (4)
57007	*Freightliner Bond*	47332	10.99	Standard	Standard	2 (3)
57008	*Freightliner Explorer*	47060	11.99	Standard	Standard	1 (4)
57009	*Freightliner Venturer*	47079	12.99	Standard	Standard	1 (4)
57010	*Freightliner Crusader*	47231	01.00	Standard	Standard	2 (3)
57011	*Freightliner Challenger*	47329	02.00	Standard	Standard	2 (3)
57012	*Freightliner Envoy*	47204	03.00	Flush	Standard	3

Key to underframe tanks (figure in brackets is style after modification): 1 - boiler water tanks (out of use), 2 - battery boxes only, 3 - long range fuel tanks, 4 - hybrid original boiler tanks and long-range tank.

before, the donors now had all suffered serious failures or were badly in need of an overhaul.

Once all 12 locos were completed, the Class 57/0s largely settled onto intermodal services in the southern half of the country. They were diagrammed to work services from Lawley Street to Tilbury and Felixstowe; Southampton Maritime/Millbrook to Cardiff Wentloog, Ripple Lane, and Trafford Park; Felixstowe to Daventry and Hams Hall plus the return workings for all the above.

Loco differences

Ostensibly, the 12 locos should have all been delivered in the same livery style. However, 57007/10/11/12 were missing some or all of their cabside Freightliner logos while the nameplates were not applied in the same positions. 57001 and 57004-12 had them both behind the secondman's doors but 57002 and 57003 had the plates applied at the No.2 end on both sides.

The conversion programme did not include the fitting of long range fuel tanks, only 57012

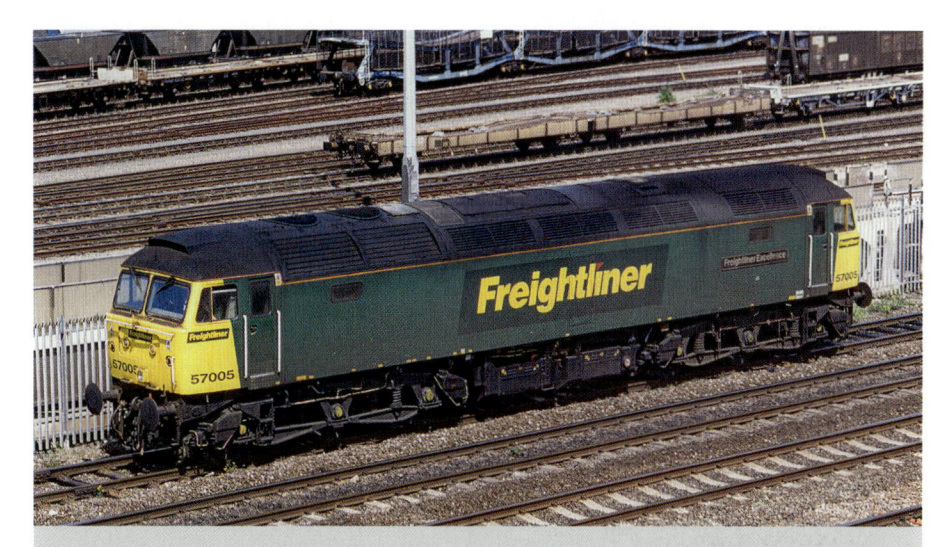

ABOVE: Now equipped with the curious hybrid design of long range fuel tank and boiler tank, 57005 *Freightliner Excellence* runs light past Washwood Heath on May 16, 2002, while heading for the container terminal at Lawley Street. External changes to the Class 57/0 sub-class were relatively minimal, the new roof silencer being the main one while sandboxes were also added to the bogies. Gareth Bayer

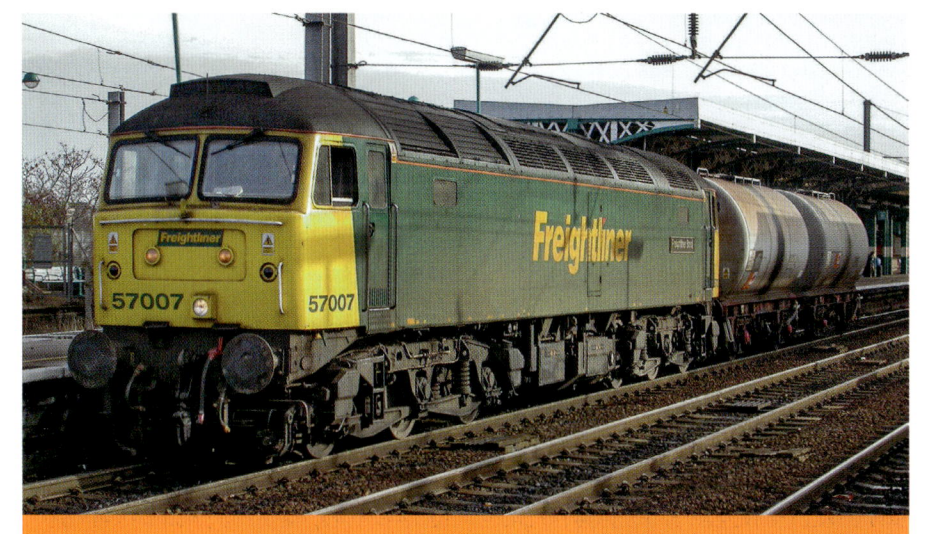

ABOVE: With no road access to the fuelling point alongside Ipswich station, the traction gas oil has long had to be delivered by rail, a situation that was still continuing in the spring of 2022. Some 19 years earlier on November 14, 2003, the superbly-named 57007 *Freightliner Bond* trips two Esso TTAs from the fuelling point to the yard for collection and onward movement to Fawley. Today, modern bogie TEA tankers fulfil this role. Bachmann produces the TTA in 4mm scale, although the springs ideally need updating to be fully accurate, while Farish does likewise in 2mm. Gareth Bayer

initially having these as they were already in place on the former 47204 when sent to Brush. As a result, it was put in a new pool of its own, DFTZ.

However, it was not long before the other 11 locos also received extended range tanks using equipment reclaimed from withdrawn Class 47s. The Class 57/0s that still carried their original and long redundant boiler water tanks only had them removed on the side where the long range tanks were fitted, resulting in an unusual combination. When Railfreight Distribution and Rail Express Systems had undertaken a similar procedure on their Class 47s, the redundant water tanks were completely removed. Following the modification, all the '57/0s' were allocated to the DFTZ pool.

By 2007, Freightliner's need for the class was much reduced, this resulting in 57007-12 being returned to Porterbrook that spring, where they were immediately taken on lease by Direct Rail Services. The other half-dozen was similarly dispensed with during the course of 2008, eventually finding their way variously to West Coast, DRS, and Advenza Freight.

Modelling BR Locomotives of the 1990s **105**

The railway reborn

Freightliner goes GM

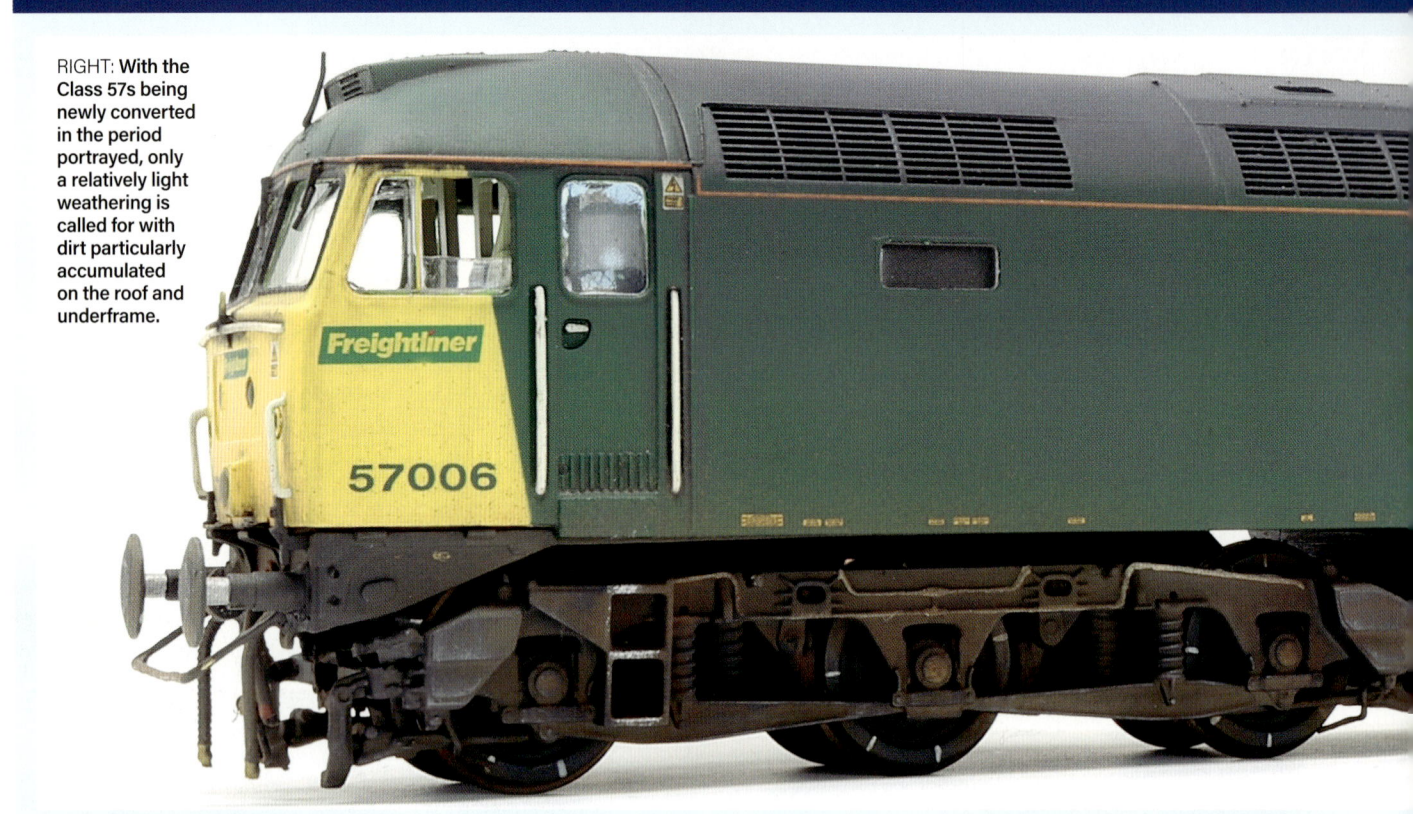

RIGHT: With the Class 57s being newly converted in the period portrayed, only a relatively light weathering is called for with dirt particularly accumulated on the roof and underframe.

The Freightliner Class 57/0s were always fascinating, seeing life-expired Class 47s fitted out with new internals and returning to service sporting a brand-new livery was enough to capture the mind of this young enthusiast in the late 1990s. It did not take long for the OO gauge models to follow with Lima's attempt soon being overtaken by Bachmann's superior take. It is this that forms the subject here, being a quick and easy exercise in taking an out of the box model and turning it into something a little more personalised.

Bachmann has released a number of Class 57s since 2005; the ones to go for are the more recent versions which brought 21-pin DCC capability, all-wheel electrical pick-ups, and a chassis with lighting independent to the bodyshell, making for easy body removal.

The first decision to make is which member of the class to model, some having flush-fronted cabs after repairs to accident damage in their previous lives. Bachmann has released models with these permutations, so it is wise to do some research before buying your donor model to save a lot of effort in the long run. In this case, Bachmann's sound-fitted 57003 release was chosen with a renumber in mind to 57006 *Freightliner Reliance*, this being an example with standard headcode recesses at both ends.

Getting started
The bodyshell was separated from the chassis and the cab interior mouldings gently removed and put to one side. In this instance, the glazing was removed but nowadays I prefer to leave it in place and mask it inside and out rather than fight with freeing the pieces from the factory glue. The roof fan grilles can be replaced with the Shawplan etched versions, these being exceptionally fine and a worthwhile improvement to the model.

A start was made on the de-branding process, rubbing carefully with a cotton bud dipped in enamel thinners the Bachmann printing lifts from the model very easily, with no damage to the green or yellow base colours. This makes removing the names and numbers a straightforward task.

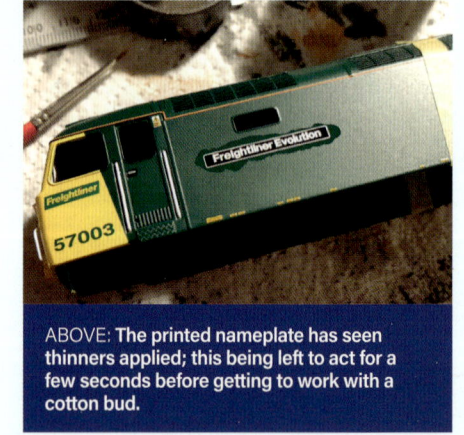

The application of the enamel thinners leaves a semi-gloss area behind where the new number decals would go. However, for the best results, it is recommended to apply an all-over coat of Railmatch gloss varnish to the bodyshell, just to avoid any risk of the carrier film on the transfers showing through once completed. With the varnish applied and having thoroughly dried, the replacement transfers were added, these can be sourced from Fox Transfers or Railtec among other suppliers, while the nameplates came from Shawplan. In line with my other loco projects, the nameplates were secured in place with matt varnish.

ABOVE: The Bachmann model of 57003 *Freightliner Evolution* out of the box and ready for work to begin. More recent releases are the best starting point as these have an upgraded chassis.

ABOVE: The printed nameplate has seen thinners applied; this being left to act for a few seconds before getting to work with a cotton bud.

Weathering
In my modelling period, the Freightliner '57s' were virtually brand new so the weathering required was minimal. It was just a case of

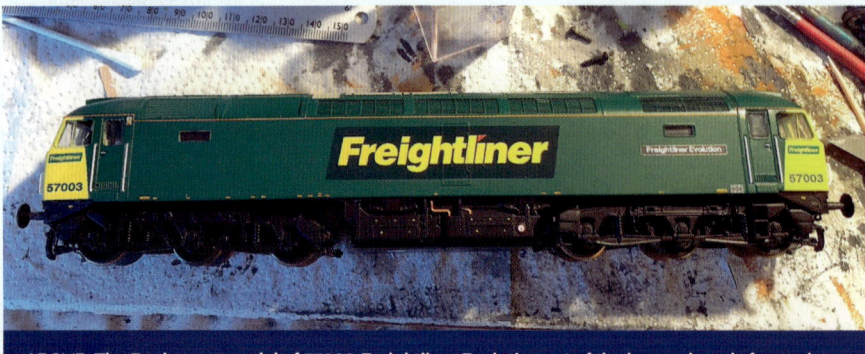

The railway reborn

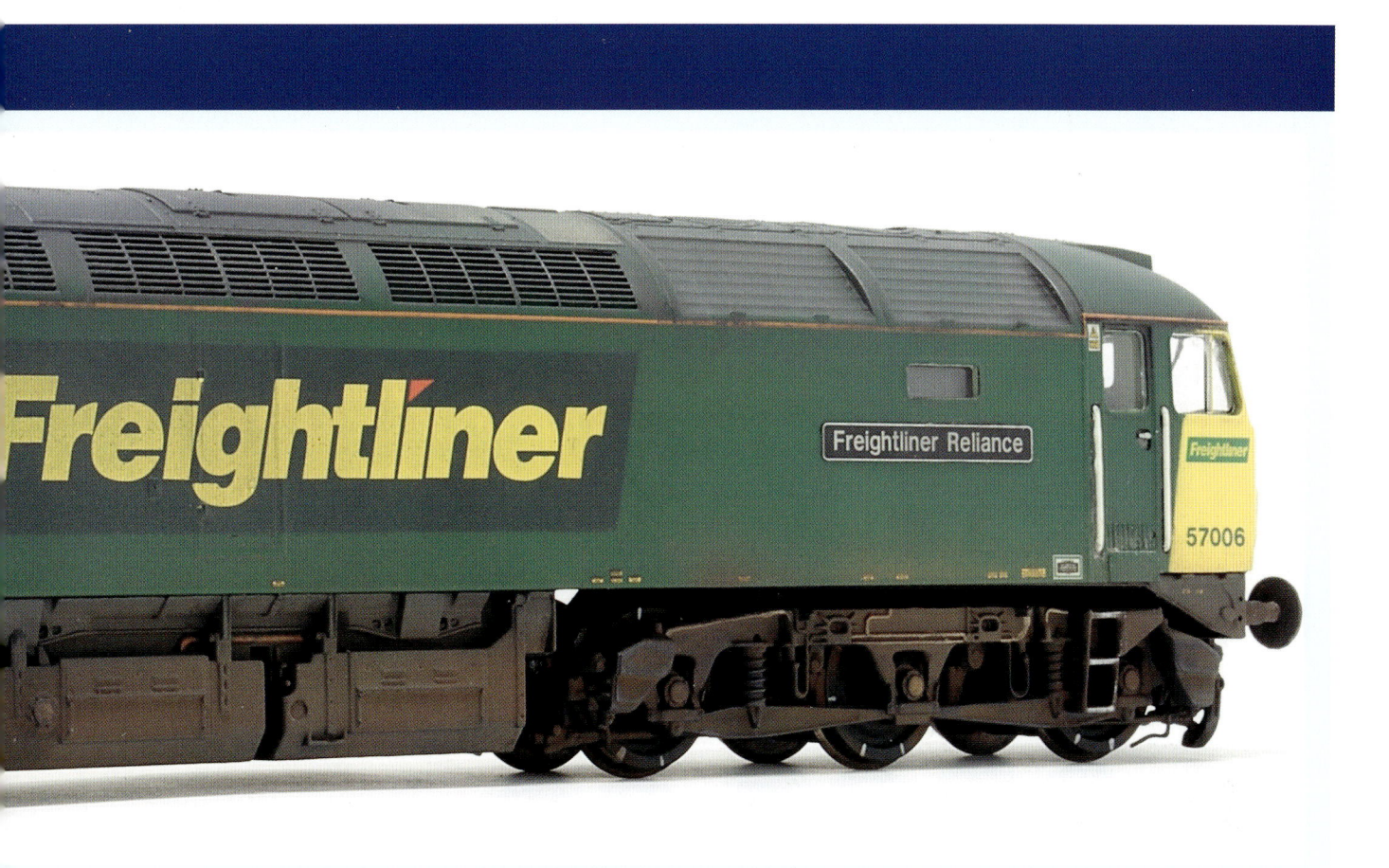

replicating the grime that had built up over the few months in traffic. The loco had already accumulated dirt in the recesses and hard-to-reach places that a washing plant could not remove, so the best way to replicate this was by doing a couple of washes of enamel paints.

Washes were applied over the bodyshell, these being a mixture of approximately 75% paint to 25% enamel thinners that were liberally painted over the body and then wiped off with kitchen towel and cotton buds dipped in thinners and working in a vertical up and down motion. Two separate washes took place, using dark brown (Humbrol No.186) and dark grey (Humbrol No.32), and the effect you are left with is a generally clean finish but with dirt deposits left in the recesses.

Neat dark grey paint, again Humbrol No. 32, was applied to the translucent roof panels to give them an extra coating, this leaving a pleasant streaky effect where the rainwater has washed some of the exhaust fumes further down to the lower parts of the roof. The initial weathering on the bodyshell was sealed in with a final coat of Railmatch

ABOVE: With the new silencer to the right of the picture, exhaust dirt has been sprayed away from this, covering the nearest roof hatches but gradually fading away over the remaining glass fibre panels.

matt varnish, applied directly from one of its aerosols to save time compared to applying with an airbrush.

On the roof, the fans that sit below the roof grilles were temporarily removed for some weathering. The moveable fans were glued in place and later painted dark grey, before being wiped away with cotton buds dipped in enamel thinners. This helped give a slightly more used appearance compared to the shiny factory finish.

Chassis work

Moving to the bufferbeams, the necessary pipework was fitted, either using the detail bag supplied with the Bachmann model or substituting 0.45mm brass handrail wire for an even finer appearance. Screw couplings were fitted, Bachmann again suppling these in the detailing pack. However, when purchasing a secondhand model, often the detailing parts are missing and here Smiths screw couplings were substituted.

A coupling loop was added to one end of the loco, which allows for operation with tension lock coupler-fitted stock while retaining the full range of bufferbeam pipe detailing. This was fashioned from 0.45mm brass wire, with small holes drilled just on the inside of each buffer shank. To get a straight and tidy loop, the brass wire was first bent to a 90-degree angle and inserted into the first hole. A black

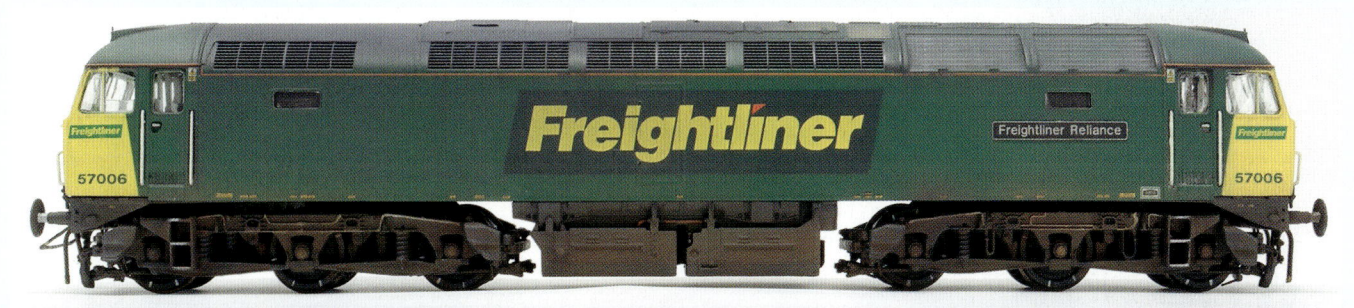

ABOVE: Despite being a sub-class of just 12 locos, there was considerable variation to be found, not only in the positioning of nameplates and presence or not of the cabside logos but also the underframe tank style.

The railway reborn

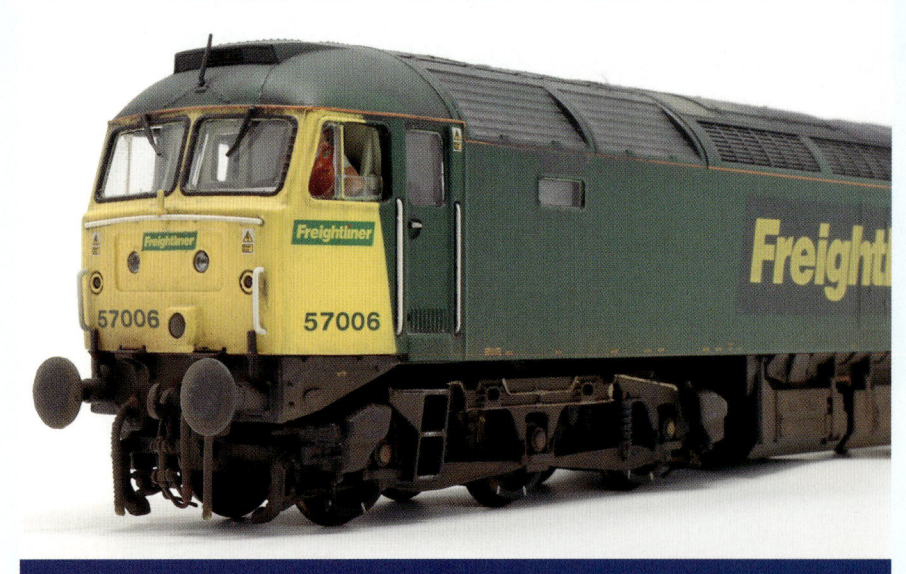

ABOVE: **Little needs to be done to the cab fronts beyond adding the supplied pipework and couplings of choice. The repainted driver figure, complete with hi-viz orange vest, can just be seen in the cab.**

and painting the floor black. All glazing was then refitted, the bogie sideframes reattached and the chassis paired back with the bodyshell.

Final tasks
With 57006 looking very smart in the chosen time period, only minimal further weathering was needed. Building on the layers applied earlier, now the dusting of grime was applied with an airbrush. Shades of paint from the Phoenix Precision weathering range were used on the chassis, primarily brake dust and track dirt, with roof dirt and dirty black employed on the roof area. This was finished off with a custom mix of Humbrol black and dark blue to give an oily finish in the immediate area of the exhaust port.

Finishing touches to the weathering then included dry-brushing gunmetal grey on the bogies to highlight raised detail and a touch of silver on the steps for some early wear and tear. With this, the loco was ready for service at the head of some late 1990s container trains.

permanent marker pen was then used to note the position of the second hole before removing the wire again to make the final 90-degree bend. The whole arrangement was secured with superglue with any extra wire bent back on itself behind the bufferbeam for a solid fit.

After the bufferbeam detailing was completed, the entire chassis was painted dark grey using Humbrol No.32, including the wheel faces, to remove the stark black finish from the Bachmann model and give a good basis for the weathering to be applied later. One detail that was replicated was the white markings on the faces of the wheels, which are used to indicate whether the outer metal tyres have slipped on the centre sections on the wheel. Painted on in white with a fine 5/0 brush, these also provide a mesmerising effect to watch when the loco is driven slowly past the viewer!

The last area to be tackled before reassembling the loco was to detail the cab interior. The driver figure was painted to more accurately represent a Freightliner driver of the period while other small cab details were added too, including painting the dials, weathering the driver's desk,

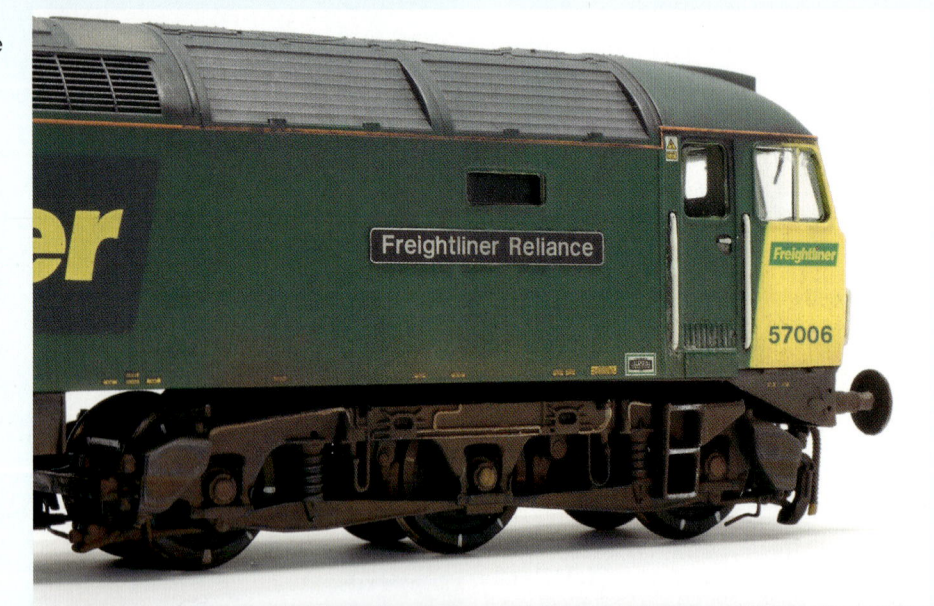

ABOVE: **The Bachmann model displays some fine small printing, including the Brush worksplate and the yellow-backed labels that indicated the positioning of various taps and valves. Weathering touches include wear on the cab steps and leaving hints of the white bogie pipework and yellow axlebox covers visible beneath the grime.**

BELOW: **The Class 57s were commonly seen on intermodal workings out of Freightliner's more southerly terminals, such as Felixstowe and Southampton, making them essential for any layouts covering routes to the Midlands and beyond. They also worked into South Wales and North Kent before being displaced by Class 66s.**

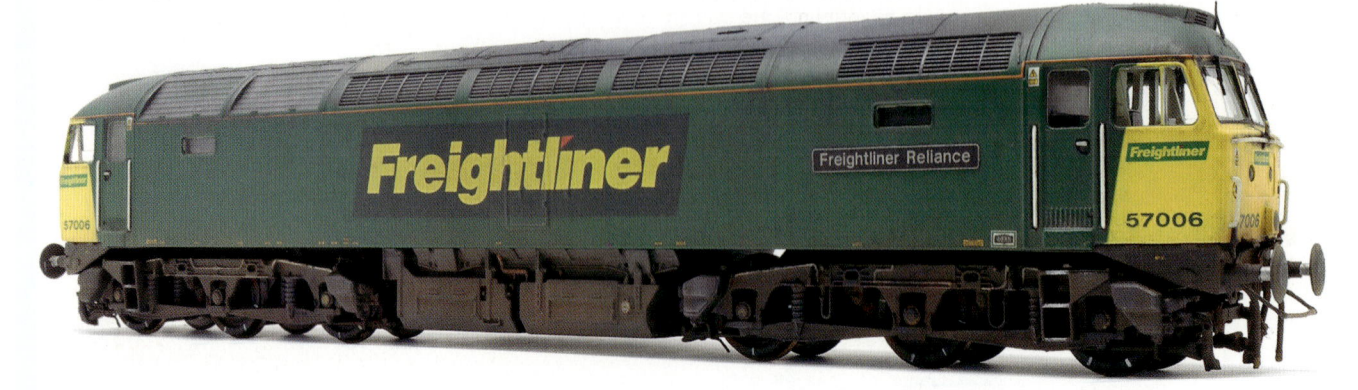

The railway reborn

RIGHT: **Depicting the loco modelled opposite,** 57006 *Freightliner Reliance* **passes Great Bourton on June 26, 2002, with the 4S59 15.12 Southampton to Coatbridge, shortly before Class 66s took over. The leading wagon set is a five-element FLA 'Lowliner', these having small wheels and a low deck to allow 9ft 6in tall containers to be conveyed within the standard loading gauge. These date from 1990/91 but a further batch of twin-sets belatedly followed in 2004 to a similar design. Realtrack Models does the latter type in OO gauge, but the original inners and outers are unavailable, as they are in N gauge. The rest of the train are FSA/FTA, soon to be released in both scales by Realtrack.** Martin Loader

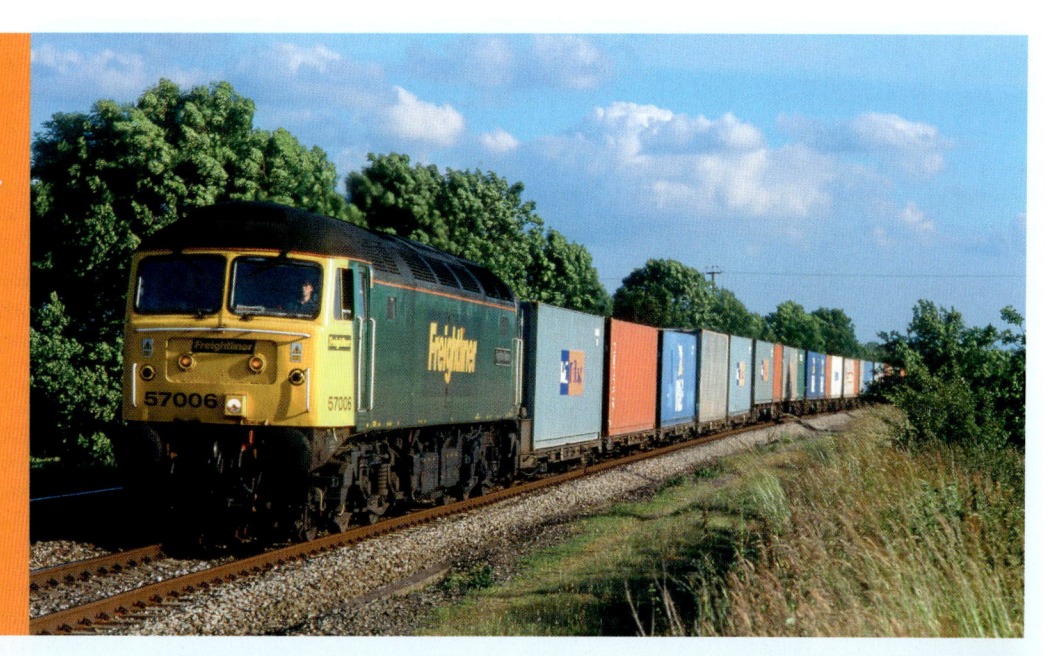

RIGHT: **Freightliner trains became more diverse in their wagon types as the 1990s ended. Illustrating this, the 4S59 15.13 Millbrook to Coatbridge was headed by 57001** *Freightliner Pioneer* **and an empty KFA at Fenny Compton on June 19, 2000, with two KQA pocket wagons standing out beyond the set of four FSA/FTA. The latter were another design that allowed 9ft 6in containers to be moved largely unrestricted. In OO gauge, Hornby produces one of the key KFA types while Dapol similarly offers the KQA. Availability is just as good in N gauge with Revolution doing the KFA and Realtrack the KQA.** Martin Loader

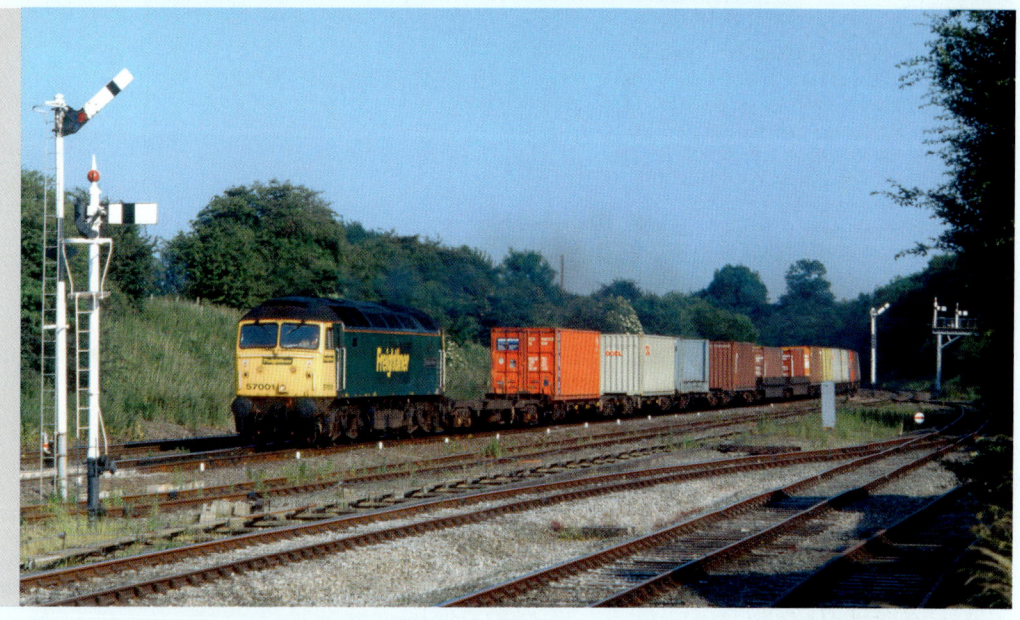

Model availability

With the Lima effort long discontinued and only partly correct anyway, Bachmann has a captive market when it comes to the Class 57/0 thanks to its OO gauge model along with the N gauge version in its Graham Farish range. More competition has existed with the Class 57/3 and Class 57/6, at least in 4mm, where Heljan once produced models of both, although the tooling has not been used for many years. While available secondhand, the Danish model is largely obsolete, leaving Bachmann free to cover more recent developments in both scales. As the Virgin Trains and First Great Western sub-classes date from after 2000, they are not covered in detail here.

RIGHT: **There have been several Freightliner releases in the Graham Farish range, this being 57008** *Freightliner Explorer***.**

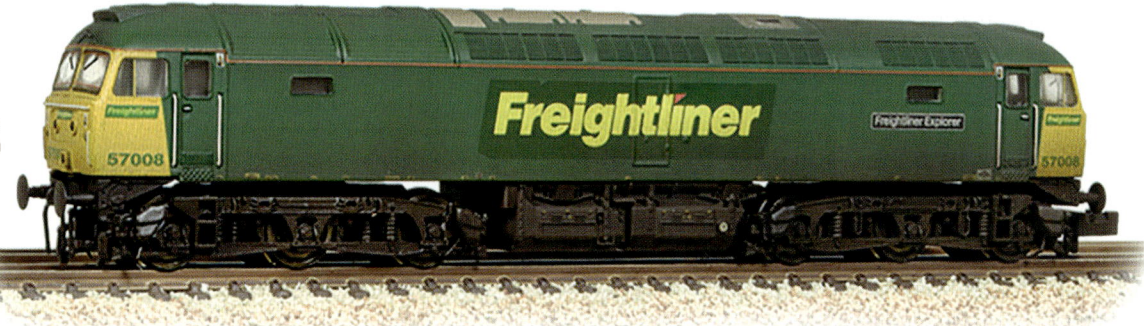

Modelling BR Locomotives of the 1990s **109**

The railway reborn

West Coast takeover

The spring of 1997 saw Virgin Trains assume control of the former InterCity services on the West Coast Main Line, quickly becoming one of the most high-profile privatised companies. **Simon Bendall** looks at the fortunes of the AC electric fleet as the decade ended while James Makin details the new generation Class 87 and Class 90 models in OO gauge.

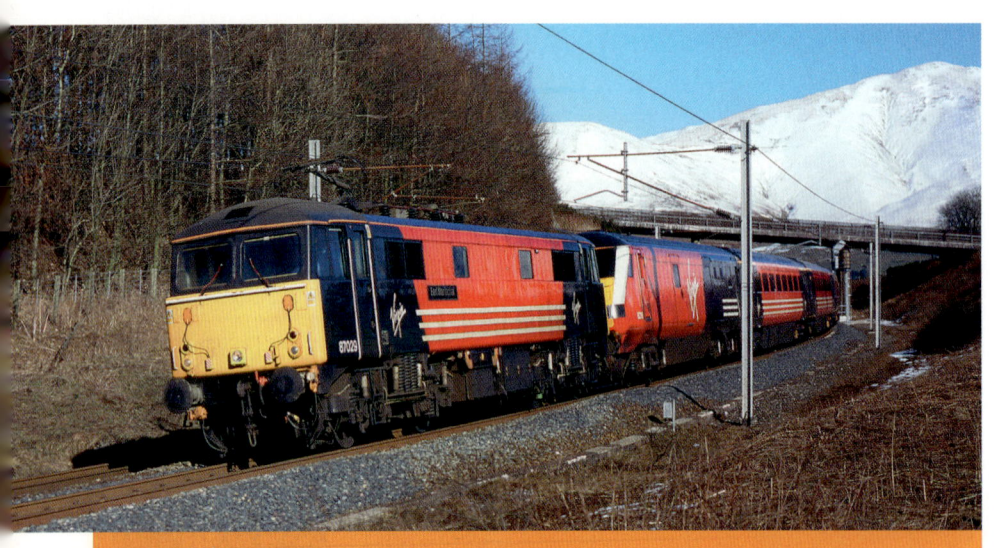

ABOVE: One of the locos modelled here, 87029 *Earl Marischal* shows of its Virgin colours at Cowperthwaite, near Shap, on March 2, 2002. The TDM system used to control the DVT from the loco at the opposite end of the train could be temperamental at times, especially in cold weather. As a result, the Class 87 has run-round to haul the Euston-bound service conventionally. Dave McAlone

The West Coast Main Line train operating unit was the last of the former InterCity routes to be passed to private control, the government giving the reigns to Virgin Trains from March 9, 1997, for a period of 15 years. The franchise was widely viewed as one of the most difficult to manage as not only was it operating at a loss, but considerable upheaval was also on the way as Railtrack prepared to conduct a complete route modernisation programme with little experience. Inevitably, this was botched, running both over schedule and budget during the next decade and with several parts of the upgrade cancelled.

As part of Virgin's bid for the franchise, it had promised complete fleet replacement with new 140mph-capable tilting EMUs set to replace the existing push-pull formations made up of a mix of Mk.2 and Mk.3 coaches and powered by Class 86s, 87s and 90s. In the event, it was another five years before the 'Pendolinos' were ready for service, leaving the former BR electrics to soldier on with assistance from classmates hired from EWS and Freightliner at various times.

Owned by Porterbrook and leased to Virgin were 87001-35 and 90001-15 while the train operator also had 86207/09/24/25/31/36/40 /42/45/48/51/53/56/58 available, the Class 86/2s all belonging to Eversholt. The latter were typically diagrammed on the Euston-Birmingham-Wolverhampton diagrams hauling the Mk.2e/f sets, while the Class 87s and Class 90s invariably headed the Mk.3a/b formations to the likes of Liverpool, Manchester, and Glasgow.

Red revolution

At the time Virgin took over, all of the AC electrics were finished in InterCity Swallow colours, the first repaint into the company's red and dark grey colours coming in March 1997. This was 90002, which was named *Mission: Impossible* in an ironic nod to the industry view of the franchise and the wider West Coast upgrade. Repaints initially focussed on the Class 90s with 90004/12/14/15 all completed during the year, but Class 87s were also underway by the autumn of 1997 with 87006/09/16 the first to be re-liveried.

As more locos and coaching stock sets were repainted, full Virgin-liveried formations became increasingly common but also it was just as likely to see an AC electric still in InterCity atop a rake of red and grey coaches and vice versa. 1998 saw the first Class 86s gain the new image in the form of 86229 and 86242 while 86245 was named *Caledonian* and painted in an approximation of that railway's historic blue shade in February, the loco retaining the dark grey cabs but with red bodyside stripes instead of white. This unique look lasted for a year until standard Virgin colours were applied.

By the end of the decade, an exchange of Class 86s between the West Coast and CrossCountry fleets meant that the former now contained 86209/29/33/45/47/59/60, although as both were Virgin controlled there was a degree of common-user to them. In addition, other locos now in Virgin colours included 86209/33/59, 87001-04/07/ 08/10/12-15/21/22/25/27/32/33/35 and 90012/13. The remaining Class 87s were finally completed in 2000 but it was the following year before the last Class 90s finally lost their InterCity colours.

One more repaint of note was in June 2002 when 86233 received BR electric blue to mark the impending demise of the Class 86s on West Coast passenger services. Thereafter the three classes were progressively run-down as the 'Pendolinos' took over, the Class 87s being the last to go, but this falls outside the scope of this feature.

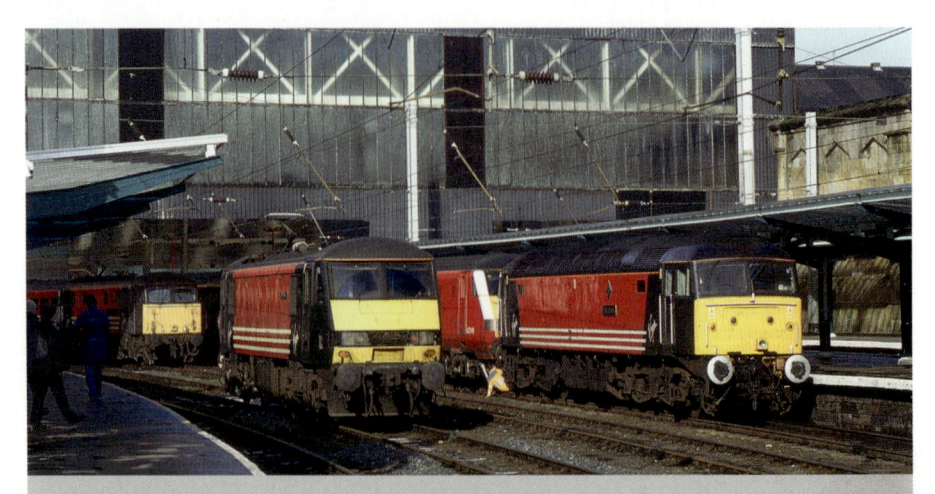

ABOVE: A busy scene at Carlisle on February 23, 2002, shows the benefits that Virgin enjoyed of having both the West Coast and CrossCountry franchises, and of these operating over a large part of the same route. With engineering work necessitating diesel-hauled diversions over the Settle and Carlisle line, the southbound 'Royal Scot' has seen 87011 *City of Wolverhampton* detached and CrossCountry's borrowed 47805 *Pride of Toton* take its place with coupling underway. In the other centre road, 90005 *Financial Times* waits for a northbound 'drag' to arrive which it will take forward. Dave McAlone

The railway reborn

West Coast workhorses

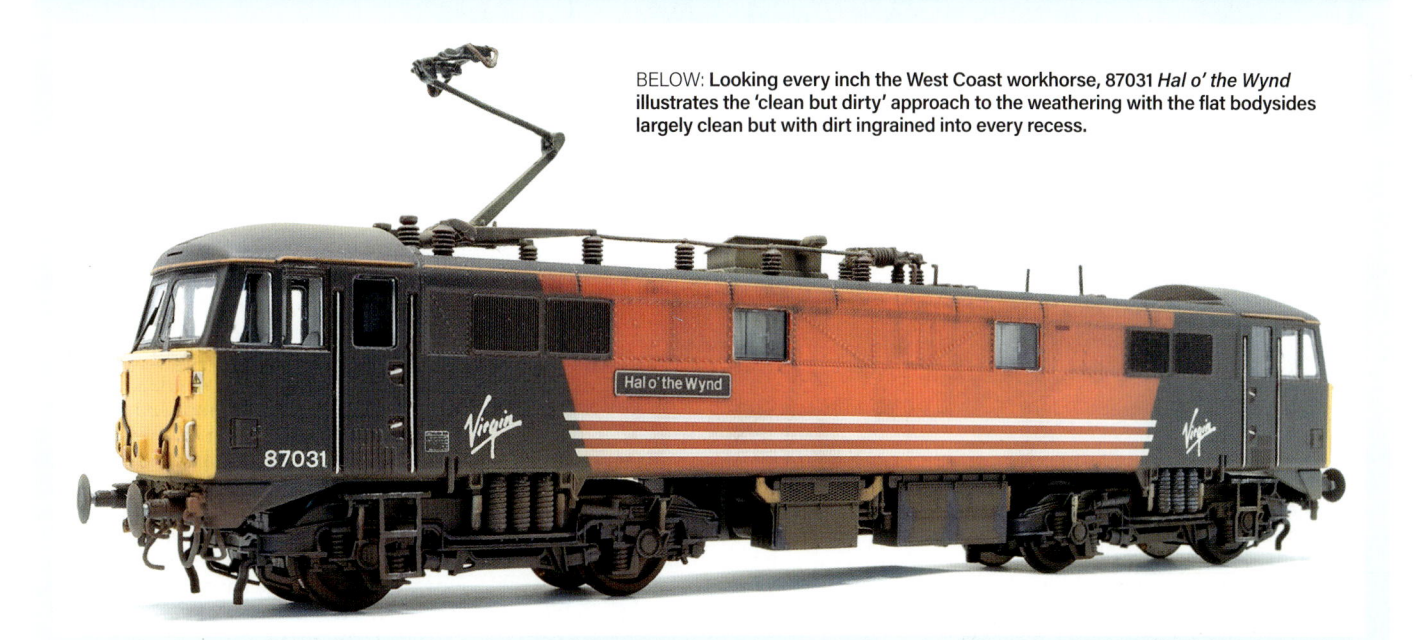

BELOW: Looking every inch the West Coast workhorse, 87031 *Hal o' the Wynd* illustrates the 'clean but dirty' approach to the weathering with the flat bodysides largely clean but with dirt ingrained into every recess.

Born as a soft southerner, travelling up north to glimpse the exotic world of overhead electrification at the dawn of the 21st century was always an amazing treat. Long days out spent at fruitful spotting locations like Birmingham New Street, Rugby and Stafford would see whole pages of locomotives ticked off in the spotting books, making for treasured memories of loco-hauled Virgin West Coast services before the 'Pendolinos' took over.

Having last dabbled in the world of AC electrics almost 20 years ago with my layout Wells Green TMD, times have changed and there is now a wide range of high-fidelity OO gauge models to choose from. Hornby's Class 87 is a great step up from the Lima model of the past, while Bachmann's Class 90 is a true gamechanger and the first UK-outline AC electric to have a DCC-operated pantograph.

Those well-thumbed trainspotting notebooks from the early 2000s were dug out and after a good dose of nostalgia, the identities were chosen; 87029 *Earl Marischal* and 87031 *Hal o' the Wynd* in Virgin colours and, accompanying them, 90010 *275 Railway Squadron (Volunteers)* still clinging to its ageing InterCity Swallow livery.

One notable difference since working on the previous generation of AC electric models is the complexity of taking them apart for reworking! Hornby's Class 87 has a simple lift-off body, but the cabs are challenging to access for dismantling, while Bachmann's Class 90 has a whole raft of screws to be unfastened, a lift-out roof section that needs securing, and a lot of care required to protect the pantograph servo mechanism during the project.

Roof detailing
Starting with the Class 87s, after consulting photos of the period, it became apparent that my chosen locos did not receive the prominent roof-mounted Inergen fire suppression equipment until 2003. As this was after my modelling period, these details need to be removed but fortunately a scalpel and screwdriver made light work of them.

The roof-mounted aerials needed to be relocated closer to the relevant cab as a result, so new holes were carefully drilled, and the details transferred across. All the remaining holes and fixing points were then filled with Humbrol model filler and sanded down afterwards. A missing pipe run was also added to connect the roof aerials and along the length of the roof, this using 0.45mm handrail wire secured with spots of superglue.

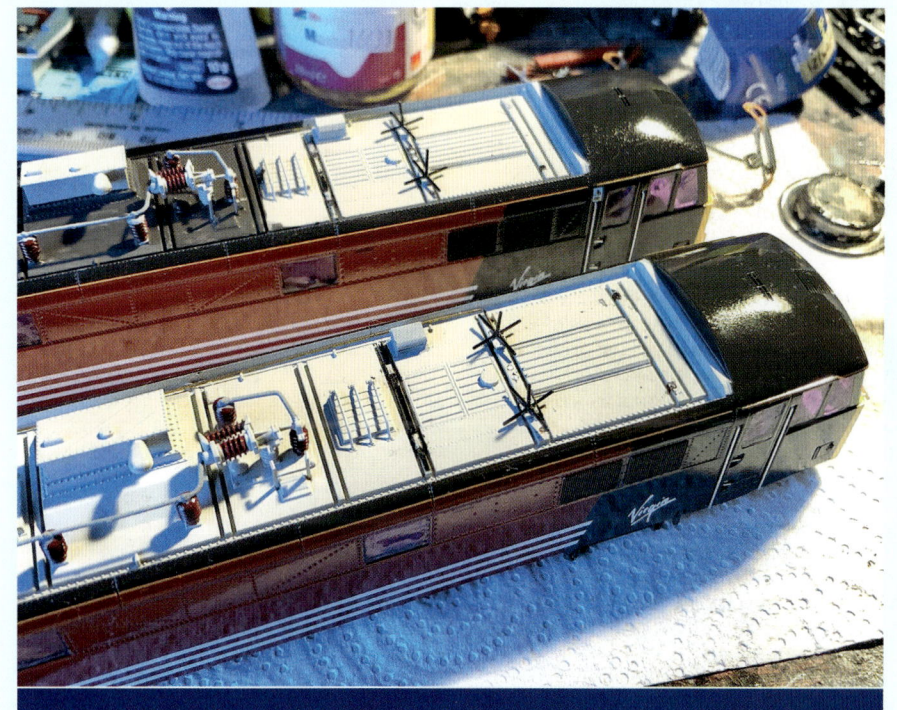

ABOVE: With the roof-mounted fire extinguisher bottles removed, the twin aerials need to be moved back to their previous position closer to the cab, which just requires new holes to be drilled.

The plastic representation of the Brecknell Willis high-speed pantograph on Hornby's model is flimsy and will likely be replaced by something from another manufacturer in due course. Perhaps a spare will be available from a Bachmann Class 90, or potentially from the forthcoming Accurascale Class 92.

Personalisation
The existing name and number printing was easily removed from each of the locos, just requiring a small amount of Humbrol enamel thinners on a cotton bud. Gentle rubbing across the desired

Modelling BR Locomotives of the 1990s 111

The railway reborn

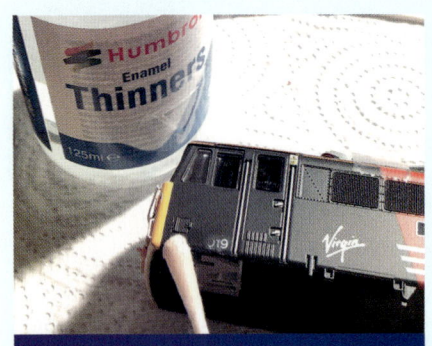

ABOVE: The printing on both models lifts easily with thinners on a cotton bud and gentle rubbing.

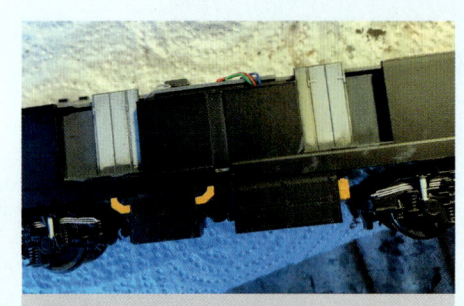

ABOVE: A simple improvement on the Class 87 is to paint the two electrical cabinets that are cast into the chassis block as these are visible through the two bodyside windows on one side.

slightly larger than scale, offer a great base for customising. Their legs and some of the torso had to be removed to fit them in the respective driver's seats, after which they were painted in the uniforms of the time.

Roof weathering

The Virgin West Coast locos would pass through a washing plant on a regular basis so would rarely be seen truly dirty, except perhaps in the depths of winter. Following photos carefully, the desired look was clean but with extensive build-up of dirt in places that the washers could not reach.

A wash of dark brown paint (Humbrol No.251) was applied over the bodysides, approximately 50:50 paint mixed to enamel thinners, and wiped down with a kitchen towel. Next, a cotton bud was dipped in neat enamel thinners and then worked vertically up and down the body, cleaning all open and flat surfaces but leaving the paint to gather in the recesses, such as in grilles and behind handrails. This was then supplemented by small further washes of other shades of brown in localised areas and again following photos for guidance.

The roof of AC electrics always collected grime, which makes for great fun to model using a combination of washes, paint mottling, dry-brushing and finally dusting with an airbrush. To start with, the main colour of the roof well on all the models needed changing. The light grey roof on the Hornby Class 87s was repainted in mid-brown (Humbrol No.113) and the same was also done to the jet black

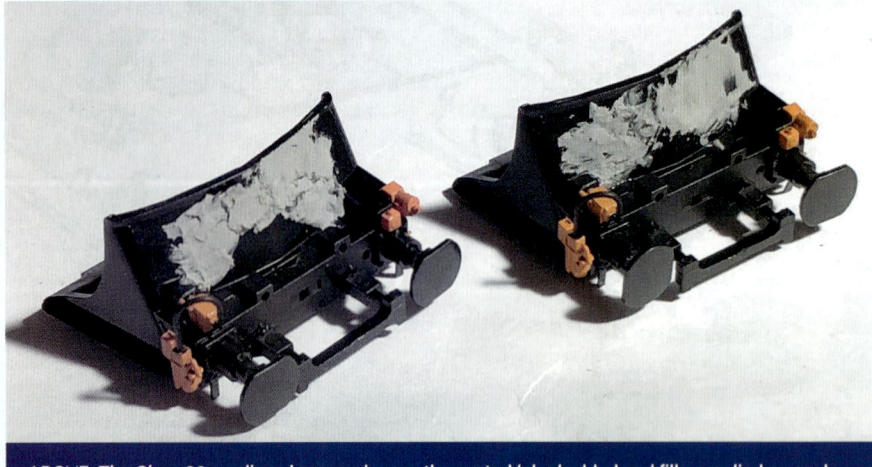

printing will see it gently lift off within approximately 30 seconds. The next stage was to add a layer of Railmatch gloss varnish, onto which the new transfers could be applied. Ahead of this, any glazing was masked using Humbrol Maskol masking fluid. Fox Transfers' Virgin Trains decals were used, and the nameplates came from Shawplan, some of which had been held in my modelling stash for almost 18 years!

Each of the Class 87s had a couple of painting details to be replicated with the outermost grille surrounds on the bodysides receiving a coat of Virgin dark grey. Additionally, the TDM cable holders on the cab fronts required the addition of thin red stripes. For 90010, one headlight surround at one end needed to be randomly painted black and some flecks of undercoat grey added to the red InterCity stripe to represent peeling paint. Some of the slats in the air horn grilles were also gently bent to replicate how the loco looked in 2000.

The bufferbeam cowling on the Class 90 was also modified at both ends to remove the cut-out section for the tension lock coupling. The 'plug' supplied with the accessory bag for each one was screwed in place and the gap then filled and sanded, after which the cowlings were fully repainted in black.

Inside the cabs, driver figures were added, these being sourced online. The 1/75 scale Chinese-made figures can be bought from eBay or Amazon for just a few pounds for 100 unpainted figures and, despite being

ABOVE: The Class 90 cowlings have each seen the central 'plug' added and filler applied around the gaps. Once dried, this will be sanded down and the parts repainted.

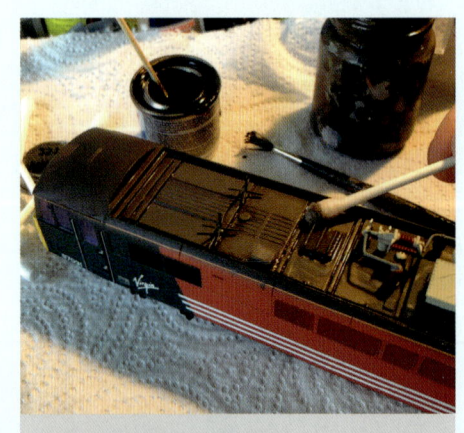

ABOVE: With the roof well already repainted on 87031, the application of the initial weathering washes is underway using the trusty cotton bud.

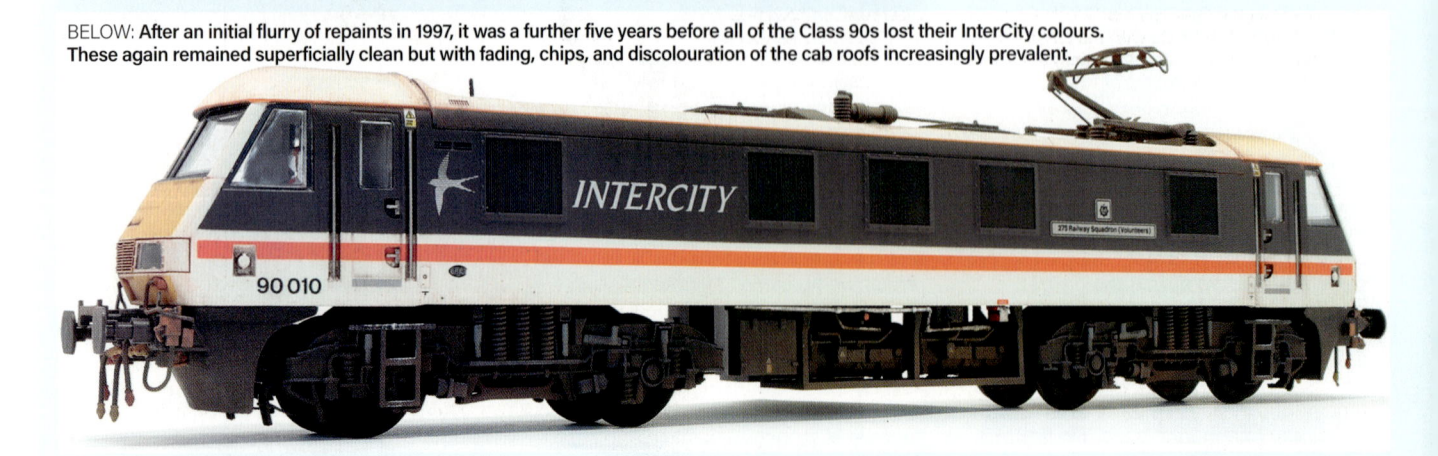

BELOW: After an initial flurry of repaints in 1997, it was a further five years before all of the Class 90s lost their InterCity colours. These again remained superficially clean but with fading, chips, and discolouration of the cab roofs increasingly prevalent.

The railway reborn

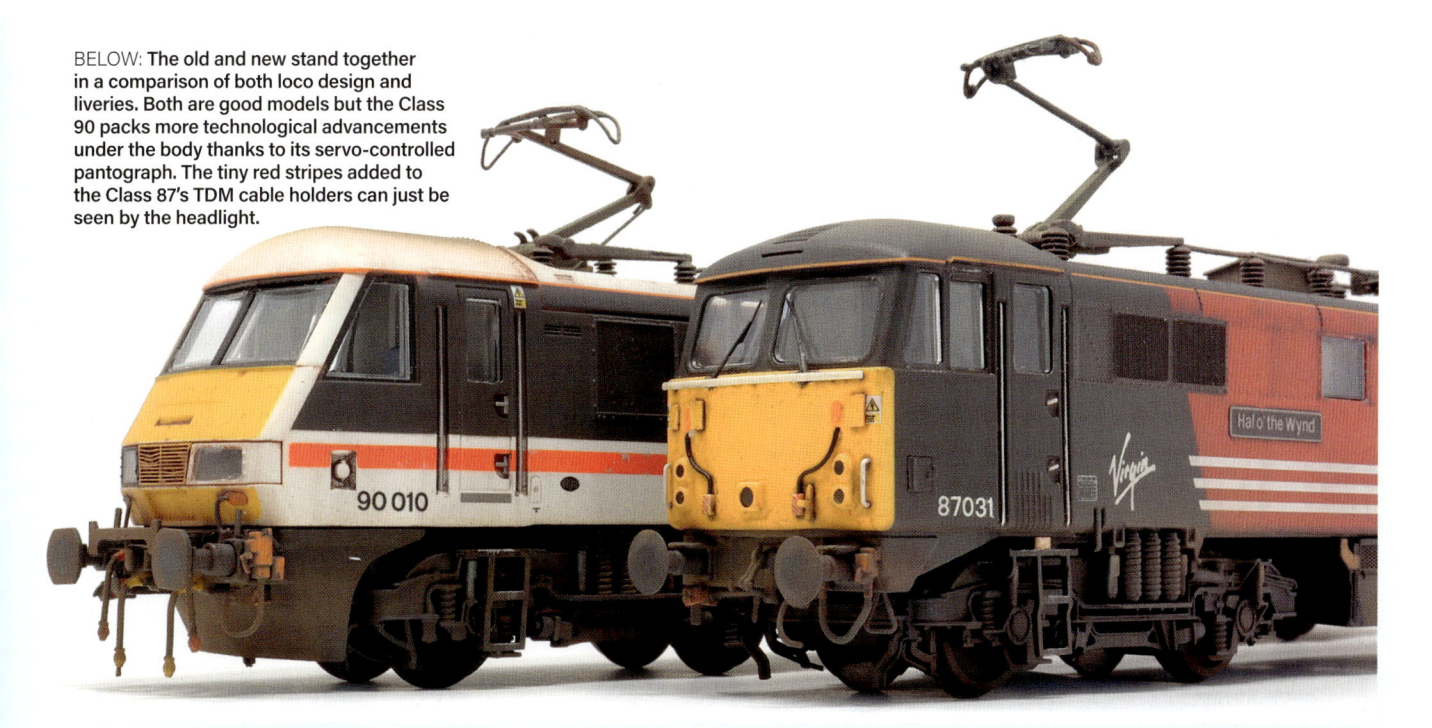

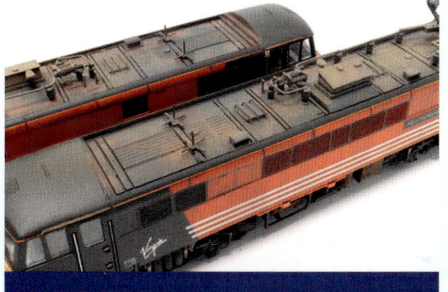

BELOW: **The old and new stand together in a comparison of both loco design and liveries. Both are good models but the Class 90 packs more technological advancements under the body thanks to its servo-controlled pantograph. The tiny red stripes added to the Class 87's TDM cable holders can just be seen by the headlight.**

ABOVE: **The Class 87s display the finished weathering of their roof wells, showing how the shades of greys and browns can be built up and varied to create a realistic look.**

factory finish of the Bachmann Class 90. After this had dried, more shades of brown were washed over the roof and rubbed back with cotton buds soaked in enamel thinners.

More shades of brown and dark grey were then mottled onto the surface using a wet brush and a small amount of paint, dabbing on the brush, and later rolling over with a cotton bud dipped in thinners to disperse the paint around on the flat recessed areas. It was then time to dry-brush on shades of sandy brown and darker greys, dipping the brush into the paint and then wiping almost all of it off with a kitchen towel, before brushing over the model to highlight raised detail on the edges of roof equipment or over the roof grilles for example.

Each loco is slightly different, so the advice is to trawl online for roof pictures of your prototype and then copy the colour palette you see. By building up a wide variety of colours and layers, the more realistic the appearance starts to become.

Final tasks
On the chassis, each model is supplied with a bright, black-painted finish and bright white pipework and bufferbeam jumpers. My chosen prototypes did not have any of this smart appearance, so the chassis were repainted dark grey and the bright orange jumper cable fittings were given a wash of dark grey to tone down the colour prior to the traffic dirt being applied.

With the airbrush out, the traffic grime layers were sprayed on, starting with Phoenix Precision's brake dust and track dirt shades across the chassis and mindful of keeping the bodysides clean. On the roof, layers of roof dirt and a variety of Humbrol sandy and green-brown shades were sprayed on, building up intensity around the pantograph to represent the carbon deposits left by the pantograph gliding along the contact wire of the overhead electrification.

As a finishing touch, the chassis were dry-brushed in Humbrol Metalcote gunmetal to emphasise the edges of the bogies and underframe equipment. The locos were now ready for some action on my depot layout Wells Green TMD, invoking memories of those early 2000s spotting adventures under the wires!

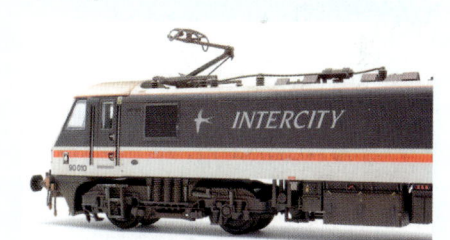

ABOVE: **Using grey to represent undercoat, flaking and chipped paint has been added to 90010, as seen particularly on the red stripe and grille.**

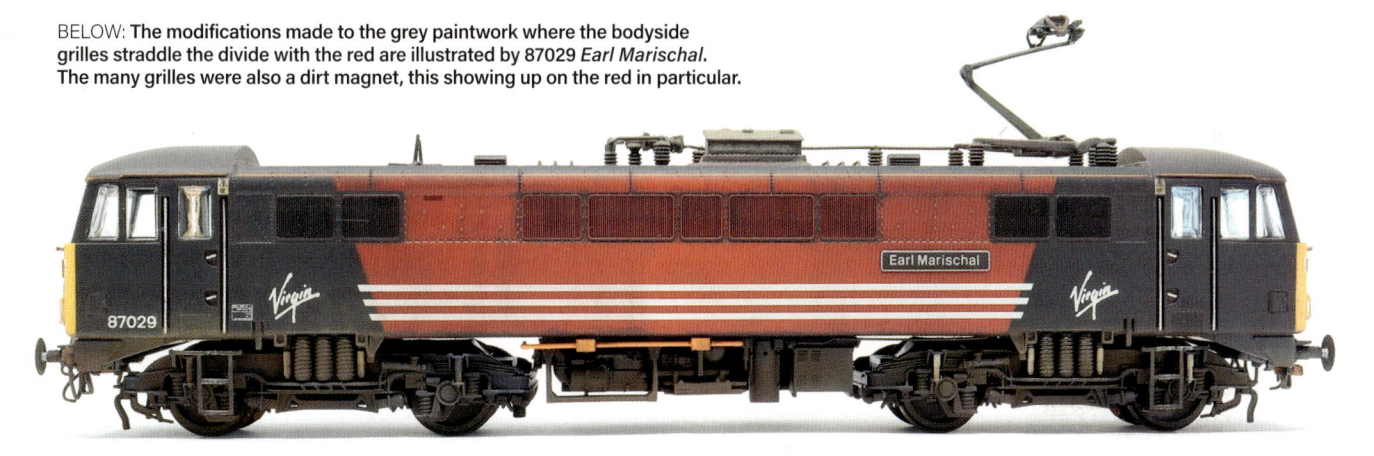

BELOW: **The modifications made to the grey paintwork where the bodyside grilles straddle the divide with the red are illustrated by 87029 *Earl Marischal*. The many grilles were also a dirt magnet, this showing up on the red in particular.**

Modelling BR Locomotives of the 1990s

The railway reborn

RIGHT: While some of its sisters retained InterCity Swallow into 2001, 90012 *British Transport Police* was a much earlier recipient of Virgin colours in 1997. On May 31, 2001, it arrives at Stafford with a northbound service formed of an all Mk.3 set, this featuring the standard Virgin formation of five TSOs, an RFM, two FOs and a DVT. In OO gauge, both Hornby and Oxford Rail have produced the passenger coaches to varying degrees of accuracy with Hornby also offering the all-important DVT. Similarly, in N gauge, both Dapol and Graham Farish have done the coaches but only Dapol markets the DVT.
John Tuner/53A Models of Hull Collection

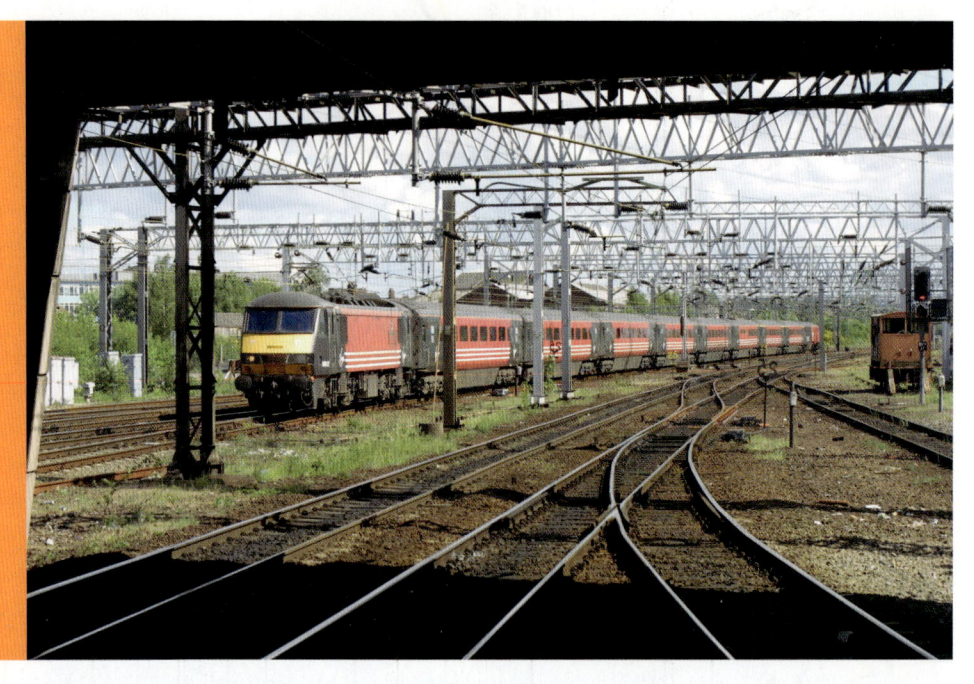

RIGHT: Like InterCity before it, Virgin Trains largely deployed its Mk.2e/f formations on the shorter distance workings between London and the West Midlands. On August 3, 2003, a power isolation for engineering work sees 47828 *Severn Valley Railway* dragging 90005 *Financial Times* north at Ansty with the 1G31 14.45 Euston-Wolverhampton, which is formed of five TSOs and three FOs either side of a Mk.3a buffet with a DVT on the rear. By this time, the Mk.2f TSOs were dominant on West Coast services with just a few of the earlier Mk.2e TSOs making up the numbers while the first class vehicles were entirely Mk.2f. As a result, the Bachmann Mk.2f coaches are the best option in OO gauge rather than the Hornby Mk.2e range, although an Oxford Rail Mk.3a RFM and Hornby DVT would also be needed. In N gauge, Graham Farish does the Mk.2f types to pair with the requisite Mk.3s.
Gareth Bayer

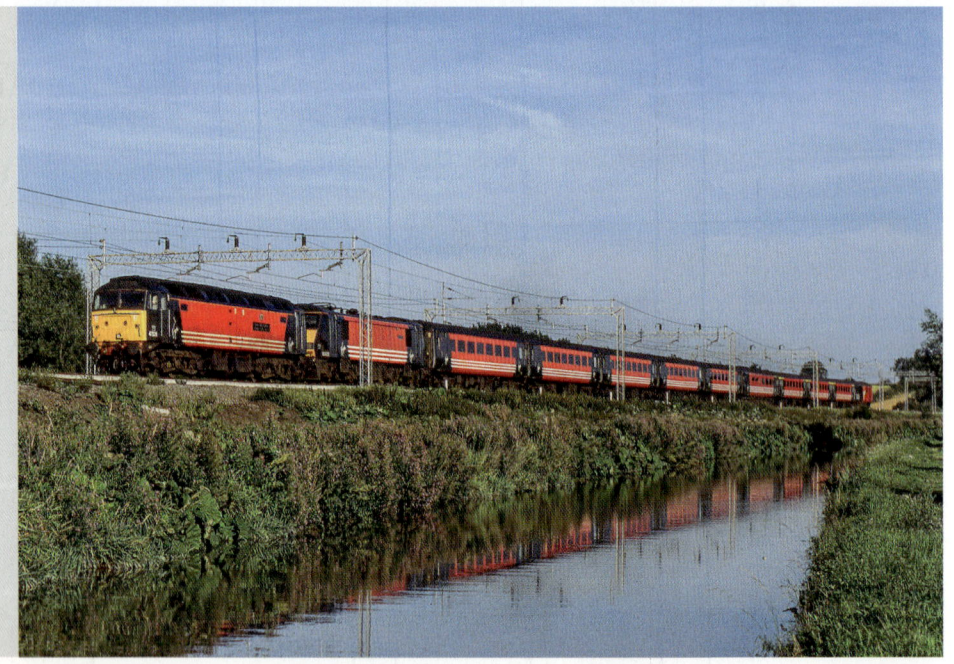

RIGHT: The uniquely-liveried 86245 *Caledonian* shows of its special blue livery at Euston on June 21, 1998. This had been unveiled four months earlier to mark the 150th anniversary of the completion of the through route from London to Scotland, the blue recalling that of the Caledonian Railway. Notably, the loco did not carry Virgin logos during its time in the colours and would revert to standard red and grey the next year. 86245 would be taken out of traffic from Willesden in October 2003. Gareth Bayer

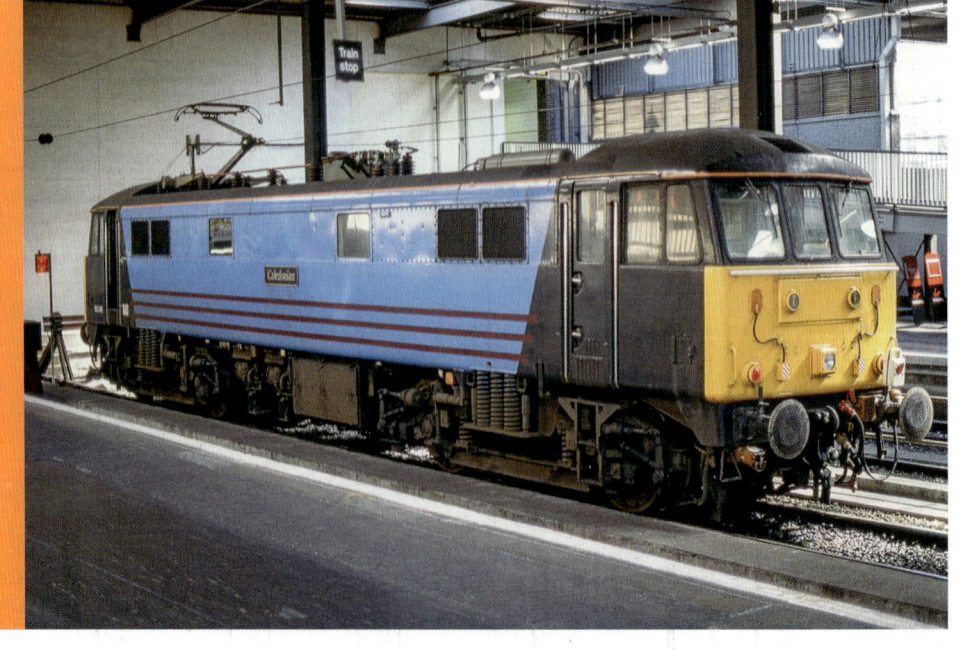